REFERENCE EDITION

ESAP™ 2022

Endocrine Society's
Endocrine Self-Assessment Program
Questions, Answers, and Discussions

Lisa R. Tannock, MD, Program Chair
Professor of Medicine
University of Kentucky and
Department of Veterans Affairs

Barbara Gisella Carranza Leon, MD
Associate Professor of Medicine
Division of Diabetes, Endocrinology,
and Metabolism
Vanderbilt University Medical Center

Alice Y. Chang, MD, MSc
Assistant Professor of Medicine
Division of Endocrinology,
Diabetes, and Nutrition
Mayo Clinic

Dima Lutfi Diab, MD
Associate Professor of Clinical Medicine
University of Cincinnati

Nicole M. Ehrhardt, MD
Assistant Professor of Medicine
University of Washington
Diabetes Institute

Nazanene H. Esfandiari, MD
Professor of Medicine
Metabolism, Endocrinology,
and Diabetes Division
University of Michigan

Mathis Grossmann, MD, PhD
Professor of Medicine
University of Melbourne
Austin Health

Mark Gurnell, MBBS, MA (Med Ed), PhD
Professor of Clinical Endocrinology
& Clinical SubDean
University of Cambridge,
Wellcome Trust-MRC Institute
of Metabolic Science &
School of Clinical Medicine

Sarah E. Mayson, MD
Associate Professor of Medicine
Director of the Endocrinology
Fellowship Program
Division of Endocrinology,
Metabolism, and Diabetes
University of Colorado School of Medicine

Kevin M. Pantalone, DO
Staff Endocrinologist
Director of Diabetes Initiatives
Department of Endocrinology
Cleveland Clinic

Deepika Reddy, MD
Assistant Professor
Division of Diabetes, Endocrinology,
and Metabolism
University of Utah Healthcare

Roberto Salvatori, MD
Professor of Medicine
Medical Director,
Johns Hopkins Pituitary Center
Johns Hopkins University

Meera Shah, MB ChB
Assistant Professor of Medicine,
Mayo Clinic College of Medicine
Consultant, Division of Endocrinology,
Mayo Clinic – Rochester

Aniket Sidhaye, MD
Assistant Professor of Medicine
Johns Hopkins University

Anand Vaidya, MD, MMSc
Associate Professor of Medicine
Brigham and Women's Hospital
Harvard Medical School

Thomas J. Weber, MD
Professor of Medicine
Division of Endocrinology,
Metabolism, and Nutrition
Duke University Medical Center

Abbie L. Young, MS, CGC, ELS(D)
Medical Editor

Endocrine Society
2055 L Street NW, Suite 600, Washington, DC 20036
1-888-ENDOCRINE • www.endocrine.org

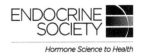

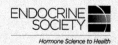

The Endocrine Society is the world's largest, oldest, and most active organization working to advance the clinical practice of endocrinology and hormone research. Founded in 1916, the Society now has more than 18,000 global members across a range of disciplines. The Society has earned an international reputation for excellence in the quality of its peer-reviewed journals, educational resources, meetings, and programs that improve public health through the practice and science of endocrinology.

For between-edition updates, visit us at:
endocrine.org/education-and-training/book-updates

Other publications:
endocrine.org/publications

The statements and opinions expressed in this publication are those of the individual authors and do not necessarily reflect the views of the Endocrine Society. The Endocrine Society is not responsible or liable in any way for the currency of the information, for any errors, omissions, or inaccuracies, or for any consequences arising therefrom. With respect to any drugs mentioned, the reader is advised to refer to the appropriate medical literature and the product information currently provided by the manufacturer to verify appropriate dosage, method and duration of administration, and other relevant information. In all instances, it is the responsibility of the treating physician or other health care professional, relying on independent experience and expertise, as well as knowledge of the patient, to determine the best treatment for the patient.

PERMISSIONS: For permission to reuse material, please visit the Copyright Clearance Center (CCC) at www.copyright.com or call 978-750-8400. CCC is a not-for-profit organization that provides licenses and registration for a variety of uses.

Copyright © 2022 by the Endocrine Society, 2055 L Street NW, Suite 600, Washington, DC 20036. All rights reserved. No part of this publication may be reproduced, stored in a retrieval system, posted on the Internet, or transmitted in any form, by any means, electronic, mechanical, photocopying, recording, or otherwise, without written permission of the publisher.

TRANSLATIONS AND LICENSING: Rights to translate and reproduce Endocrine Society publications internationally are extended through a licensing agreement on full or partial editions. To request rights for a local edition, please visit: endocrine.org/products-and-services/licensing.

ISBN: 978-1-943550-11-1

Library of Congress Control Number: 2021950586

On the Cover: @ Pexels. Person Holding Pen Writing on Paper (by Ivan Samkov).

OVERVIEW

The Endocrine Self-Assessment Program (ESAP™) is a self-study curriculum aimed at physicians wanting a self-assessment and a broad review of endocrinology. The ESAP Reference Edition consists of 120 brand-new multiple-choice questions in all areas of endocrinology, diabetes, and metabolism. There is extensive discussion of each correct answer, a comprehensive syllabus, and references. ESAP is updated annually with new questions.

The ESAP reference book is intended primarily for consultation and self-assessment of knowledge relating to endocrinology. As a reference book, educational credits are not available upon completion of the multiple-choice questions included. For information on educational products that include educational credit, please visit endocrine.org/store.

LEARNING OBJECTIVES

ESAP 2022 will allow learners to assess their knowledge of all aspects of endocrinology, diabetes, and metabolism.

Completion of this educational activity enables learners to accomplish key objectives:

- Recognize clinical manifestations of endocrine and metabolic disorders and select among current options for diagnosis, management, and therapy.
- Identify risk factors for endocrine and metabolic disorders and develop strategies for prevention.
- Evaluate endocrine and metabolic manifestations of systemic disorders.
- Use existing resources pertaining to clinical guidelines and treatment recommendations for endocrine and related metabolic disorders to guide diagnosis and treatment.

TARGET AUDIENCE

ESAP is a self-study curriculum aimed at physicians seeking initial certification or recertification in endocrinology, program directors interested in a testing and training instrument, and clinicians simply wanting a self-assessment and broad review of endocrinology.

STATEMENT OF INDEPENDENCE

The Endocrine Society has a policy of ensuring that the content and quality of this educational activity are balanced, independent, objective, and scientifically rigorous. The scientific content of this activity was developed under the supervision of the Endocrine Society's ESAP Faculty Working Group.

DISCLOSURE POLICY

The faculty, committee members, and staff who are in position to control the content of this activity are required to disclose to the Endocrine Society and to learners any relevant financial relationship(s) of the individual or spouse/partner that have occurred within the last 12 months with any commercial interest(s) whose products or services are related to the CME content. Financial relationships are defined by remuneration in any amount from the commercial interest(s) in the form of grants; research support; consulting fees; salary; ownership interest (eg, stocks, stock options, or ownership interest excluding diversified mutual funds); honoraria or other payments for participation in speakers' bureaus, advisory boards, or boards of directors; or other financial benefits. The intent of this disclosure is not to prevent CME planners with relevant financial relationships from planning or delivering content, but rather to provide learners with information that allows them to make their own judgments of whether these financial relationships may have influenced the educational activity with regard to exposition or conclusion. The Endocrine Society has reviewed all disclosures and resolved or managed all identified conflicts of interest, as applicable.

The following faculty reported relevant financial relationship(s): **Roberto Salvatori, MD**, receives grant funds from Roche, NIH, and the Department of Defense. He is on the advisory board of NovoNordisk, Ipsen, and Strongbridge Biopharma. He serves as a clinical trial investigator for Corcept Therapeutics, Chiasma (now Amryt), and Crinetics Pharmaceuticals. **Anand Vaidya, MD, MMSc**, is a consultant for Mineralys, HRA Pharma, and Corcept. **Thomas J. Weber, MD**, is a consultant for Ultragenyx Pharmaceutical, Pharmacosmos, and Lakeside Life Science. He is also a primary investigator for Ultragenyx Pharmaceutical. His spouse is a primary investigator for AstraZeneca, Sanofi, and Robling Pharmaceutical. **Kevin M. Pantalone, DO**, is a consultant for AstraZeneca, Bayer, Corcept, Diasome, Eli Lilly, Merck, Novo Nordisk, Sanofi, and Twin Health. He is a speaker for AstraZeneca, Corcept, Merck, and Novo Nordisk. He also receives research support from Bayer, Merck, Novo Nordisk, and Twin Health. **Barbara Gisella Carranza Leon, MD**, is a coinvestigator for clinical trials and/or research studies for Novartis, IONIS Pharmaceutical Inc, NIH, FH Foundation, and Regenxbio, Inc. **Meera Shah, MB ChB**, is a research collaborator for Pendulum Therapeutics, Inc. The compensation is paid to Mayo Clinic in lieu of her time. **Nicole M. Ehrhardt, MD**, is a consultant for Novo Nordisk and Dexcom. She is the recipient of educational grants from Novo Nordisk and Merck and the recipient of an investigator-initiated grant from Dexcom. **Mathis Grossmann, MD, PhD**, receives research support for investigator-initiated studies from Bayer AG and Otsuka, and speaker honoraria from Bayer AG, Besins Health Care, and Novartis.

The following committee members reported no relevant financial relationships: **Lisa R. Tannock, MD; Alice Y. Chang, MD, MSc; Dima Lutfi Diab, MD; Nazanene H. Esfandiari, MD; Mark Gurnell, MBBS, MA (Med Ed), PhD; Deepika Reddy, MD; Aniket Sidhaye, MD; Sarah E. Mayson, MD.**

The medical editor for this program, **Abbie L. Young, MS, CGC, ELS(D)**, reported no relevant financial relationships.

The Endocrine Society staff associated with the development of content for this activity reported no relevant financial relationships.

DISCLAIMERS

The information presented in this activity represents the opinion of the faculty and is not necessarily the official position of the Endocrine Society.

USE OF PROFESSIONAL JUDGMENT:

The educational content in this self-assessment test relates to basic principles of diagnosis and therapy and does not substitute for individual patient assessment based on the health care provider's examination of the patient and consideration of laboratory data and other factors unique to the patient. Standards in medicine change as new data become available.

DRUGS AND DOSAGES:

When prescribing medications, the physician is advised to check the product information sheet accompanying each drug to verify conditions of use and to identify any changes in drug dosage schedule or contraindications.

POLICY ON UNLABELED/OFF-LABEL USE

The Endocrine Society has determined that disclosure of unlabeled/off-label or investigational use of commercial product(s) is informative for audiences and therefore requires this information to be disclosed to the learners at the beginning of the presentation. Uses of specific therapeutic agents, devices, and other products discussed in this educational activity may not be the same as those indicated in product labeling approved by the Food and Drug Administration (FDA). The Endocrine Society requires that any discussions of such "off-label" use be based on scientific research that conforms to generally accepted standards of experimental design, data collection, and data analysis. Before recommending or prescribing any therapeutic agent or device, learners should review the complete prescribing information, including indications, contraindications, warnings, precautions, and adverse events.

ACKNOWLEDGMENT OF COMMERCIAL SUPPORT

This activity is not supported by educational grant(s) or other funds from any commercial supporter.

PUBLICATION DATE: February 2022

Laboratory Reference Ranges

Reference ranges vary among laboratories. The listed reference ranges should be used when interpreting laboratory values presented in ESAP™. Conventional units are listed first with SI units in parentheses.

Lipid Values

High-density lipoprotein (HDL) cholesterol
- Optimal — >60 mg/dL (SI: >1.55 mmol/L)
- Normal — 40-60 mg/dL (SI: 1.04-1.55 mmol/L)
- Low — <40 mg/dL (SI: <1.04 mmol/L)

Low-density lipoprotein (LDL) cholesterol
- Optimal — <100 mg/dL (SI: <2.59 mmol/L) (for primary prevention); <70 mg/dL (SI: <1.81 mmol/L) (for secondary prevention)
- Low — 100-129 mg/dL (SI: 2.59-3.34 mmol/L)
- Borderline-high — 130-159 mg/dL (SI: 3.37-4.12 mmol/L)
- High — 160-189 mg/dL (SI: 4.14-4.90 mmol/L)
- Very high — ≥190 mg/dL (SI: ≥4.92 mmol/L)

Non-HDL cholesterol
- Optimal — <130 mg/dL (SI: <3.37 mmol/L)
- Borderline-high — 130-159 mg/dL (SI: 3.37-4.12 mmol/L)
- High — ≥240 mg/dL (SI: ≥6.22 mmol/L)

Total cholesterol
- Optimal — <200 mg/dL (SI: <5.18 mmol/L)
- Borderline-high — 200-239 mg/dL (SI: 5.18-6.19 mmol/L)
- High — ≥240 mg/dL (SI: ≥6.22 mmol/L)

Triglycerides
- Optimal — <150 mg/dL (SI: <1.70 mmol/L)
- Borderline-high — 150-199 mg/dL (SI: 1.70-2.25 mmol/L)
- High — 200-499 mg/dL (SI: 2.26-5.64 mmol/L)
- Very high — ≥500 mg/dL (SI: ≥5.65 mmol/L)

Lipoprotein (a) — ≤30 mg/dL (SI: ≤1.07 µmol/L)
Apolipoprotein B — 50-110 mg/dL (SI: 0.5-1.1 g/L)

Hematologic Values

Erythrocyte sedimentation rate — 0-20 mm/h
Haptoglobin — 30-200 mg/dL (SI: 300-2000 mg/L)
Hematocrit — 41%-51% (SI: 0.41-0.51) (male); 35%-45% (SI: 0.35-0.45) (female)
Hemoglobin A_{1c} — 4.0%-5.6% (20-38 mmol/mol)
Hemoglobin — 13.8-17.2 g/dL (SI: 138-172 g/L) (male); 12.1-15.1 g/dL (SI: 121-151 g/L) (female)
International normalized ratio — 0.8-1.2
Mean corpuscular volume (MCV) — 80-100 µm³ (SI: 80-100 fL)
Platelet count — 150-450 × 10³/µL (SI: 150-450 × 10⁹/L)
Protein (total) — 6.3-7.9 g/dL (SI: 63-79 g/L)
Reticulocyte count — 0.5%-1.5% of red blood cells (SI: 0.005-0.015)
White blood cell count — 4500-11,000/µL (SI: 4.5-11.0 × 10⁹/L)

Thyroid Values

Thyroglobulin — 3-42 ng/mL (SI: 3-42 µg/L) (after surgery and radioactive iodine treatment: <1.0 ng/mL [SI: <1.0 µg/L])
Thyroglobulin antibodies — ≤4.0 IU/mL (SI: ≤4.0 kIU/L)
Thyrotropin (TSH) — 0.5-5.0 mIU/L
Thyrotropin-receptor antibodies (TRAb) — ≤1.75 IU/L
Thyroid-stimulating immunoglobulin — ≤120% of basal activity
Thyroperoxidase (TPO) antibodies — <2.0 IU/mL (SI: <2.0 kIU/L)
Thyroxine (T_4) (free) — 0.8-1.8 ng/dL (SI: 10.30-23.17 pmol/L)
Thyroxine (T_4) (total) — 5.5-12.5 µg/dL (SI: 94.02-213.68 nmol/L)
Free thyroxine (T_4) index — 4-12
Triiodothyronine (T_3) (free) — 2.3-4.2 pg/mL (SI: 3.53-6.45 pmol/L)
Triiodothyronine (T_3) (total) — 70-200 ng/dL (SI: 1.08-3.08 nmol/L)
Triiodothyronine (T_3), reverse — 10-24 ng/dL (SI: 0.15-0.37 nmol/L)
Triiodothyronine uptake, resin — 25%-38%
Radioactive iodine uptake — 3%-16% (6 hours); 15%-30% (24 hours)

Endocrine Values

Serum

Aldosterone — 4-21 ng/dL (SI: 111.0-582.5 pmol/L)
Alkaline phosphatase — 50-120 U/L (SI: 0.84-2.00 µkat/L)
Alkaline phosphatase (bone-specific) — ≤20 µg/L (adult male); ≤14 µg/L (premenopausal female); ≤22 µg/L (postmenopausal female)
Androstenedione — 65-210 ng/dL (SI: 2.27-7.33 nmol/L) (adult male); 30-200 ng/dL (SI: 1.05-6.98 nmol/L) (adult female)
Antimullerian hormone — 0.7-19.0 ng/mL (SI: 5.0-135.7 pmol/L) (male, >12 years); 0.9-9.5 ng/mL (SI: 6.4-67.9 pmol/L) (female, 13-45 years); <1.0 ng/mL (SI: <7.1 pmol/L) (female, >45 years)
Calcitonin — <16 pg/mL (SI: <4.67 pmol/L) (basal, male); <8 pg/mL (SI: <2.34 pmol/L) (basal, female); ≤130 pg/mL (SI: ≤37.96 pmol/L) (peak calcium infusion, male); ≤90 pg/mL (SI: ≤26.28 pmol/L) (peak calcium infusion, female)
Carcinoembryonic antigen — <2.5 ng/mL (SI: <2.5 µg/L)
Chromogranin A — <93 ng/mL (SI: <93 µg/L)
Corticosterone — 53-1560 ng/dL (SI: 1.53-45.08 nmol/L) (>18 years)
Corticotropin (ACTH) — 10-60 pg/mL (SI: 2.2-13.2 pmol/L)
Cortisol (8 AM) — 5-25 µg/dL (SI: 137.9-689.7 nmol/L)
Cortisol (4 PM) — 2-14 µg/dL (SI: 55.2-386.2 nmol/L)
C-peptide — 0.5-2.0 ng/mL (SI: 0.17-0.66 nmol/L)
C-reactive protein — 0.8-3.1 mg/L (SI: 7.62-29.52 nmol/L)
Cross-linked N-telopeptide of type 1 collagen — 5.4-24.2 nmol BCE/mmol creat (male); 6.2-19.0 nmol BCE/mmol creat (female)

Dehydroepiandrosterone sulfate (DHEA-S)

Patient Age	Female	Male
18-29 years	44-332 µg/dL (SI: 1.19-9.00 µmol/L)	89-457 µg/dL (SI: 2.41-12.38 µmol/L)
30-39 years	31-228 µg/dL (SI: 0.84-6.78 µmol/L)	65-334 µg/dL (SI: 1.76-9.05 µmol/L)
40-49 years	18-244 µg/dL (SI: 0.49-6.61 µmol/L)	48-244 µg/dL (SI: 1.30-6.61 µmol/L)
50-59 years	15-200 µg/dL (SI: 0.41-5.42 µmol/L)	35-179 µg/dL (SI: 0.95-4.85 µmol/L)
≥60 years	15-157 µg/dL (SI: 0.41-4.25 µmol/L)	25-131 µg/dL (SI: 0.68-3.55 µmol/L)

Deoxycorticosterone ------ <10 ng/dL (SI: <0.30 nmol/L) (>18 years)
1,25-Dihydroxyvitamin D$_3$ ----- 16-65 pg/mL (SI: 41.6-169.0 pmol/L)
Estradiol --------------- 10-40 pg/mL (SI: 36.7-146.8 pmol/L) (male);
 10-180 pg/mL (SI: 36.7-660.8 pmol/L) (follicular, female);
 100-300 pg/mL (SI: 367.1-1101.3 pmol/L) (midcycle, female);
 40-200 pg/mL (SI: 146.8-734.2 pmol/L) (luteal, female);
 <20 pg/mL (SI: <73.4 pmol/L) (postmenopausal, female)
Estrone --------------- 10-60 pg/mL (SI: 37.0-221.9 pmol/L) (male);
 17-200 pg/mL (SI: 62.9-739.6 pmol/L) (premenopausal female);
 7-40 pg/mL (SI: 25.9-147.9 pmol/L) (postmenopausal female)
α-Fetoprotein ---------------------------------- <6 ng/mL (SI: <6 µg/L)
Follicle-stimulating hormone (FSH) ----------------------------------
 1.0-13.0 mIU/mL (SI: 1.0-13.0 IU/L) (male);
 <3.0 mIU/mL (SI: <3.0 IU/L) (prepuberty, female);
 2.0-12.0 mIU/mL (SI: 2.0-12.0 IU/L) (follicular, female);
 4.0-36.0 mIU/mL (SI: 4.0-36.0 IU/L) (midcycle, female);
 1.0-9.0 mIU/mL (SI: 1.0-9.0 IU/L) (luteal, female);
 >30.0 mIU/mL (SI: >30.0 IU/L) (postmenopausal, female)
Free fatty acids ---------------- 10.6-18.0 mg/dL (SI: 0.4-0.7 nmol/L)
Gastrin --------------------------------- <100 pg/mL (SI: <100 ng/L)
Growth hormone (GH) -- 0.01-0.97 ng/mL (SI: 0.01-0.97 µg/L) (male);
 0.01-3.61 ng/mL (SI: 0.01-3.61 µg/L) (female)
Homocysteine ------------------------- ≤1.76 mg/L (SI: ≤13 µmol/L)
β-Human chorionic gonadotropin (β-hCG) --------------------------
 <3.0 mIU/mL (SI: <3.0 IU/L) (nonpregnant female);
 >25 mIU/mL (SI: >25 IU/L) indicates a positive pregnancy test
β-Hydroxybutyrate ------------------- <3.0 mg/dL (SI: <288.2 µmol/L)
17-Hydroxypregnenolone ------ 29-189 ng/dL (SI: 0.87-5.69 nmol/L)
17α-Hydroxyprogesterone <220 ng/dL (SI: <6.67 nmol/L) (adult male);
 <80 ng/dL (SI: <2.42 nmol/L) (follicular, female);
 <285 ng/dL (SI: <8.64 nmol/L) (luteal, female);
 <51 ng/dL (SI: <1.55 nmol/L) (postmenopausal, female)
25-Hydroxyvitamin D ---- <20 ng/mL (SI: <49.9 nmol/L) (deficiency);
 21-29 ng/mL (SI: 52.4-72.4 nmol/L) (insufficiency);
 30-80 ng/mL (SI: 74.9-199.7 nmol/L) (optimal levels);
 >80 ng/mL (SI: >199.7 nmol/L) (toxicity possible)
Inhibin B --------------------------- 15-300 pg/mL (SI: 15-300 ng/L)

Insulinlike growth factor 1 (IGF-1)

Patient Age	Female	Male
18 years	162-541 ng/mL (SI: 21.2-70.9 nmol/L)	170-640 ng/mL (SI: 22.3-83.8 nmol/L)
19 years	138-442 ng/mL (SI: 18.1-57.9 nmol/L)	147-527 ng/mL (SI: 19.3-69.0 nmol/L)
20 years	122-384 ng/mL (SI: 16.0-50.3 nmol/L)	132-457 ng/mL (SI: 17.3-59.9 nmol/L)
21-25 years	116-341 ng/mL (SI: 15.2-44.7 nmol/L)	116-341 ng/mL (SI: 15.2-44.7 nmol/L)
26-30 years	117-321 ng/mL (SI: 15.3-42.1 nmol/L)	117-321 ng/mL (SI: 15.3-42.1 nmol/L)
31-35 years	113-297 ng/mL (SI: 14.8-38.9 nmol/L)	113-297 ng/mL (SI: 14.8-38.9 nmol/L)
36-40 years	106-277 ng/mL (SI: 13.9-36.3 nmol/L)	106-277 ng/mL (SI: 13.9-36.3 nmol/L)
41-45 years	98-261 ng/mL (SI: 12.8-34.2 nmol/L)	98-261 ng/mL (SI: 12.8-34.2 nmol/L)
46-50 years	91-246 ng/mL (SI: 11.9-32.2 nmol/L)	91-246 ng/mL (SI: 11.9-32.2 nmol/L)
51-55 years	84-233 ng/mL (SI: 11.0-30.5 nmol/L)	84-233 ng/mL (SI: 11.0-30.5 nmol/L)
56-60 years	78-220 ng/mL (SI: 10.2-28.8 nmol/L)	78-220 ng/mL (SI: 10.2-28.8 nmol/L)
61-65 years	72-207 ng/mL (SI: 9.4-27.1 nmol/L)	72-207 ng/mL (SI: 9.4-27.1 nmol/L)
66-70 years	67-195 ng/mL (SI: 8.8-25.5 nmol/L)	67-195 ng/mL (SI: 8.8-25.5 nmol/L)
71-75 years	62-184 ng/mL (SI: 8.1-24.1 nmol/L)	62-184 ng/mL (SI: 8.1-24.1 nmol/L)
76-80 years	57-172 ng/mL (SI: 7.5-22.5 nmol/L)	57-172 ng/mL (SI: 7.5-22.5 nmol/L)
>80 years	53-162 ng/mL (SI: 6.9-21.2 nmol/L)	53-162 ng/mL (SI: 6.9-21.2 nmol/L)

Insulinlike growth factor binding protein 3 -------------- 2.5-4.8 mg/L
Insulin -------------------------- 1.4-14.0 µIU/mL (SI: 9.7-97.2 pmol/L)
Islet-cell antibody assay ------- 0 Juvenile Diabetes Foundation units
Luteinizing hormone (LH) --- 1.0-9.0 mIU/mL (SI: 1.0-9.0 IU/L) (male);
 <1.0 mIU/mL (SI: <1.0 IU/L) (prepuberty, female);
 1.0-18.0 mIU/mL (SI: 1.0-18.0 IU/L) (follicular, female);
 20.0-80.0 mIU/mL (SI: 20.0-80.0 IU/L) (midcycle, female);
 0.5-18.0 mIU/mL (SI: 0.5-18.0 IU/L) (luteal, female);
 >30.0 mIU/mL (SI: >30.0 IU/L) (postmenopausal, female)
Metanephrines (plasma fractionated)
 Metanephrine ----------------------- <99 pg/mL (SI: <0.50 nmol/L)
 Normetanephrine ---------------- <165 pg/mL (SI: <0.90 nmol/L)
75-g oral glucose tolerance test blood glucose values ---------------
 60-100 mg/dL (SI: 3.3-5.6 mmol/L) (fasting);
 <200 mg/dL (SI: <11.1 mmol/L) (1 hour);
 <140 mg/dL (SI: <7.8 mmol/L) (2 hour); between 140-200 mg/dL (SI: 7.8-11.1 mmol/L) is considered impaired glucose tolerance or prediabetes; greater than 200 mg/dL (SI: >11.1 mmol/L) is a sign of diabetes mellitus

50-g oral glucose tolerance test for gestational diabetes ----------
<140 mg/dL (SI: <7.8 mmol/L) (1 hour)
100-g oral glucose tolerance test for gestational diabetes ----------
<95 mg/dL (SI: <5.3 mmol/L) (fasting);
<180 mg/dL (SI: <10.0 mmol/L) (1 hour);
<155 mg/dL (SI: <8.6 mmol/L) (2 hour);
<140 mg/dL (SI: <7.8 mmol/L) (3 hour)
Osteocalcin ---------------------- 9.0-42.0 ng/mL (SI: 9.0-42.0 µg/L)
Parathyroid hormone, intact (PTH) ---- 10-65 pg/mL (SI: 10-65 ng/L)
Parathyroid hormone–related protein (PTHrP) ----------<2.0 pmol/L
Progesterone -------------------≤1.2 ng/mL (SI: ≤3.8 nmol/L) (male)
≤1.0 ng/mL (SI: ≤3.2 nmol/L) (follicular, female);
2.0-20.0 ng/mL (SI: 6.4-63.6 nmol/L) (luteal, female);
≤1.1 ng/mL (SI: ≤3.5 nmol/L) (postmenopausal, female);
>10.0 ng/mL (SI: >31.8 nmol/L) (evidence of ovulatory adequacy)
Proinsulin ------------------- 26.5-176.4 pg/mL (SI: 3.0-20.0 pmol/L)
Prolactin ----------------- 4-23 ng/mL (SI: 0.17-1.00 nmol/L) (male);
4-30 ng/mL (SI: 0.17-1.30 nmol/L) (nonlactating female);
10-200 ng/mL (SI: 0.43-8.70 nmol/L) (lactating female)
Prostate-specific antigen (PSA) -----------------------------------
<2.0 ng/mL (SI: <2.0 µg/L) (≤40 years);
<2.8 ng/mL (SI: <2.8 µg/L) (≤50 years);
<3.8 ng/mL (SI: <3.8 µg/L) (≤60 years);
<5.3 ng/mL (SI: <5.3 µg/L) (≤70 years);
<7.0 ng/mL (SI: <7.0 µg/L) (≤79 years);
<7.2 ng/mL (SI: <7.2 µg/L) (≥80 years)
Renin activity, plasma, sodium replete, ambulatory ----------------
0.6-4.3 ng/mL per h
Renin, direct concentration ---------- 4-44 pg/mL (SI: 0.1-1.0 pmol/L)
Sex hormone–binding globulin (SHBG) --------------- 1.1-6.7 µg/mL
(SI: 10-60 nmol/L) (male);
2.2-14.6 µg/mL (SI: 20-130 nmol/L) (female)
α-Subunit of pituitary glycoprotein hormones ---------------------
<1.2 ng/mL (SI: <1.2 µg/L)
Testosterone (bioavailable) ----- 0.8-4.0 ng/dL (SI: 0.03-0.14 nmol/L)
(20-50 years, female on oral estrogen);
0.8-10.0 ng/dL (SI: 0.03-0.35 nmol/L)
(20-50 years, female not on oral estrogen);
83.0-257.0 ng/dL (SI: 2.88-8.92 nmol/L) (male 20-29 years);
72.0-235.0 ng/dL (SI: 2.50-8.15 nmol/L) (male 30-39 years);
61.0-213.0 ng/dL (SI: 2.12-7.39 nmol/L) (male 40-49 years);
50.0-190.0 ng/dL (SI: 1.74-6.59 nmol/L) (male 50-59 years);
40.0-168.0 ng/dL (SI: 1.39-5.83 nmol/L) (male 60-69 years)
Testosterone (free) ----- 9.0-30.0 ng/dL (SI: 0.31-1.04 nmol/L) (male);
0.3-1.9 ng/dL (SI: 0.01-0.07 nmol/L) (female)
Testosterone (total) ---- 300-900 ng/dL (SI: 10.4-31.2 nmol/L) (male);
8-60 ng/dL (SI: 0.3-2.1 nmol/L) (female)
Vitamin B_{12} -------------------- 180-914 pg/mL (SI: 133-674 pmol/L)

Chemistry Values

Alanine aminotransferase ---------- 10-40 U/L (SI: 0.17-0.67 µkat/L)
Albumin----------------------------------3.5-5.0 g/dL (SI: 35-50 g/L)
Amylase --------------------------- 26-102 U/L (SI: 0.43-1.70 µkat/L)
Aspartate aminotransferase ------- 20-48 U/L (SI: 0.33-0.80 µkat/L)
Bicarbonate ------------------------ 21-28 mEq/L (SI: 21-28 mmol/L)
Bilirubin (total) ------------------- 0.3-1.2 mg/dL (SI: 5.1-20.5 µmol/L)
Blood gases
    Po_2, arterial blood ----------- 80-100 mm Hg (SI: 10.6-13.3 kPa)
    Pco_2, arterial blood ---------------- 35-45 mm Hg (SI: 4.7-6.0 kPa)
Blood pH--7.35-7.45
Calcium ----------------------- 8.2-10.2 mg/dL (SI: 2.1-2.6 mmol/L)
Calcium (ionized) -------------- 4.60-5.08 mg/dL (SI: 1.2-1.3 mmol/L)
Carbon dioxide --------------------- 22-28 mEq/L (SI: 22-28 mmol/L)
CD_4 cell count--------------------- 500-1400/µL (SI: 0.5-1.4 × 10^9/L)
Chloride------------------------- 96-106 mEq/L (SI: 96-106 mmol/L)
Creatine kinase -------------------- 50-200 U/L (SI: 0.84-3.34 µkat/L)
Creatinine------------- 0.7-1.3 mg/dL (SI: 61.9-114.9 µmol/L) (male);
0.6-1.1 mg/dL (SI: 53.0-97.2 µmol/L) (female)
Ferritin ----------------------- 15-200 ng/mL (SI: 33.7-449.4 pmol/L)
Folate-------------------------------------≥4.0 ng/mL (SI: ≥4.0 µg/L)
Glucose -------------------------- 70-99 mg/dL (SI: 3.9-5.5 mmol/L)
γ-Glutamyltransferase ---------------2-30 U/L (SI: 0.03-0.50 µkat/L)
Iron -----------------------50-150 µg/dL (SI: 9.0-26.8 µmol/L) (male);
35-145 µg/dL (SI: 6.3-26.0 µmol/L) (female)
Lactate dehydrogenase ----------- 100-200 U/L (SI: 1.7-3.3 µkat/L)
Lactic acid ---------------------- 5.4-20.7 mg/dL (SI: 0.6-2.3 mmol/L)
Lipase ---------------------------- 10-73 U/L (SI: 0.17-1.22 µkat/L)
Magnesium ---------------------- 1.5-2.3 mg/dL (SI: 0.6-0.9 mmol/L)
Osmolality --------------- 275-295 mOsm/kg (SI: 275-295 mmol/kg)
Phosphate---------------------- 2.3-4.7 mg/dL (SI: 0.7-1.5 mmol/L)
Potassium --------------------------3.5-5.0 mEq/L (SI: 3.5-5.0 mmol/L)
Prothrombin time ------------------------------------- 8.3-10.8 s
Serum urea nitrogen--------------- 8-23 mg/dL (SI: 2.9-8.2 mmol/L)
Sodium ----------------------- 136-142 mEq/L (SI: 136-142 mmol/L)
Transferrin saturation --------------------------------- 14%-50%
Troponin I----------------------------------<0.6 ng/mL (SI: <0.6 µg/L)
Tryptase ------------------------------ <11.5 ng/mL (SI: <11.5 µg/L)
Uric acid --------------------- 3.5-7.0 mg/dL (SI: 208.2-416.4 µmol/L)

Urine

Albumin------------- 30-300 µg/mg creat (SI: 3.4-33.9 µg/mol creat)
Albumin-to-creatinine ratio ------------------------- <30 mg/g creat
Aldosterone---------------------- 3-20 µg/24 h (SI: 8.3-55.4 nmol/d)
(should be <12 µg/24 h [SI: <33.2 nmol/d] with oral sodium
loading—confirmed with 24-hour urinary sodium >200 mEq)
Calcium ----------------------- 100-300 mg/24 h (SI: 2.5-7.5 mmol/d)
Catecholamine fractionation
    Normotensive normal ranges:
        Dopamine-------------------<400 µg/24 h (SI: <2610 nmol/d)
        Epinephrine-------------------<21 µg/24 h (SI: <115 nmol/d)
        Norepinephrine---------------<80 µg/24 h (SI: <473 nmol/d)

Citrate -------------------- 320-1240 mg/24 h (SI: 16.7-64.5 mmol/d)
Cortisol --------------------------- 4-50 µg/24 h (SI: 11-138 nmol/d)
Cortisol following dexamethasone-suppression test (low-dose:
    2 day, 2 mg daily) ----------------- <10 µg/24 h (SI: <27.6 nmol/d)
Creatinine---------------------- 1.0-2.0 g/24 h (SI: 8.8-17.7 mmol/d)
Glomerular filtration rate (estimated) ------->60 mL/min per 1.73 m^2
5-Hydroxyindole acetic acid----- 2-9 mg/24 h (SI: 10.5-47.1 µmol/d)
Iodine (random)--- >100 µg/L
17-Ketosteroids ---- 6.0-21.0 mg/24 h (SI: 20.8-72.9 µmol/d) (male);
    4.0-17.0 mg/24 h (SI: 13.9-59.0 µmol/d) (female)
Metanephrine fractionation
    Normotensive normal ranges:
        Metanephrine -------- <261 µg/24 h (SI: <1323 nmol/d) (male);
            <180 µg/24 h (SI: <913 nmol/d) (female)
        Normetanephrine --------------------- age and sex dependent
        Total metanephrine ------------------- age and sex dependent
Osmolality ------------- 150-1150 mOsm/kg (SI: 150-1150 mmol/kg)
Oxalate ----------------------------- <40 mg/24 h (SI: <456 mmol/d)
Phosphate --------------------- 0.9-1.3 g/24 h (SI: 29.1-42.0 mmol/d)
Potassium --------------------- 17-77 mEq/24 h (SI: 17-77 mmol/d)
Sodium ---------------------- 40-217 mEq/24 h (SI: 40-217 mmol/d)
Uric acid -------------------------------<800 mg/24 h (SI: <4.7 mmol/d)

Saliva

Cortisol (salivary), midnight ------------ <0.13 µg/dL (SI: <3.6 nmol/L)

Semen

Semen analysis ---------------- >20 million sperm/mL; >50% motility

Abbreviations

ACTH -- corticotropin
ACE inhibitor--------------- angiotensin-converting enzyme inhibitor
ALT -- alanine aminotransferase
AST --------------------------------------- aspartate aminotransferase
BMI -- body mass index
CNS -- central nervous system
CT-- computed tomography
DHEA -- dehydroepiandrosterone
DHEA-S----------------------------- dehydroepiandrosterone sulfate
DNA --- deoxyribonucleic acid
DPP-4 inhibitor ----------------------- dipeptidyl-peptidase 4 inhibitor
DXA------------------------------- dual-energy x-ray absorptiometry
FDA------------------------------------- Food and Drug Administration
FGF-23 ------------------------------------ fibroblast growth factor 23
FNA-- fine-needle aspiration
FSH --- follicle-stimulating hormone
GH --- growth hormone
GHRH--------------------------- growth hormone–releasing hormone
GLP-1 receptor agonist----- glucagonlike peptide 1 receptor agonist
GnRH ----------------------------- gonadotropin-releasing hormone
hCG ----------------------------------- human chorionic gonadotropin
HDL--- high-density lipoprotein
HIV------------------------------------ human immunodeficiency virus
HMG-CoA reductase inhibitor ---------- 3-hydroxy-3-methylglutaryl
    coenzyme A reductase inhibitor
IGF-1------------------------------------- insulinlike growth factor 1
LDL ---low-density lipoprotein
LH --- luteinizing hormone
MCV --- mean corpuscular volume
MIBG------------------------------------ meta-iodobenzylguanidine
MRI --------------------------------------- magnetic resonance imaging
NPH insulin --------------------- neutral protamine Hagedorn insulin
PCSK9 inhibitor ---- proprotein convertase subtilisin/kexin 9 inhibitor
PET -------------------------------------positron emission tomography
PSA -- prostate-specific antigen
PTH ---parathyroid hormone
PTHrP------------------------- parathyroid hormone–related protein
SGLT-2 inhibitor ----------sodium-glucose cotransporter 2 inhibitor
SHBG --------------------------------- sex hormone–binding globulin
T$_3$ --- triiodothyronine
T$_4$ --- thyroxine
TPO antibodies -------------------------- thyroperoxidase antibodies
TRH--------------------------------------- thyrotropin-releasing hormone
TRAb -- TSH-receptor antibodies
TSH --- thyrotropin
VLDL------------------------------------ very low-density lipoprotein

ENDOCRINE SELF-ASSESSMENT PROGRAM 2022

Part I

1 A 24-year-old medical student presents for further evaluation of hyperglycemia. One night 6 weeks ago, he was on a night shift at the hospital when he missed dinner and ate a generous piece of cake instead. About 30 minutes later, he felt "lousy," with symptoms including headache, dizziness, and sweating. He checked his blood glucose by fingerstick, and the value was 220 mg/dL (12.2 mmol/L).

His primary care physician measured his hemoglobin A$_{1c}$, which was 7.7% (61 mmol/mol). He was prescribed insulin glargine, 8 units once daily, and insulin aspart with meals, 2 units per meal. He has since reduced the insulin glargine dose to 4 units due to nocturnal hypoglycemia. He limits carbohydrates with meals and rarely takes mealtime insulin. He has no relevant medical history.

During a rotation in endocrinology, he learned about autoimmune and monogenic causes of diabetes. He wants to know whether he has maturity-onset diabetes of the young or perhaps type 1 diabetes and is in the honeymoon period since his insulin needs have dropped.

Review of family history documents type 2 diabetes in his paternal grandfather and father. Although he does not know whether his grandfather had diabetes-related complications, his father has neuropathy and a mildly elevated urine albumin-to-creatinine ratio (57 mg/g creat). His father has no structural kidney problems such as cysts.

On physical examination, the patient's blood pressure is 112/72 mm Hg and pulse rate is 68 beats/min. His height is 71 in (180 cm), and weight is 165 lb (75 kg) (BMI = 23 kg/m^2). He appears well. There are no skin findings such as acanthosis nigricans. His thyroid gland appears normal, and the rest of the examination findings are unremarkable.

Laboratory test results:
Hemoglobin A$_{1c}$ = 7.4% (4.0%-5.6%) (57 mmol/mol [20-38 mmol/mol])
C-peptide = 2.6 ng/mL (0.9-4.3 ng/mL) (SI: 0.86 nmol/L [0.30-1.42 nmol/L])
Glucose = 165 mg/dL (70-99 mg/dL) (SI: 9.2 mmol/L [3.9-5.5 mmol/L])
Glutamic acid decarboxylase 65 antibodies, undetectable

This patient most likely has a pathogenic variant in which of the following genes?
A. *HNF1A* (HNF1 homeobox A)
B. *NEUROD1* (neuronal differentiation 1)
C. *GCK* (glucokinase)
D. *HNF1B* (HNF1 homeobox B)
E. *PDX1* (pancreatic and duodenal homeobox 1)

2 A 59-year-old woman is referred for endocrine evaluation after a suspected pituitary macroadenoma was identified on CT performed to investigate right-sided headaches. She reports tiredness and fatigue, which she attributes to poor-quality sleep. She has type 2 diabetes mellitus and hypertension. Her medications are metformin, 850 mg twice daily; empagliflozin, 10 mg daily; ramipril, 10 mg daily; and atorvastatin, 80 mg daily.

On physical examination, her height is 68 in (173 cm) and weight is 203 lb (92.3 kg) (BMI = 31 kg/m^2). Her resting pulse rate is 64 beats/min and regular, and blood pressure is 145/85 mm Hg. Visual acuity is 20/20 (6/6) in both eyes. Formal visual field assessment demonstrates no abnormality.

Laboratory test results:
Prolactin = 69.5 ng/mL (4-30 ng/mL) (SI: 3.02 nmol/L [0.17-1.30 nmol/L]) (confirmed following dilution studies)
TSH = 0.7 mIU/L (0.5-5.0 mIU/L)
Free T$_4$ = 0.65 ng/dL (0.8-1.8 ng/dL) (SI: 8.37 pmol/L [10.30-23.17 pmol/L])
Cortisol (8 AM) = 24.5 μg/dL (5-25 μg/dL) (SI: 675.9 nmol/L [137.9-689.7 nmol/L])
ACTH = 52 pg/mL (10-60 pg/mL) (SI: 11.4 pmol/L [2.2-13.2 pmol/L])
IGF-1 = 125 ng/mL (78-220 ng/mL) (SI: 16.4 nmol/L [10.2-28.8 nmol/L])
FSH = 2.1 mIU/mL (>30.0 mIU/mL) (SI: 2.1 IU/L [>30.0 IU/L])
LH = 1.9 mIU/mL (>30.0 mIU/mL) (SI: 1.9 IU/L [>30.0 IU/L])
Estradiol = 15 pg/mL (<20 pg/mL) (SI: 55.1 pmol/L [<73.4 pmol/L])

MRI of the sella is shown (*see images*).

T1 coronal (postcontrast)   **T1 sagittal (postcontrast)**   **T2 sagittal**

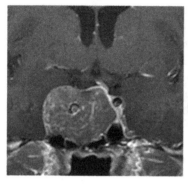 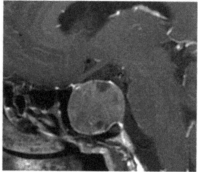 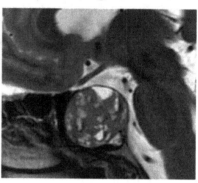

The patient is referred for transsphenoidal surgical decompression.

Which of the following immunohistochemical stains is most likely to be positive in the resected tumor?
- A. ACTH
- B. FSH β-subunit
- C. GH
- D. Prolactin
- E. TSH β-subunit

3 A 47-year-old woman is found to have a 2.8-cm right adrenal mass on abdominal CT performed for evaluation of left iliac fossa pain, which is subsequently attributed to diverticulitis. She has a history of rheumatoid arthritis that is well controlled on a combination of methotrexate and adalimumab. Following resolution of the diverticulitis, she is referred for endocrine assessment.

On physical examination, her blood pressure is 145/85 mm Hg and pulse rate is 76 beats/min and regular. Her height is 67 in (170.2 cm), and weight is 179 lb (81.4 kg) (BMI = 28 kg/m^2). Examination findings are unremarkable, and no specific endocrine stigmata are observed.

Laboratory test results:
    Serum potassium = 3.6 mEq/L (3.5-5.0 mEq/L) (SI: 3.6 mmol/L [3.5-5.0 mmol/L])
    Plasma renin activity = 1.8 ng/mL per h (0.6-4.3 ng/mL per h)
    Plasma aldosterone = 11.2 ng/dL (4-21 ng/dL) (SI: 311 pmol/L [111.0-582.5 pmol/L])
    Serum cortisol following 1-mg dexamethasone-suppression test = 3.8 µg/dL (SI: 105 nmol/L)
    Serum DHEA-S = 205 µg/dL (18-244 µg/dL) (SI: 5.56 µmol/L [0.49-6.61 µmol/L])
    Plasma ACTH = 33 pg/mL (10-60 pg/mL) (SI: 7.3 pmol/L [2.2-13.2 pmol/L])

Adrenal CT shows a 2.8-cm homogeneous right adrenal lesion. The unenhanced density is 8 Hounsfield units. The left adrenal gland is normal.

Which of the following is the most likely explanation for these findings?
- A. Adrenocortical carcinoma
- B. Cortisol-secreting adrenal adenoma
- C. Cushing disease
- D. Ectopic ACTH syndrome with adrenal metastasis
- E. Nonfunctioning adrenal adenoma

4 A 65-year-old man with hypertension, prediabetes, irritable bowel syndrome, and coronary artery disease status post coronary artery bypass grafting is referred for management of hypercholesterolemia. A cholesterol disorder was diagnosed when he had open-heart surgery 5 years ago. Since then, he has tried several statins at different dosages and frequencies and has only been able to tolerate atorvastatin, 20 mg daily. A few months ago, ezetimibe was added to his regimen because his LDL-cholesterol level was not at goal (<70 mg/dL [<1.81 mmol/L]). However, he developed adverse effects related to this medication and stopped taking it. He follows a plant-based diet. His medications include lisinopril, metoprolol, atorvastatin, aspirin, and furosemide.

On physical examination, his blood pressure is 122/77 mm Hg, and pulse rate is 88 beats/min. His height is 69 in (175.3 cm), and weight is 185 lb (84.1 kg) (BMI = 27 kg/m^2). He has a well-healed midline scar on his chest. His breathing effort is normal, and his lungs are clear to auscultation bilaterally. On cardiac examination, his heart sounds are normal with a regular rate and rhythm. His abdomen is soft and nontender.

The patient is aware that adding a second agent to his cholesterol-lowering regimen will decrease his risk of having another cardiovascular event. However, he is interested in a medication that will not affect his other comorbidities.

Laboratory test results:
    Hemoglobin A$_{1c}$ = 6.0% (4.0%-5.6%) (42 mmol/mol [20-38 mmol/mol])
    Creatinine = 0.9 mg/dL (0.7-1.3 mg/dL) (SI: 79.6 μmol/L [61.9-114.9 μmol/L])
    Total cholesterol = 152 mg/dL (<200 mg/dL [optimal]) (SI: 3.94 mmol/L [<5.18 mmol/L])
    Triglycerides = 103 mg/dL (<150 mg/dL [optimal]) (SI: 1.16 mmol/L [<1.70 mmol/L])
    HDL cholesterol = 47 mg/dL (>60 mg/dL [optimal]) (SI: 1.22 mmol/L [>1.55 mmol/L])
    LDL cholesterol = 84 mg/dL (<100 mg/dL [optimal]) (SI: 2.18 mmol/L [<2.59 mmol/L])

Which of the following medications should be added next to this patient's regimen?
    A. Niacin
    B. Colesevelam
    C. Bempedoic acid
    D. Fenofibrate
    E. Icosapent ethyl

5 A 66-year-old woman with a history of muscular dystrophy returns for a follow-up visit for osteoporosis. Osteoporosis was diagnosed at age 58 years when DXA revealed T-scores of −3.2 in the right total hip and −3.3 in the left total hip. She took alendronate very briefly and stopped it due to upper gastrointestinal adverse effects. She then took teriparatide for 2 years, followed by 2 annual intravenous zoledronic acid infusions. Because of declining bone mineral density despite therapy, her regimen was switched to denosumab injections 1 year ago. She now reports that she was recently diagnosed with stage 1 osteonecrosis of the jaw. She has no history of fragility fractures. Her intake of calcium and vitamin D is adequate. She had a myocardial infarction 6 months ago.

Physical examination reveals a 2-cm area of mucosal ulceration with minimal bone exposure in her hard palate at the location of a maxillary torus. She is unable to stand without assistance.

Laboratory test results:
    Serum calcium = 10.1 mg/dL (8.2-10.2 mg/dL) (SI: 2.5 mmol/L [2.1-2.6 mmol/L])
    Serum phosphate = 3.7 mg/dL (2.3-4.7 mg/dL) (SI: 1.2 mmol/L [0.7-1.5 mmol/L])
    Serum creatinine = 0.3 mg/dL (0.6-1.1 mg/dL) (SI: 26.5 μmol/L [53.0-97.2 μmol/L])
    Serum 25-hydroxyvitamin D = 48 ng/mL (30-80 ng/mL [optimal]) (SI: 119.8 nmol/L [74.9-199.7 nmol/L])
    Serum albumin = 4.6 g/dL (3.5-5.0 g/dL) (SI: 46 g/L [35-50 g/L])
    Serum alkaline phosphatase = 66 U/L (50-120 U/L) (SI: 1.10 μkat/L [0.84-2.00 μkat/L])

Another DXA scan documents improving bone mineral density readings in both hips, with T-scores of −2.9 in the right total hip and −3.0 in the left total hip.

Which of the following is the best recommendation regarding this patient's medical management?
- A. Discontinue denosumab
- B. Switch from denosumab to raloxifene
- C. Switch from denosumab to abaloparatide
- D. Switch from denosumab to romosozumab
- E. Continue denosumab

6

A 51-year-old man presents to discuss a new diagnosis of diabetes mellitus. Two weeks ago, he saw his primary care provider because of polyuria, polydipsia, and a 15-lb (6.8-kg) weight loss over the last 3 months. His hemoglobin A_{1c} value at that time was 12.2% (110 mmol/mol). He was told he had diabetes and was prescribed metformin, 500 mg XR twice daily.

His point-of-care glucose value today is 512 mg/dL (28.4 mmol/L), 90 minutes after eating lunch. He still has significant thirst and urination but no abdominal pain, nausea, muscle pain, or light-headedness and no gastrointestinal distress from metformin.

On physical examination, his height is 70 in (177.8 cm) and weight is 232 lb (105.5 kg) (BMI = 33 kg/m²). His blood pressure is 142/83 mm Hg, and pulse rate is 88 beats/min. He appears to be comfortable and in no acute distress. There is no epigastric tenderness and no skin turgor, but acanthosis nigricans is present in the neck creases. Distal pulses are 2+.

Initial laboratory test results from the primary care clinic:
Hemoglobin A_{1c} = 12.2% (4.0%-5.6%) (110 mmol/mol [20-38 mmol/mol])
Creatinine = 1.0 mg/dL (0.7-1.3 mg/dL) (SI: 88.4 µmol/L [61.9-114.9 µmol/L])
Serum urea nitrogen = 36 mg/dL (8-23 mg/dL) (SI: 12.9 mmol/L [2.9-8.2 mmol/L])
Plasma glucose = 301 mg/dL (70-99 mg/dL) (SI: 16.7 mmol/L [3.9-5.5 mmol/L])
Sodium = 132 mEq/L (136-142 mEq/L) (SI: 132 mmol/L [136-142 mmol/L])

Which of the following is the best next step in this patient's management?
- A. Send him to the emergency department for fluids and acute glucose management
- B. Increase metformin dosage to 1000 mg twice daily
- C. Increase metformin dosage to 1000 mg twice daily and add glimepiride
- D. Increase metformin dosage to 1000 mg twice daily and add basal insulin
- E. Increase metformin dosage to 1000 mg twice daily and add glimepiride and sitagliptin

7

A 32-year-old man seeks evaluation for infertility after a semen analysis performed via his primary care provider demonstrated azoospermia. He attends the appointment with his wife, aged 34 years, who leads the discussion. They have been married for 3 years and have regular sexual intercourse. She is healthy and reports regular menses. He describes normal puberty, has no significant medical history, and reports no regular medication use. He does not smoke cigarettes or drink alcohol.

On physical examination, his height is 68 in (173 cm), and weight is 170 lb (77.3 kg) (BMI = 26 kg/m²). His blood pressure is 149/83 mm Hg, and resting pulse rate is 68 beats/min. He is muscular and has pustular acne on his upper back and midline chest. Phallus is normal, and testicular volume is 5 mL bilaterally, without masses.

Current laboratory test results (drawn in the morning, in the fasting state):
Serum testosterone = 50 ng/dL (300-900 ng/dL) (SI: 1.7 nmol/L [10.4-31.2 nmol/L])
SHBG = 0.8 µg/mL (1.1-6.7 µg/mL) (SI: 7.1 nmol/L [10-60 nmol/L])
LH = 0.2 mIU/mL (1.0-9.0 mIU/mL) (SI: 0.2 IU/L [1.0-9.0 IU/L])
FSH = 0.3 mIU/mL (1.0-13.0 mIU/mL) (SI: 0.3 IU/L [1.0-13.0 IU/L])
Hemoglobin = 18.3 g/dL (13.8-17.2 g/dL) (SI: 183 g/L [138-172 g/L])
Thyroid function, normal
Prolactin, normal

A repeated serum testosterone measurement (sample drawn 1 week later) is 40 ng/dL (1.4 nmol/L).

Which of the following is the best next step in this patient's management?
A. Perform pituitary-directed MRI
B. Take a careful drug and supplement history
C. Perform testicular ultrasonography
D. Measure serum hCG
E. Measure serum DHEA-S

8 A 72-year-old woman is referred following a recent vertebral fracture. She reports the onset of acute midback pain after lifting her mattress 6 weeks ago. Evaluation by her primary care physician included a plain x-ray that showed a new moderate compression fracture (~30% anterior height loss) at the eighth thoracic vertebrae without evidence of retropulsion. At today's appointment, she reports mild, dull midback pain (3/10) that is worse with standing. There is no radiation of pain and no other associated symptoms. Her medical history is notable for osteoporosis based on DXA without history of low-trauma fractures, for which she has not been treated with pharmacotherapy to date. Family history is negative for osteoporosis or hip fracture. Current medications include tramadol, ibuprofen, and calcium with vitamin D. She is allergic to penicillin and whitefish.

On physical examination, she is approximately 2 in (5.1 cm) shorter than her self-reported maximum adult height. She has tenderness to palpation and percussion over the midthoracic spine without deformity. Her spine is minimally kyphotic. The rib-to-pelvis distance is diminished at 1 fingerbreadth bilaterally.

Laboratory test results are all within acceptable limits, including measurements of calcium, albumin, creatinine, TSH, phosphate, and 25-hydroxyvitamin D. DXA from 6 months ago shows osteoporosis, with a lumbar spine T-score of –2.8. The left hip is osteopenic based on femoral neck and total hip T-scores of –2.2 and –1.6, respectively.

In addition to prescribing an oral bisphosphonate, which of the following is the recommended next step in the management of this patient's osteoporosis?
A. Referral to interventional radiology for kyphoplasty
B. Strict bedrest for 4 weeks
C. Oxycodone for pain control
D. Referral to physical therapy for acute fracture management
E. Nasal calcitonin

9 A 42-year-old woman presents with a chief concern of neck fullness for the last 2 to 3 weeks. She also has intermittent difficulty swallowing calcium tablets and metformin. She has had no weight loss or dysphonia. She has a history of polycystic ovary syndrome.

On physical examination, her blood pressure is 125/68 mm Hg and pulse rate is 70 beats/min and regular. Her height is 62 in (157.5 cm), and weight is 171 lb (77.5 kg) (BMI = 31 kg/m^2). Her thyroid gland is not palpable and no thyroid nodules are felt. There is no lower-extremity edema. The rest of the examination findings are normal.

Laboratory test results:
TSH = 1.6 mIU/L (0.5-5.0 mIU/L)
Basic metabolic panel, normal

Thyroid ultrasonography reveals a right thyroid nodule (1.2 cm [anteroposterior] × 1.3 cm [transverse] × 1.45 cm [longitudinal]) with the feature noted by the arrow (*see images*). The left lobe is unremarkable.

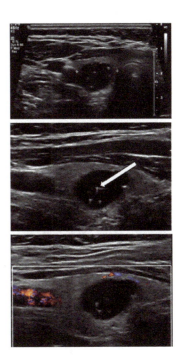

Which of the following is the best next step in this patient's management?
- A. FNA biopsy of the nodule
- B. Thyroid ultrasonography again in 12 months
- C. Neck CT to evaluate dysphagia
- D. Barium esophagography to evaluate dysphagia
- E. Alcohol ablation of the nodule

10 A 46-year-old woman with type 2 diabetes mellitus, hypertension, and hyperlipidemia presents for a follow-up appointment. Since her diagnosis of type 2 diabetes 4 years ago, her hemoglobin A_{1c} levels have been in the range of 7.0% to 8.0% (53-64 mmol/mol).

Her hemoglobin A_{1c} level today is 7.5% (58 mmol/mol) despite trying to maintain a strict diet (<100 g carbohydrate per 24 hours), an exercise regimen (moderately intense exercise 30 minutes a day, 6 days a week), and metformin therapy. Current medications are metformin, 1000 mg twice daily; lisinopril, 10 mg daily; and atorvastatin, 40 mg daily. She has no history of significant alcohol or acetaminophen use.

On physical examination, her blood pressure is 128/72 mm Hg and pulse rate is 50 beats/min. Her height is 65 in (165 cm), and weight is 175 lb (79.5 kg) (BMI = 29 kg/m²). She has skin tags and acanthosis nigricans. No violacious striae are visible. The rest of the examination findings are normal.

Laboratory test results:
    Comprehensive metabolic panel, normal (except for AST and ALT)
    AST = 80 U/L (20-48 U/L) (SI: 1.34 µkat/L [0.33-0.80 µkat/L])
    ALT = 25 U/L (10-40 U/L) (SI: 0.42 µkat/L [0.17-0.67 µkat/L])
    γ-Glutamyltransferase = 20 U/L (2-30 U/L) (SI: 0.33 µkat/L [0.03-0.50 µkat/L])
    Viral hepatitis screen, negative
    Antinuclear antibodies, normal
    Albumin = 4.0 g/dL (3.5-5.0 g/dL) (SI: 70 g/L [35-50 g/L])
    Platelet count = 300 × 10³/µL (150-450 × 10³/µL) (SI: 300 × 10⁹/L [150-450 × 10⁹/L])
    Estimated glomerular filtration rate = 92 mL/min per 1.73 m² (>60 mL/min per 1.73 m²)
    Albumin-to-creatinine ratio = 14 mg/g creat (<30 mg/g creat)

Her Fibrosis-4 (FIB-4) score is 2.45. She undergoes liver biopsy, which confirms nonalcoholic steatohepatitis with moderate fibrosis.

On the basis of this patient's presentation, which of the following medications should be added as the best next step in her management?
- A. Obeticholic acid
- B. Canagliflozin
- C. Vitamin E
- D. Sitagliptin
- E. Pioglitazone

11 A 36-year-old woman presents for evaluation of weight gain and fatigue. Her weight had been steady for several years prior to an unexplained weight gain of 20 lb (9.1 kg) in the last 3 months, despite no obvious change in physical activity or dietary intake. She has a history of migraine headaches that have been well managed on topiramate. However, 6 months prior to this visit, she described intermittent fingertip tingling to her primary care physician who discontinued topiramate and started gabapentin, 300 mg 3 times daily, with subsequent symptom improvement. Topiramate was reintroduced about 1 week ago because of worsening headaches.

The patient has taken an oral contraceptive pill for several years. In addition, she has depression that is well managed with bupropion and fluoxetine.

On physical examination, her height is 64 in (163 cm) and weight is 142 lb (64.4 kg) (BMI = 24 kg/m²). She has no facial rounding or supraclavicular fullness. Her weight is symmetrically distributed, and there is no peripheral edema. She has a large, firm thyroid on examination.

Laboratory test results:
    Fasting glucose = 98 mg/dL (70-99 mg/dL) (SI: 5.4 mmol/L [3.9-5.5 mmol/L])
    TSH = 6.1 mIU/L (0.5-5.0 mIU/L)
    Free T_4 = 1.0 ng/dL (0.8-1.8 ng/dL) (SI: 12.87 pmol/L [10.30-23.147 pmol/L])
    Serum cortisol (8 AM) = 22 μg/dL (5-25 μg/dL) (SI: 607 nmol/L [137.9-689.1 nmol/L])

Which of the following is the most likely explanation for this patient's weight gain?
    A. Primary hypothyroidism
    B. Starting gabapentin
    C. Oral contraceptive pill
    D. Hypercortisolism
    E. Combination therapy with bupropion and fluoxetine

12

A 66-year-old man with type 2 diabetes mellitus returns to clinic for a follow-up visit. His diabetes has been well controlled for the past 5 years on once-weekly exenatide LAR and insulin glargine, and his most recent hemoglobin A_{1c} value is 6.5% (48 mmol/mol). He has not noticed any hypoglycemia. His weight has been stable.

He has had peripheral neuropathy for several years, and the associated pain is treated with gabapentin, 300 mg 3 times daily. Over the past year, he has had increased numbness and decreased sensation in his feet. He recently noticed some weakness in his lower extremities and subsequently in his hands. He has also had difficulty getting dressed and standing from the seated position and has fallen twice. He reports mild worsening of the burning sensation in his feet, particularly when lying in bed.

He has a history of Crohn disease and underwent total colectomy 20 years ago. He has not been able to tolerate metformin. He has hypertension treated with lisinopril and hydrochlorothiazide and hyperlipidemia treated with atorvastatin.

On physical examination, his blood pressure is 126/76 mm Hg and pulse rate is 78 beats/min. His height is 74.5 in (189.2 cm), and weight is 264 lb (120 kg) (BMI = 33 kg/m²). On 10-g monofilament testing, he has decreased sensation on the plantar aspect of his feet and fingertips (most prominent distally). He has atrophy of the thenar eminence, as well as the dorsal web space of the hands. He has to push on the arms of the chair to rise from the seated position. Muscle strength at the hip flexors is +3/5. He has trouble raising his arms above his head.

Laboratory test results:
    Hemoglobin A_{1c} = 6.5% (4.0%-5.6%) (48 mmol/mol [20-38 mmol/mol])
    Protein (total) = 7.7 g/dL (6.3-7.9 g/dL) (SI: 77 g/L [63-79 g/L])
    Albumin = 4.0 g/dL (3.5-5.0 g/dL) (SI: 40 g/L [35-50 g/L])
    Creatinine = 1.2 mg/dL (0.7-1.3 mg/dL) (SI: 106.1 μmol/L [61.9-114.9 μmol/L])
    Calcium = 9.2 mg/dL (8.5-10.2 mg/dL)
    Albumin-to-creatinine ratio = 84 mg/g creat (<30 mg/g creat)
    Hemoglobin = 13.9 g/dL (13.8-17.2 g/dL) (SI: 139 g/L [138-172 g/L])
    Hematocrit = 42% (39.0%-51.0%) (SI: 0.42 [0.41-0.51])
    Vitamin B_{12} = 322 pg/mL (180-914 pg/mL) (SI: 238 pmol/L [133-674 pmol/L])
    Glutamic acid decarboxylase 65 antibodies, undetectable

Which of the following is the best next step in this patient's management?
    A. Increase the gabapentin dosage to 600 mg 3 times daily
    B. Stop gabapentin and start duloxetine
    C. Measure rheumatoid factor
    D. Consult neurology
    E. Perform serum protein electrophoresis/urine protein electrophoresis

13

A 25-year-old woman with classic congenital adrenal hyperplasia presents for preconception counseling. Congenital adrenal hyperplasia was diagnosed when she had an adrenal crisis shortly after birth. She had clitoromegaly and labial changes and underwent minor surgery as a child. She was treated with prednisone in childhood and switched to hydrocortisone when she transitioned to adult endocrinology. Oral contraceptives were started shortly after menarche to help manage hirsutism. She had some menstrual irregularity although she never skipped any cycles. She takes no other medications aside from the oral contraceptive and hydrocortisone, 15 mg in the morning, and 5 mg in the evening with fludrocortisone, 0.1 mg daily. She and her husband would like to start trying to conceive within the next year. She has no pain with intercourse and no sexual dysfunction.

On physical examination, her blood pressure is 118/82 mm Hg. Her height is 64 in (162.5 cm), and weight is 140 lb (63.6 kg) (BMI = 24 kg/m^2). She has terminal hair growth on her chin, abdomen, and thighs with an elevated Ferriman-Gallwey score of 9. The rest of her examination findings are unremarkable.

Laboratory test results:
Total testosterone = 72 ng/dL (8-60 ng/dL) (SI: 2.5 nmol/L [0.3-2.1 nmol/L])
DHEA-S = 413 µg/dL (44-332 µg/dL) (SI: 11.15 µmol/L [1.19-9.00 µmol/L])
Androstenedione = 401 ng/dL (30-200 ng/dL) (SI: 13.99 nmol/L [1.05-6.98 nmol/L])

Which of the following is the best next step in this patient's management?
A. Switch hydrocortisone to dexamethasone
B. Discontinue the oral contraceptive and start trying to conceive
C. Discuss the potential value of genetic counseling/testing for the parents and fetus
D. Measure 17-hydroxyprogesterone
E. Measure progesterone in the follicular phase

14

A 32-year-old woman is referred for further investigation of recurrent hypokalemia. She has a 2-year history of hypertension, initially diagnosed during routine medical assessment. Her current medications are amlodipine, 10 mg; doxazosin, 8 mg; and ramipril, 10 mg daily. She also takes potassium chloride, 2 tablets (470 mg potassium per tablet) twice daily. Her medical history is otherwise unremarkable, and there is no relevant family history.

On physical examination, her height is 66 in (167.6 cm) and weight is 154 lb (70 kg) (BMI = 25 kg/m^2). Her blood pressure is 155/92 mm Hg, and pulse rate is 74 beats/min and regular. Examination findings are unremarkable.

Laboratory test results:
Serum potassium = 3.4 mEq/L (3.5-5.0 mEq/L) (SI: 3.4 mmol/L [3.5-5.0 mmol/L])
Plasma renin activity = 0.05 ng/mL per h (0.6-4.3 ng/mL per h)
Serum aldosterone = 39.5 ng/dL (4-21 ng/dL) (SI: 1095.7 pmol/L [111-582.5 pmol/L])
Serum cortisol following 1-mg dexamethasone-suppression test = 1.0 µg/dL (SI: 27.6 nmol/L)

CT of the adrenal glands (triple-phase) shows a 2.5-cm nodule in the right adrenal (baseline = 20 Hounsfield units; 1 minute following contrast = 50 Hounsfield units; 15 minutes following contrast = 25 Hounsfield units). The left adrenal gland has a normal appearance.

Which of the following is the most appropriate next step in this patient's evaluation and management?
A. Adrenal venous sampling
B. Genetic testing for glucocorticoid-remediable aldosteronism
C. MRI of the adrenal glands
D. Right adrenalectomy
E. Saline-suppression test

15 A 72-year-old woman with osteoporosis presents for follow-up. Osteoporosis was diagnosed 5 years ago when she sought evaluation for a 2-month history of atraumatic, subacute onset of lower back pain and was found to have a moderate compression fracture at the third lumbar vertebra. DXA at that time showed the following results:

Lumbar spine T-score = –3.0
Femoral neck T-score = –3.2
Total hip T-score = –2.9

Alendronate, 70 mg weekly, was initiated and she has tolerated this well and continues the same regimen. She has not had interval low-trauma fractures, and her height has been stable on serial follow-up. Her medical history is notable for hypertension, cerebrovascular accident without sequelae, and hypothyroidism. Medications include a stable dosage of levothyroxine, losartan, atorvastatin, and aspirin. Family history is notable for hip fracture in her mother at age 75 years. The patient does not smoke cigarettes or drink alcohol.

On physical examination, she is normotensive. Her height is 65 in (165 cm), which is 2.5 in (6.4 cm) shorter than her self-reported maximum adult height. The thyroid gland is nonpalpable. Spine examination shows minimal midthoracic kyphosis, no elicitable vertebral tenderness, and a reduced rib-to-pelvis distance of 1 fingerbreadth.

Laboratory studies are notable for normal chemistries, including measurements of calcium, albumin, phosphate, creatinine, TSH, and 25-hydroxyvitamin D.

An updated DXA scan performed today on the same instrument as previous studies documents the following:
Lumbar spine T-score = –2.2
Femoral neck T-score = –2.5
Total hip T-score = –2.2

FRAX-determined 10-year risks of hip and major osteoporotic fractures are 6.5% and 24%, respectively.

On the basis of her skeletal history and current clinical status, which of the following is the best next step in this patient's management?

A. Continue alendronate
B. Measure fasting serum C-telopeptide
C. Discontinue alendronate and start teriparatide
D. Discontinue alendronate and begin a drug holiday
E. Discontinue alendronate and start raloxifene

16 A 41-year-old woman with fibromyalgia, migraine headache, hypothyroidism, and history of lung transplant is referred for management of a new cholesterol problem. Before lung transplant, her lipid profile was normal. She has not taken any cholesterol-lowering medications. She has no personal history of atherosclerotic cardiovascular disease, and there is no family history of premature heart disease. She uses a stationary bike for 20 minutes 3 times daily. She avoids red meat and fried foods. Review of systems is notable for weight gain of 4 lb (1.8 kg) in the past year and fatigue. Before lung transplant, her only medication was levothyroxine. Her current medications are cyclosporine, prednisone, levothyroxine, sulfamethoxazole-trimethoprim, azithromycin, and topiramate.

On physical examination, her blood pressure is 118/83 mm Hg and pulse rate is 86 beats/min. Her height is 64 in (162.5 cm), and weight is 145 lb (65.9 kg) (BMI = 25 kg/m^2). She is in no distress and is well developed. Her thyroid gland is normal in size and has no palpable nodules. Heart sounds have a normal rate and regular rhythm. On respiratory examination, she has normal work of breathing on room air and her lungs are clear to auscultation bilaterally. Her abdomen is soft and nontender with no hepatomegaly or splenomegaly.

In addition to a TSH measurement of 6.8 mIU/L (0.5-5.0 mIU/L), her laboratory test results include the following:

Lipid profile	Before transplant	Current
Total cholesterol	171 mg/dL (SI: 4.43 mmol/L)	210 mg/dL (SI: 5.44 mmol/L)
Triglycerides	98 mg/dL (SI: 1.11 mmol/L)	88 mg/dL (SI: 0.99 mmol/L)
HDL cholesterol	65 mg/dL (SI: 1.68 mmol/L)	50 mg/dL (SI: 1.30 mmol/L)
LDL cholesterol	86 mg/dL (SI: 2.23 mmol/L)	143 mg/dL (SI: 3.70 mmol/L)

Reference ranges: total cholesterol, <200 mg/dL (SI: <5.18 mmol/L); triglycerides, <150 mg/dL (SI: <1.70 mmol/L); HDL cholesterol, >60 mg/dL (SI: >1.55 mmol/L); LDL cholesterol, <100 mg/dL (SI: <2.59 mmol/L).

Which of the following explains the change in this patient's lipid profile?
 A. Hypothyroidism
 B. Weight gain
 C. Topiramate
 D. Prednisone
 E. Cyclosporine

17 A 28-year-old man returns for follow-up of type 1 diabetes mellitus, diagnosed at age 8 years. His weight is 195.8 lb (89 kg). He has been on insulin pump therapy since age 19 years, and over the last 2 years his hemoglobin A_{1c} values have ranged from 5.9% to 6.5% (41-48 mmol/mol). He recently started using a partially closed-loop system pump and continuous glucose monitoring. His current hemoglobin A_{1c} level is 5.9% (41 mmol/mol). He has noticed some hypoglycemia around 5 to 6 PM, which is when he gets off work and plays with his son. Three weeks ago, he had 1 severely low glucose value (<54 mg/dL [<3.0 mmol/L]) at 4 AM when his sensor malfunctioned overnight.

A 2-week download of continuous glucose monitoring and pump delivery documents are available. The ambulatory glucose profile is shown (*see image*).

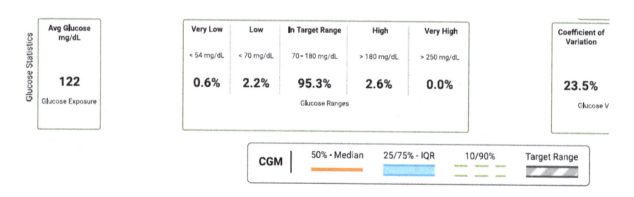

Review of his pump settings shows pump use in automode 93% of the time. The correction factor is 1 unit per 25 mg/dL (1.4 mmol/L) with an insulin-to-carbohydrate ratio of 1 unit per 12.0 g carbohydrate.

Manual device settings for the basal rate are shown (*see table*).

Start time	Basal rate
Midnight	1.100 units/h
4:00 AM	1.050 units/h
8:00 AM	1.125 units/h
1:00 PM	1.300 units/h
Calculated total daily basal	28.53 units

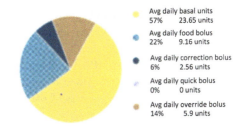

The insulin delivery summary (*see image*) shows that the average daily basal units is 23.65.

Which of the following is the best next step in managing this patient's insulin regimen?
- A. Maintain current settings
- B. Modify the insulin-to-carbohydrate ratio from 1:12 to 1:13
- C. Place the pump in exercise mode while he plays with his son
- D. Reduce the hourly rate from 1 PM to midnight from 1.3 unit/h to 1.1 unit/h
- E. Review the daily insulin delivery data for further information

18 A 78-year-old woman with polymyalgia rheumatica presents with acute back pain and is found to have T12 and L2 compression fractures. She has been taking weekly alendronate consistently for the past 8 years. DXA reveals declining bone mineral density, with a T-score of −3.5 in the spine. She has been on long-term intermittent prednisone but is currently off glucocorticoid therapy. She had an ischemic stroke 6 months ago, which resulted in right-sided weakness. She has a history of recurrent kidney stones.

She has limited dietary calcium intake and does not take any calcium supplements, but she does take over-the-counter cholecalciferol, 1000 IU daily.

On physical examination, she has point tenderness on palpation of her thoracolumbar spine at the site of the fractures. She has mild right-sided hemiparesis.

Laboratory test results:
Serum calcium = 10.3 mg/dL (8.2-10.2 mg/dL) (SI: 2.6 mmol/L [2.1-2.6 mmol/L])
Serum phosphate = 3.0 mg/dL (2.3-4.7 mg/dL) (SI: 1.0 mmol/L [0.7-1.5 mmol/L])
Serum creatinine = 1.3 mg/dL (0.6-1.1 mg/dL) (SI: 114.9 μmol/L [53.0-97.2 μmol/L])
Glomerular filtration rate (estimated) = 35 mL/min per 1.73 m² (>60 mL/min per 1.73 m²)
Serum intact PTH = 65 pg/mL (10-65 pg/mL) (SI: 65 ng/L [10-65 ng/L])
Serum 25-hydroxyvitamin D = 39 ng/mL (30-80 ng/mL [optimal]) (SI: 97.3 nmol/L [74.9-199.7 nmol/L])
Serum albumin = 4.3 g/dL (3.5-5.0 g/dL) (SI: 43 g/L [35-50 g/L])
Serum alkaline phosphatase = 61 U/L (50-120 U/L) (SI: 1.02 μkat/L [0.84-2.00 μkat/L])
Serum C-telopeptide = 401 pg/mL (34-1037 pg/mL)
Urinary calcium = 280 mg/24 h (100-300 mg/24 h) (SI: 7.0 mmol/d [2.5-7.5 mmol/d])

Which of the following should be recommended in addition to adequate calcium and vitamin D intake?
- A. Continue alendronate
- B. Switch to zoledronic acid
- C. Switch to denosumab
- D. Switch to teriparatide
- E. Switch to romosozumab

19 A 65-year-old man is referred for evaluation of a multinodular goiter. On examination, several thyroid nodules are palpated, up to 3 cm in size. Incidentally, marked bilateral gynecomastia is observed. When asked, the patient is vague but states that gynecomastia has been present for many years and it does not bother him. He reports good health and states that he takes no regular medications, apart from a variety of dietary supplements. He is married and has fathered 2 children, now in their 30s. He recalls normal pubertal development.

On physical examination, he appears well. In addition to what is noted above, his height is 68 in (173 cm), and weight is 196 lb (89.1 kg) (BMI = 30 kg/m^2). His blood pressure is 152/85 mm Hg, and resting pulse rate is 70 beats/min. On palpation, firm symmetric enlargement of glandular breast tissue is evident, corresponding to a C bra cup size (3 in [7.6 cm]). There is no axillary lymphadenopathy or distinct breast mass lesions. Testicular volume is 10 mL bilaterally and no masses are detected. There is no clinical visual field defect, and he has full range of eye movements.

Laboratory test results (sample drawn at 8 AM while fasting):
  TSH = 1.0 mIU/L (0.5-5.0 mIU/L)
  Free T$_4$ = 1.7 ng/dL (0.8-1.8 ng/dL) (SI: 21.88 pmol/L [10.30-23.17 pmol/L])
  Total testosterone = 50 ng/dL (300-900 ng/dL) (SI: 1.7 nmol/L [10.4-31.2 nmol/L]) (repeated measurement 1 week later = 60 ng/dL [SI: 2.1 nmol/L])
  SHBG = 12.3 µg/mL (1.1-6.7 µg/mL) (SI: 109 nmol/L [10-60 nmol/L])
  LH = 0.2 mIU/mL (1.0-9.0 mIU/mL) (SI: 0.2 IU/L [1.0-9.0 IU/L])
  Complete blood cell count, normal
  Electrolytes, normal
  Liver function, normal

Recent bone mineral density assessment shows a lumbar spine T-score of +1.6 and a femoral neck T-score of +1.8.

Which of the following is the most important diagnostic test to order now to evaluate his gynecomastia?
  A. Serum prolactin measurement
  B. Serum DHEA-S measurement
  C. Testicular ultrasonography
  D. Karyotype analysis
  E. Serum estradiol measurement

20 A 39-year-old woman seeks evaluation for hypoglycemia. She has a history of type 2 diabetes mellitus and elevated BMI, and she underwent Roux-en-Y gastric bypass surgery 4 years ago. During the first year after surgery, she lost 85 lb (38.6 kg) and had remission of diabetes.

Six months ago, she began having episodes of sweating, shaking, and confusion. Her husband reports that at these times, her speech is unclear, she has difficulty focusing on conversations, and her blood glucose is often low. During the most recent episode, her fingerstick glucose concentration was 43 mg/dL (2.4 mmol/L). Her symptoms improve in 15 to 30 minutes if she eats carbohydrates. She has noticed that her symptoms mostly occur in the fasting state, and she sometimes wakes in the early-morning hours with symptoms of hypoglycemia. Her blood glucose levels also drop with physical activity. She has had 10-lb (4.5-kg) weight regain since these episodes began.

Careful review of medication use reveals she is taking only postbariatric multivitamin tablets and nutritional supplements. No other medications or over-the-counter product use is reported. The patient reports no history of alcohol use, and no household member has diabetes.

Which of the following is the best next step in this patient's management?
  A. Perform a mixed-meal challenge
  B. Perform a 72-hour fast
  C. Perform a 75-g oral glucose tolerance test
  D. Measure insulin antibodies
  E. Recommend a carbohydrate-restricted diet

21 An 82-year-old woman is referred for evaluation of possible adrenal insufficiency. Her internist recorded a low morning serum cortisol concentration of 2.9 μg/dL (80.0 nmol/L) during the workup of recently worsening tiredness. She has a history of hypertension, hypercholesterolemia, migraine headaches, and microscopic collagenous colitis diagnosed by colonoscopy 5 months ago. Her current medications are listed:

    Chlorthalidone, 25 mg daily
    Diltiazem, 180 mg daily
    Lisinopril, 20 mg daily
    Metoprolol succinate, 25 mg daily
    Budesonide, 9 mg every other day (reduced from 9 mg daily 2 months ago)
    Methenamine hippurate, 500 mg twice daily with meals
    Nortriptyline, 10 mg nightly
    Pantoprazole, 40 mg twice daily
    Potassium chloride, 20 mEq daily
    Rosuvastatin, 5 mg daily
    Ketoconazole, 2% cream to scalp daily

On physical examination, she is a thin, elderly woman in no acute distress. She has mild fullness of her cheeks. Her blood pressure is 133/67 mm Hg, and pulse rate is 74 beats/min. Her height is 59 in (150 cm), and weight is 121.2 lb (55 kg) (BMI = 24 kg/m^2). There is no mucosal hyperpigmentation. Her abdomen is not protuberant and is mildly tense to palpation. There are no purplish striae. Her skin appears thin.

Laboratory test results:
    Repeated serum cortisol (8 AM) = 2.4 μg/dL (5-25 μg/dL) (SI: 66.2 nmol/L [137.9-689.7 nmol/L])
    Plasma ACTH = 5 pg/mL (10-60 pg/mL) (SI: 1.1 pmol/L [2.2-13.2 pmol/L])
    TSH = 2.3 mIU/L (0.5-5.0 mIU/L)
    Free T$_4$ = 1.0 ng/dL (0.8-1.8 ng/dL) (SI: 12.87 pmol/L [10.30-23.17 pmol/L])
    FSH = 38.0 mIU/mL (>30.0 mIU/mL [postmenopausal]) (SI: 38.0 IU/L [>30.0 IU/L])
    Prolactin = 12 ng/mL (4-30 ng/mL) (SI: 0.52 nmol/L [0.17-1.30 nmol/L])

In addition to starting hydrocortisone therapy, which of the following is the most appropriate next step?
    A. Measure adrenal antibodies
    B. Stop ketoconazole cream
    C. Perform pituitary-directed MRI
    D. Stop methenamine
    E. Recommend no additional action now

22 A 45-year-old woman seeks evaluation for diffuse abdominal pain. Abdominal ultrasonography reveals a possible left suprarenal mass. Abdominal CT documents a 1.6 × 1.7-cm left adrenal mass. The unenhanced attenuation of the mass is 22 Hounsfield units. One minute following contrast injection, the enhanced attenuation is 77 Hounsfield units. Fifteen minutes later, the delayed enhancement is 66 Hounsfield units. The absolute contrast washout is 20%, and the relative contrast washout is 14%.

Her abdominal pain spontaneously resolves, and she has no overt signs or symptoms of Cushing syndrome. She has no hirsutism or weight gain. She has no hyperadrenergic symptoms such as palpitations, sweating, or anxiety. Her blood pressure is normal. Her only medications are venlafaxine, 37.5 mg daily, and vitamin D, 1000 IU daily.

Laboratory test results:
    Cortisol after overnight 1-mg dexamethasone-suppression test = 1.7 μg/dL (SI: 46.9 nmol/L)
    Plasma normetanephrine = 329.7 pg/mL (<165 pg/mL) (SI: 1.80 nmol/L [<0.90 nmol/L])
    Plasma metanephrine = 59.2 pg/mL (<99 pg/mL) (SI: 0.30 nmol/L [<0.50 nmol/L])
    Morning DHEA-S, normal
    Total testosterone, normal

24-hour urine collection:
  Volume = 2.1 L/24 h
  Creatinine = 0.9 g/24 h (1.0-2.0 g/24 h) (SI: 79.6 mmol/d [8.8-17.7 mmol/d])
  Urinary normetanephrine = 1709 µg/24 h (<451 µg/24 h) (SI: 9331 nmol/d [<2463 nmol/d])
  Urinary metanephrine = 292 µg/24 h (<180 µg/24 h) (SI: 1480 nmol/d [<913 nmol/d])

Which of the following is this patient's most likely diagnosis?
  A. Adrenocortical carcinoma
  B. Adrenomedullary cyst
  C. Lipid-rich adrenocortical adenoma
  D. Lipid-poor adrenocortical adenoma
  E. Pheochromocytoma

23

A 59-year-old woman with hypertension and stage 3 chronic kidney disease is referred after her primary care provider documented elevated triglycerides. Her triglyceride concentration is greater than 1000 mg/dL (>11.3 mmol/L). She has no history of type 2 diabetes mellitus, hypothyroidism, or nephrotic syndrome. She has not had pancreatitis and does not use steroids or oral estrogen. There is no family history of elevated triglycerides or pancreatitis. She reports drinking 2 to 3 beers daily, 36 oz of regular soda per day, and 32 oz of sweet tea per day. Her medications include lisinopril, 20 mg daily, and atorvastatin, 20 mg daily. She is advised to decrease the intake of alcoholic and sugary beverages.

The patient returns 3 months later and is pleased to report that she was able to stop her alcohol and sweet tea intake. She currently drinks 1 can of soda weekly.

On physical examination, her blood pressure is 105/74 mm Hg and pulse rate is 70 beats/min. Her height is 66 in (167.5 cm), and weight is 192 lb (87.3 kg) (BMI = 31 kg/m^2). She is alert, oriented, and in no distress. She has no eruptive xanthomas. Her lungs are clear to auscultation bilaterally, and heart sounds are regular. On abdominal examination, bowel sounds are present and there is no tenderness to palpation.

Laboratory test results (fasting):
  Creatinine = 1.6 mg/dL (0.6-1.1 mg/dL) (SI: 141.4 µmol/L [53.0-97.2 µmol/L])
  Estimated glomerular filtration rate = 35 mL/min per 1.73 m^2 (>60 mL/min per 1.73 m^2)
  Liver function, normal
  Total cholesterol = 274 mg/dL (<200 mg/dL [optimal]) (SI: 7.10 mmol/L [<5.18 mmol/L])
  Triglycerides = 645 mg/dL (<150 mg/dL [optimal]) (SI: 7.29 mmol/L [<1.70 mmol/L])
  HDL cholesterol = 38 mg/dL (>60 mg/dL [optimal]) (SI: 0.98 mmol/L [>1.55 mmol/L])
  Direct LDL cholesterol = 83 mg/dL (<100 mg/dL [optimal]) (SI: 2.15 mmol/L [<2.59 mmol/L])

Which of the following should be recommended to treat her hypertriglyceridemia?
  A. Switch atorvastatin to pravastatin, 40 mg daily
  B. Start ezetimibe, 10 mg daily
  C. Start fenofibrate, 145 mg daily
  D. Start gemfibrozil, 600 mg twice daily
  E. Start colestipol, 2 g daily

24

A 45-year-old man with a history of attention-deficit/hyperactivity disorder presents for the initial evaluation and management of breast enlargement. The patient describes symmetric breast enlargement beginning 3 to 4 months ago. This is associated with nipple sensitivity but no breast pain or discharge. Review of systems is notable for increasing anxiety over the past year and a 20-lb (9.1-kg) weight loss, which the patient attributes to increased gym participation. His libido is normal and he has no erectile dysfunction. He takes no medications or supplements. Family history is notable for hypothyroidism secondary to Hashimoto thyroiditis in his sister.

On physical examination, his temperature is 98°F (36.7°C), blood pressure is 135/82 mm Hg, and pulse rate is 100 beats/min. His height is 72 in (183 cm), and weight is 215 lb (97.7 kg) (BMI = 29 kg/m^2). The patient has normal male distribution of facial and body hair and no acne. The thyroid gland is nontender and is approximately

25 g without nodules. A fine tremor of the upper extremities is present. Chest examination reveals bilateral, nontender, palpable masses of tissue in the subareolar region measuring 2 cm. Testicular volume is 25 mL bilaterally. No testicular or abdominal masses are palpated.

Results of a complete metabolic panel are normal.

Which of the following is the most likely cause of this patient's gynecomastia?
A. Hypogonadism
B. Hyperthyroidism
C. Germ-cell tumor
D. Breast cancer
E. Anabolic androgenic steroid use

25

A 75-year-old woman is referred for assistance with osteoporosis treatment. Osteoporosis was diagnosed following recent baseline DXA, but she has no history of low-trauma fractures as an adult. She underwent menopause at age 50 years and has been on long-term hormone replacement therapy (compounded cream), but she has never taken an FDA-approved antifracture therapy. Her medical history is notable for varicose veins status post venous stripping, as well as recurrent nephrolithiasis requiring lithotripsy bilaterally. Her family history is positive for osteoporosis and hip fracture in her mother at age 72 years. Current medications include hydrochlorothiazide and cholecalciferol.

On physical examination, she is normotensive. Her height is 67 in (170.2 cm), which is only 1.0 in (2.5 cm) shorter than her self-reported maximum adult height. Her weight is 132 lb (60 kg) (BMI = 21 kg/m²). The oropharynx appears normal. The thyroid gland is not palpable. Findings on spine examination are unremarkable; there is no kyphosis, scoliosis, or elicitable vertebral tenderness to palpation or percussion.

Laboratory test results:
Calcium = 9.5 mg/dL (8.2-10.2 mg/dL) (SI: 2.4 mmol/L [2.1-2.6 mmol/L])
Phosphate = 3.5 mg/dL (2.3-4.7 mg/dL) (SI: 1.1 mmol/L [0.7-1.5 mmol/L])
Creatinine = 0.7 mg/dL (0.6-1.1 mg/dL) (SI: 61.9 μmol/L [53.0-97.2 μmol/L])
Albumin = 4.0 g/dL (3.5-5.0 g/dL) (SI: 40 g/L [35-50 g/L])
Intact PTH = 45 pg/mL (10-65 pg/mL) (SI: 45 ng/L [10-65 ng/L])
25-Hydroxyvitamin D = 42 ng/mL (30-80 ng/mL [optimal]) (SI: 104.8 nmol/L [74.9-199.7 nmol/L])
Urinary calcium excretion = 250 mg/24 h (100-300 mg/24 h) (SI: 6.3 mmol/d [2.5-7.5 mmol/d])
Urinary creatinine excretion = 1.0 g/24 h (1.0-2.0 g/24 h) (SI: 8.8 mmol/d [8.8-17.7 mmol/d])

Recent DXA bone density results are shown (*see images*).

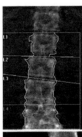

Region	Area, cm²	Bone mineral density, g/cm²	T-score
L1	12.47	0.468	−4.2
L2	12.82	0.503	−4.8
L3	15.76	0.577	−4.6
Total	41.05	0.520	−4.5

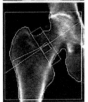

Region	Area, cm²	Bone mineral density, g/cm²	T-score
Neck	5.32	0.512	−3.0
Troch	21.67	0.438	−2.6
Inter	21.67	0.762	−2.2
Total	37.96	0.633	−2.5

FRAX-determined 10-year risks of hip and major osteoporotic fractures are 20% and 26%, respectively.

On the basis of the available data, which of the following is the best treatment choice for this patient's osteoporosis?
- A. Alendronate
- B. Raloxifene
- C. Teriparatide
- D. Denosumab
- E. Romosozumab

26

A 33-year-old woman with type 2 diabetes mellitus returns for consultation. Diabetes was diagnosed during the second month of her recent pregnancy based on a fasting glucose concentration of 371 mg/dL (20.6 mmol/L) identified on routine blood testing. Initially, she was treated with NPH and regular insulin, but she had recurrent hypoglycemia and her regimen was transitioned to metformin, 1000 mg twice daily. Her baby, delivered 13 months ago, had congenital cardiac malformations. Since she gave birth, she has lost 60 lb (27.2 kg), and her current weight is 143.9 lb (65.3 kg) (BMI = 22.6 kg/m²). Her weight before pregnancy was 222.6 lb (101 kg).

At today's appointment, her point-of-care hemoglobin A_{1c} level is 5.0% (31 mmol/mol) and she continues to take metformin, 1000 mg in the morning and 500 mg in the evening. If she stops metformin, she notes that she has postprandial hyperglycemia (160-180 mg/dL [8.9-10.0 mmol/L]). If she eats a carbohydrate-heavy meal, she takes an extra 500 mg of metformin. She is puzzled by the persistence of diabetes despite losing so much weight and maintaining a high activity level (30 minutes of cardio 6 days per week and weightlifting 4 days per week).

Her medical history is notable for hypothyroidism. Medications include metformin as noted. Family history is notable for rheumatoid arthritis in her brother, rheumatoid arthritis and thyroid disease in her paternal grandmother, and thyroid disease in both parents. There are no family members with diabetes.

Physical examination findings are unremarkable.

Which of the following blood tests would help identify a potential explanation for her persistent hyperglycemia?
- A. C-peptide measurement
- B. Glutamic acid decarboxylase 65 antibody assessment
- C. *HNF1A* genetic testing
- D. Insulin autoantibody assessment
- E. *GCK* genetic testing

27

A 49-year-old woman is diagnosed with hyperthyroidism and is referred for further evaluation and management. She reports 2 months of tachycardia and anxiety, and she has lost 15 lb (6.5 kg) in this same period. She has the feeling of sand in her eyes and pain with eye movement. Before this visit, her primary care physician ordered thyroid ultrasonography, which confirmed an enlarged thyroid gland and no evidence of nodules.

Her medical history is notable for attention-deficit/hyperactivity disorder and she is status post appendectomy. She takes no medication. She smokes cigarettes (1 pack per day for the last 10 years).

On physical examination, her blood pressure is 140/76 mm Hg and pulse rate is 100 beats/min and regular. Her height is 63 in (160 cm), and weight is 130 lb (59 kg) (BMI = 23 kg/m²). She appears thin and very anxious. She has bilateral proptosis with lid retraction (≥2 mm), periorbital edema, chemosis, and diplopia. Her thyroid gland is visible upon swallowing and is 80 g in size. Lungs are clear to auscultation bilaterally. There is tremor in both hands.

Laboratory test results:
TSH = <0.01 mIU/L (0.5-5.0 mIU/L)
Free T_4 = 4.2 ng/dL (0.8-1.8 ng/dL) (SI: 54.05 pmol/L [10.30-23.17 pmol/L])
Free T_3 = 11.2 pg/mL (2.3-4.2 pg/mL) (SI: 17.20 pmol/L [3.53-6.45 pmol/L])
Thyroid-stimulating immunoglobulin = 220% (≤120% of basal activity)
Complete blood count, normal
Comprehensive metabolic panel, normal

In addition to starting a β-adrenergic blocker, which of the following is the best next step in the management of this patient's Graves disease?
- A. Order neck CT to check for compression
- B. Achieve euthyroidism with antithyroid drugs and then recommend radioiodine treatment
- C. Achieve euthyroidism with antithyroid drugs and then recommend total thyroidectomy
- D. Recommend SSKI drops for 10 days
- E. Order thyroid scan to better delineate the etiology of her hyperthyroidism

28

A 54-year-old man is currently hospitalized for surgical complications following coronary artery bypass grafting. He has a 10-year history of type 2 diabetes mellitus that was managed with oral antidiabetes agents before his surgery. However, postoperatively, he has required insulin therapy to maintain glycemic control. He has been receiving continuous tube feeding for nutritional support. He is currently at his goal rate, receiving 55 mL/h of enteral nutrition (216 g carbohydrate per 1000 mL). He is receiving a continuous intravenous infusion of insulin (total daily dose = 50 units), and his blood glucose values range between 130 and 190 mg/dL (7.2-10.5 mmol/L). The plan is to transition his regimen to subcutaneous insulin therapy. His current weight is 209 lb (95 kg).

Laboratory test results:
Serum creatinine = 1.1 mg/dL (0.7-1.3 mg/dL) (SI: 97.2 μmol/L [61.9-114.9 μmol/L])
Estimated glomerular filtration rate = 65 mL/min per 1.73 m² (>60 mL/min per 1.73 m²)

Which of the following is the best insulin regimen to start in the management of this patient's hyperglycemia?
- A. Insulin glargine, 50 units subcutaneously once daily
- B. Insulin glargine, 50 units once daily, and insulin aspart, correction dosing every 6 hours
- C. Insulin glargine, 20 units once daily, and regular insulin, 8 units every 6 hours
- D. Insulin glargine, 25 units subcutaneously twice daily
- E. Insulin glargine, 50 units once daily, and insulin aspart, 6 units every 6 hours

29

A 33-year-old woman presents for evaluation of secondary amenorrhea via telemedicine. She has a history of transsphenoidal resection of a 2-cm, nonsecreting gonadotroph pituitary adenoma when she presented for evaluation of secondary amenorrhea 6 years ago. Menses became regular after surgery. However, she had residual tumor that continued to grow over the first year of follow-up. She decided to proceed with radiosurgery as recommended by her neurosurgeon. Follow-up MRI after radiosurgery demonstrated no growth of residual disease. She has 2 children; the first child was born when she was 23 years old, and the second child was born 2 years ago, 4.4 years after surgery.

She reports that her period has still not returned after weaning her second child 6 months ago. She has no vaginal dryness, but she has noticed a decrease in libido that she attributes to parenting 2 young children. She has had no skin or hair changes, constipation, or weight gain or loss. There is no family history of pituitary tumors.

On the video visit, the patient appears well. Her primary care provider ordered the following laboratory tests:
TSH = 1.7 mIU/L (0.5-5.0 mIU/L)
Free T₄ = 1.1 ng/dL (0.8-1.8 ng/dL) (SI: 14.2 pmol/L [10.30-23.17 pmol/L])
Prolactin = 5 ng/mL (4-30 ng/mL) (SI: 0.22 nmol/L [0.17-1.30 nmol/L])
FSH = 5.0 mIU/mL (2.0-12.0 mIU/mL [follicular]) (SI: 5.0 IU/L [2.0-12.0 IU/L])
β-hCG, negative

Which of the following is the best next step in this patient's evaluation?
- A. Measure FSH and estradiol
- B. Perform pituitary MRI
- C. Perform pelvic ultrasonography
- D. Perform a progesterone withdrawal test
- E. Prescribe a combined oral contraceptive to induce a period

30 A 32-year-old woman reports a 4-month history of intermittent palpitations, weight loss (5 lb [2.3 kg]) despite increased appetite, and menstrual irregularity. An anxiety disorder was diagnosed 18 months ago, and she is currently treated with citalopram. Her mother has primary hypothyroidism.

On physical examination, her height is 67 in (170 cm) and weight is 142 lb (64.4 kg) (BMI = 22 kg/m^2). Her blood pressure is 130/85 mm Hg, and resting pulse rate is 115 beats/min and regular. She has a fine resting tremor and warm peripheral extremities. There is a small, symmetric goiter but no signs of dysthyroid eye disease.

Initial laboratory test results:
TSH = 2.1 mIU/L (0.5-5.0 mIU/L)
Free T$_4$ = 2.3 ng/dL (0.8-1.8 ng/dL) (SI: 29.60 pmol/L [10.30-23.17 pmol/L])
Free T$_3$ = 5.2 pg/mL (2.3-4.2 pg/mL) (SI: 7.99 pmol/L [3.53-6.45 pmol/L])
TRAb = 0.3 IU/L (≤1.75 IU/L)

There is no evidence of laboratory assay interference in the free T$_4$ or TSH assays.

Additional laboratory test results:
SHBG = 16.5 µg/mL (2.2-14.6 µg/mL) (SI: 147 nmol/L [20-130 nmol/L])
α-Subunit of pituitary glycoprotein hormones = 0.8 ng/mL (<1.2 ng/mL) (SI: 0.8 µg/L [<1.2 µg/L])

Results of thyrotropin-releasing hormone–stimulation testing (200 mcg intravenously):

Time, min	TSH
0	2.3 mIU/L
20	2.5 mIU/L
60	2.1 mIU/L

MRI of the sella (*see images*).

T1 coronal (precontrast)   **T1 coronal (postcontrast)**   **T2 coronal**

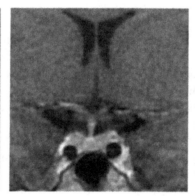
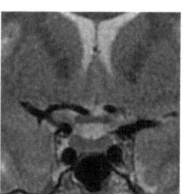

Which of the following diagnoses is the most likely explanation for this patient's presentation?
A. Surreptitious ingestion of thyroid hormone
B. Familial dysalbuminemic hyperthyroxinemia
C. Resistance to thyroid hormone (*THRB*)
D. Thyrotropinoma
E. Toxic multinodular goiter

31 A 45-year-old woman who underwent Roux-en-Y gastric bypass 3 years ago presents with shortness of breath on exertion and fatigue. She has been taking daily oral iron supplementation containing 65 mg of elemental iron in addition to a mineral-containing multivitamin twice daily; cholecalciferol, 5000 IU daily; vitamin B12 injections monthly; and calcium citrate, 500 mg 3 times daily. She does not report dyspepsia or epigastric discomfort. She has no blood in her stool or urine and there is no history of nosebleeds. She continues to have monthly menstrual periods, which are described as having moderate flow and lasting 4 days.

On physical examination, her height is 61.5 in (156 cm) and weight is 176 lb (80 kg) (BMI = 33 kg/m^2). Examination findings are notable for conjunctival pallor and dry oral mucosa.

Laboratory test results confirm the diagnosis of anemia:
    Hemoglobin = 10.5 g/dL (12.1-15.1 g/dL) (SI: 105 g/L [121-151 g/L])
    Mean corpuscular volume = 80 μm^3 (80-100 μm^3) (SI: 80 fL [80-100 fL])
    Ferritin = 4 ng/mL (15-200 ng/mL) (SI: 9.0 pmol/L [33.7-449.4 pmol/L])

Laboratory tests obtained just before surgery documented a hemoglobin concentration of 12.5 g/dL (125 g/L) and a mean corpuscular volume of 89 μm^3 (89 fL).

Which of the following is the best next step in this patient's management?
    A. Increase oral iron supplementation and advise her to separate this from when she takes calcium supplements
    B. Refer for upper endoscopy and colonoscopy to screen for occult blood loss
    C. Refer for intravenous iron infusion
    D. Prescribe thiamine supplementation
    E. Prescribe folate supplementation

32 A 45-year-old man with a history of intravenous illicit drug use presents for initial evaluation of thyrotoxicosis. Three weeks ago, he noted the acute onset of fevers and mild flulike symptoms, including sore throat, malaise, and myalgias, as well as right neck and jaw pain. His flulike symptoms resolved over the next few days, but he has continued to have daily fever with a temperature as high as 102°F (38.9°C). Starting 2 weeks ago, the patient also began experiencing tachycardia, tremors, and anxiety. One week ago, his primary care physician prescribed metoprolol succinate, 25 mg daily, and he titrated the dosage to 50 mg daily yesterday. The patient has been taking ibuprofen and acetaminophen for his neck and jaw pain, and this improves but does not resolve the discomfort. His sister has Graves disease.

On physical examination, his temperature is 99.4°F (37.4°C), blood pressure is 117/74 mm Hg, and pulse rate is 85 beats/min. His height is 66 in (167.6 cm), and weight is 141 lb (64 kg) (BMI = 23 kg/m^2). The thyroid gland is mildly enlarged (~25 g) and tender to palpation, particularly on the right side. A fine tremor of the upper extremities is present. The rest of his examination findings are normal.

Laboratory test results:
    White blood cell count = 12,800/μL (4500-11,000/μL) (SI: 12.8 × 10^9/L [4.5-11.0 × 10^9/L])
    Hemoglobin = 12.7 g/dL (13.8-17.2 g/dL) (SI: 127 g/L [138-172 g/L])
    Platelet count = 489 × 10^3/μL (150-450 × 10^3/μL) (SI: 489 × 10^9/L [150-450 × 10^9/L])
    Erythrocyte sedimentation rate = 60 mm/h (0-20 mm/h)
    TSH = <0.01 mIU/L (0.5-5.0 mIU/L)
    Free T$_4$ = 2.6 ng/dL (0.8-1.8 ng/dL) (SI: 33.5 pmol/L [10.30-23.17 pmol/L])
    Total T$_3$ = 180 ng/dL (70-200 ng/dL) (SI: 2.8 nmol/L [1.08-3.08 nmol/L])

Neck ultrasonography is shown (*see images*). Mildly enlarged lymph nodes with fatty hila are present bilaterally.

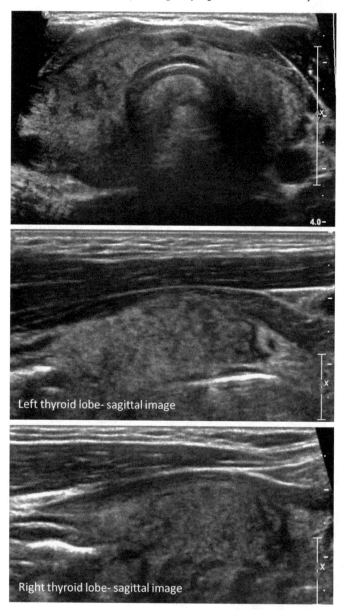

Which of the following is this patient's most likely diagnosis?
A. Graves disease
B. Autoimmune thyroiditis
C. Subacute thyroiditis
D. Suppurative thyroiditis
E. Thyroid lymphoma

33 A 44-year-old man with a 4-year history of type 2 diabetes mellitus presents with symptoms of nausea, vomiting, abdominal discomfort, and lethargy. The symptoms have been progressively worsening over the past 5 days. He has no dysuria or hematuria. His blood glucose levels have been in the usual range (fasting 100-120 mg/dL [5.6-6.7 mmol/L]; random values later in the day <180 mg/dL [<10.0 mmol/L]). His last 2 hemoglobin A_{1c} measurements were 6.7% and 6.9% (50 and 52 mmol/mol). His treatment regimen has been the stable for the past 2 years: glimepiride, 4 mg once daily; metformin, 1000 mg twice daily; and empagliflozin, 10 mg daily.

He reports struggling with his weight for many years. He has tried numerous dietary programs and most recently began following a ketogenic diet (<30 g carbohydrate daily). He has been pleased with the results so far, having lost 32 lb (14.5 kg) over the past 3 months.

On physical examination, his blood pressure is 118/74 mm Hg and pulse rate is 96 beats/min. His height is 72 in (182.9 cm), and weight is 278 lb (126.4 kg) (BMI = 38 kg/m^2). He has 1+ pitting edema in both lower extremities. The rest of the examination findings are normal.

Which of the following is the best next step to evaluate this patient's symptoms?
- A. Basic metabolic panel and serum β-hydroxybutyrate measurement
- B. C-peptide measurement
- C. CT of the abdomen and pelvis
- D. Urine analysis
- E. Point-of-care blood glucose measurement

34

A 58-year-old man is referred for further evaluation of hypertension and hypokalemia. Hypertension was diagnosed at age 38 years, but he was not treated with medication. At age 43 years, his blood pressure was noted to be 200/100 mm Hg, and lisinopril was prescribed. By age 58 years, he had been evaluated in an emergency department and admitted to a hospital more than 3 times for hypertensive urgency and hypokalemia. Electrocardiography and echocardiography confirmed left ventricular hypertrophy. He is currently treated with lisinopril, 40 mg daily; nifedipine, 60 mg daily; and carvedilol, 50 mg daily. His blood pressure ranges from 135-156/80-90 mm Hg. However, his serum potassium concentration has continued to range from 3.1 to 3.4 mEq/L (3.1-3.4 mmol/L), and his serum bicarbonate concentration ranges from 25 to 30 mEq/L (25-30 mmol/L).

Testing for secondary causes of hypertension reveals the following:
Cortisol after overnight 1-mg dexamethasone-suppression test = 1.1 µg/dL (SI: 30.3 nmol/L)
Plasma renin activity = <0.6 ng/mL per h (0.6-4.3 ng/mL per h)
Plasma aldosterone = 5.2 ng/dL (4-21 ng/dL) (SI: 144.2 pmol/L [111.0-582.5 pmol/L])
Serum potassium = 3.4 mEq/L (3.5-5.0 mEq/L) (SI: 3.4 mmol/L [3.5-5.0 mmol/L])
Plasma metanephrines, normal

Which of the following most likely explains this patient's presentation?
- A. Consumption of licorice (glycyrrhetinic acid)
- B. Idiopathic resistant hypertension
- C. Liddle syndrome
- D. Primary aldosteronism
- E. Syndrome of apparent mineralocorticoid excess

35

A 55-year-old woman is referred for assessment and recommendations regarding recently identified hypercalcemia. At her annual examination, routine laboratory studies documented elevated serum calcium and concomitantly elevated PTH. She has had generalized fatigue for the past 12 to 18 months, but she has otherwise felt well without musculoskeletal pain, fevers, sweats, or weight loss. She has no history of low-trauma fractures, nephrolithiasis, head and neck irradiation, or family history of calcium disorders. Her medical history includes hypertension and bipolar disorder. Current medications include lisinopril, atenolol, and lithium carbonate. She does not take calcium supplements. She does not smoke cigarettes and drinks alcohol rarely.

On physical examination, she appears well. Her blood pressure is 110/65 mm Hg, and pulse rate is 75 beats/min. Her height is 66 in (167.5 cm) (0.5 in [1.3 cm] shorter than self-reported maximum adult height), and weight is 154 lb (70 kg) (BMI = 25 kg/m^2). There are no corneal calcifications on eye examination. She has no thyromegaly or palpable nodules. Spine examination shows normal curvature without kyphosis or vertebral tenderness to palpation. The rest of the examination findings are normal.

Laboratory test results:
- Calcium = 11.2 mg/dL (8.2-10.2 mg/dL) (SI: 2.8 mmol/L [2.1-2.6 mmol/L])
- Phosphate = 3.2 mg/dL (2.3-4.7 mg/dL) (SI: 1.0 mmol/L [0.7-1.5 mmol/L])
- Magnesium = 1.9 mg/dL (1.5-2.3 mg/dL) (SI: 0.8 mmol/L [0.6-0.9 mmol/L])
- Creatinine = 0.9 mg/dL (0.6-1.1 mg/dL) (SI: 79.6 µmol/L [53.0-97.2 µmol/L])
- Albumin = 4.2 g/dL (3.5-5.0 g/dL) (SI: 42 g/L [35-50 g/L])
- Intact PTH = 110 pg/mL (10-65 pg/mL) (SI: 110 ng/L [10-65 ng/L])
- 25-Hydroxyvitamin D = 32 ng/mL (30-80 ng/mL [optimal]) (SI: 79.9 nmol/L [74.9-199.7 nmol/L])
- Urinary calcium = 320 mg/24 h (100-300 mg/24 h) (SI: 8.0 mmol/d [2.5-7.5 mmol/d])
- Urinary creatinine = 1.0 g/24 h (1.0-2.0 g/24 h) (SI: 8.8 mmol/d [8.8-17.7 mmol/d])

DXA scan reveals normal bone mineral density (T-score >–1.0) at the lumbar spine, right femoral neck, total hip, and nondominant proximal one-third radius. Thyroid ultrasonography reveals an ovoid 0.6 × 0.5-cm mass in the neck adjacent to the inferior aspect of the left thyroid lobe.

Which of the following is the best next step in the management of this patient's hypercalcemia?

A. Refer to endocrine surgery for minimally invasive parathyroidectomy
B. Refer to endocrine surgery for bilateral neck exploration
C. Refer for genetic testing of the *CASR* gene (encoding the calcium-sensing receptor)
D. Start alendronate
E. Monitor calcium, albumin, and PTH levels every 6 months

36

A 24-year-old White woman seeks evaluation for hypoglycemia. She was in good health until about 2 years ago when she started having episodes of tingling in her arms and legs and blurred vision if she skipped a meal. Over the past 6 months, her symptoms have worsened, and she wakes up at least twice nightly with symptoms of hypoglycemia and finds that her blood glucose values are less than 60 mg/dL (<3.3 mmol/L). She cannot run or go on long walks like she used to. On one occasion, she was speaking with her husband on the phone and he reported she sounded confused. When she has these symptoms, her blood glucose values have been in the range of 40 to 50 mg/dL (2.2-2.8 mmol/L). If she eats a bowl of cereal, symptoms resolve in 20 to 30 minutes.

The patient has no history of gastrointestinal procedures, use of steroids or over-the-counter medications, or liver or kidney dysfunction. Although there is no history of insulinoma or multiple endocrine neoplasia in the family, she reports that her father has hypoglycemia that is currently being evaluated.

On physical examination, her blood pressure is 108/68 mm Hg and pulse rate is 70 beats/min. Her height is 63 in (160 cm), and weight is 132 lb (60 kg) (BMI = 23 kg/m²). She is alert and oriented and appears well. Examination of the skin reveals no areas of hypopigmentation or hyperpigmentation. The rest of the examination findings are normal.

Laboratory test results (sample drawn at 8 AM after a 12-hour fast; the patient reports she had sweating and blurred vision at this time):
- Blood glucose = 32 mg/dL (70-99 mg/dL) (SI: 1.8 mmol/L [3.9-5.5 mmol/L])
- C-peptide = 1.7 ng/mL (0.9-4.3 ng/mL) (SI: 0.56 nmol/L [0.30-1.42 nmol/L])
- Insulin = 5.1 µIU/mL (1.4-14.0 µIU/mL) (SI: 35.4 pmol/L [9.7-97.2 pmol/L])
- β-Hydroxybutyrate = 0.4 mg/dL (<3.0 mg/dL) (SI: 38.4 µmol/L [<288.2 µmol/L])
- Cortisol = 16 µg/dL (5-25 µg/dL) (SI: 441.4 nmol/L [137.9-689.7 nmol/L])
- IGF-1 = 175 ng/mL (116-341 ng/mL) (SI: 22.9 nmol/L [15.2-44.7 nmol/L])
- Meglitinide and sulfonylurea screen, negative

Which of the following is this patient's most likely diagnosis?

A. Non–islet-cell tumor
B. Endogenous excess insulin production
C. Adrenal insufficiency
D. Insulin autoimmune syndrome
E. Surreptitious insulin use

37 A 30-year-old transgender man (G2P2) seeks advice regarding initiation of gender-affirming hormone therapy. After his second pregnancy, gender dysphoria was diagnosed by a behavioral health provider and endocrinologist using standards of care (v7) from the World Professional Association for Transgender Health. Dysphoria began at puberty (age 10 years), but he realized his transgender identity during a high school psychology project on gender dysphoria.

After delivering his first baby, he provided milk both by direct feeding and expressing milk for 2.5 years. His second baby was born 13 months ago, and he has been directly chestfeeding this child since birth. Symptoms of gender dysphoria have increased, and his behavioral health provider/gender therapist has recommended discussing risks and benefits of initiating gender-affirming testosterone therapy while continuing to chestfeed. His son feeds 2 or 3 times daily while also receiving nutrition from other solid food and liquids. He does not feel that alternative methods of feeding human milk would be enough to alleviate dysphoria. He emphasizes that he wants to continue chestfeeding until his son is ready to wean because of the benefits of nursing and human comfort. He is not planning any additional pregnancies.

On physical examination, his height is 66 in (167.6 cm) and weight is 198.5 lb (90.2 kg) (BMI = 32 kg/m^2). His blood pressure is 125/82 mm Hg. There is terminal hair growth on the upper lip, chin, abdomen, and thighs with a Ferriman-Gallwey score of 12. There is no acanthosis and no other pertinent findings on examination.

If the patient chooses to continue chestfeeding and also start testosterone therapy, which of the following is most likely to occur?
- A. Reduction in milk production
- B. Masculinization of the baby
- C. Increased testosterone concentrations in the milk
- D. Correlation of testosterone concentrations in milk with circulating testosterone concentrations in the infant
- E. Decreased masculinization risk for the baby with transdermal vs injectable therapy

38 A 52-year-old woman with bipolar disorder and hypertension is referred for weight gain of 8 lb (3.6 kg) over the last 2 months. She also has fatigue and feels unmotivated. She has no nocturia. Three months ago, her psychiatrist increased her lithium dosage from 300 mg twice daily to 600 mg twice daily. She also takes lisinopril and a multivitamin. She does not smoke cigarettes or drink alcohol. She has stopped going to work because of her symptoms.

On physical examination, her blood pressure is 140/70 mm Hg and pulse rate is 56 beats/min and regular. Her height is 64 in (162.6 cm), and weight is 165 lb (74.8 kg) (BMI = 28 kg/m^2). Her affect is flat. Her thyroid gland is palpable and twice normal size with no nodularity. Her heart has a regular rate and rhythm. Lungs are clear to auscultation. There is no lower-extremity edema. The rest of the examination findings are normal.

Laboratory test results 3 months ago:
   TSH = 2.2 mIU/L (0.5-5.0 mIU/L)
   Free T$_4$ = 1.0 ng/dL (0.8-1.8 ng/dL) (SI: 12.87 pmol/L [10.30-23.17 pmol/L])

Basic metabolic panel last week was normal.

Which of the following is the best next step in this patient's management?
- A. Measure serum TSH
- B. Measure urine osmolality
- C. Measure TPO antibodies
- D. Measure serum PTH and calcium levels
- E. Perform thyroid ultrasonography

39 An 86-year-old woman with hypertension, chronic kidney disease, congestive heart failure (ejection fraction = 35%), and chronic obstructive pulmonary disease is referred for evaluation of chronic hypercalcemia. Her calcium concentrations over the past 5 years have been in the range of 11.5 to 13.5 mg/dL (2.9-3.4 mmol/L). She reports joint pain, memory loss, decreased appetite, constipation, polyuria, and muscle weakness. She has no history of fractures or kidney stones. Recent DXA reveals a T-score of −2.3 in the left one-third radius. Her dietary calcium intake is approximately 600 mg daily, and she does not take any calcium or vitamin D supplements. She has no known family history of calcium or parathyroid disease.

On physical examination, she is in a wheelchair. She is wearing a nasal cannula for oxygen supplementation; her respiratory effort is normal. Her height is 63 in (160 cm), and weight is 114 lb (51.8 kg) (BMI = 20 kg/m^2).

Laboratory test results:
    Serum calcium = 12.0 mg/dL (8.2-10.2 mg/dL) (SI: 3.0 mmol/L [2.1-2.6 mmol/L])
    Serum phosphate = 2.6 mg/dL (2.3-4.7 mg/dL) (SI: 0.8 mmol/L [0.7-1.5 mmol/L])
    Serum creatinine = 1.3 mg/dL (0.6-1.1 mg/dL) (SI: 114.9 μmol/L [53.0-97.2 μmol/L])
    Glomerular filtration rate (estimated) = 25 mL/min per 1.73 m^2 (>60 mL/min per 1.73 m^2)
    Serum intact PTH = 195 pg/mL (10-65 pg/mL) (SI: 195 ng/L [10-65 ng/L])
    Serum 25-hydroxyvitamin D = 21 ng/mL (30-80 ng/mL [optimal]) (SI: 52.4 nmol/L [74.9-199.7 nmol/L])
    Serum albumin = 3.8 g/dL (3.5-5.0 g/dL) (SI: 38 g/L [35-50 g/L])
    Urinary calcium = 238 mg/24 h (100-300 mg/24 h) (SI: 6.0 mmol/d [2.5-7.5 mmol/d])

Which of the following is the most appropriate next step in the management of this patient's hypercalcemia?
    A. Initiate subcutaneous calcitonin therapy
    B. Initiate oral cinacalcet therapy
    C. Initiate subcutaneous denosumab therapy
    D. Treat with intravenous pamidronate
    E. Refer for parathyroid surgery

40 A 76-year-old man with a history of macroprolactinoma presents for follow-up. A 3.2-cm macroprolactinoma was diagnosed 1 year ago, and his prolactin concentration was documented to be 3200 ng/mL (139 nmol/L). He had central adrenal insufficiency, central hypothyroidism, and central hypogonadism. At that time, the following medications were initiated: levothyroxine, 125 mcg daily; hydrocortisone, 15 mg in the morning and 5 mg in the evening; and cabergoline, 0.5 mg twice weekly.

Laboratory test results after 1 month of therapy:
    Prolactin = 110 ng/mL (4-23 ng/mL) (SI: 4.8 nmol/L [0.17-1.00 nmol/L])
    Free T$_4$ = 1.8 ng/dL (0.8-1.8 ng/dL) (SI: 23.2 pmol/L [10.30-23.17 pmol/L])

After 6 months of therapy, his prolactin concentration had further decreased to 14 ng/mL (0.6 nmol/L) and MRI showed significant tumor shrinkage. Because his testosterone was still low, testosterone replacement therapy was initiated.

Current laboratory test results:
    Prolactin = 14 ng/mL (4-23 ng/mL) (SI: 0.61 nmol/L [0.17-1.00 nmol/L])
    Total testosterone = 632 ng/dL (300-900 ng/dL) (SI: 21.9 nmol/L [10.4-31.2 nmol/L])
    Free T$_4$ = 1.9 ng/dL (0.8-1.8 ng/dL) (SI: 24.5 pmol/L [10.30-23.17 pmol/L])

At some point since his last visit, his primary care physician switched his hydrocortisone to prednisone without changing the milligram dosage.

On physical examination, his height is 72 in (183 cm) and weight is 220 lb (99.8 kg) (BMI = 30 kg/m^2). He has gained 15 lb (6.8 kg) over the past few months.

Cabergoline and testosterone therapy are recommended to be continued. The levothyroxine dosage is reduced to 112 mcg daily. A prescription is written for the correct hydrocortisone dosage. His wife asks to speak with you in private. She is teary and says that during the recent months her husband has been frequenting prostitutes. On 2 different occasions, he told her that he had lost or misplaced money, but she suspects that this is not true. This behavior is new for him.

Which of the following is the most likely cause of this behavior?
- A. Excessive thyroid hormone replacement dosage
- B. Excessive glucocorticoid dosage
- C. Cabergoline therapy
- D. Excessive testosterone dosage
- E. New presentation of bipolar disorder

41 A 28-year-old woman comes for a follow-up appointment after recent hospital admission for diabetic ketoacidosis and newly diagnosed diabetes. Her mother has rheumatoid arthritis and hypothyroidism, and her paternal grandfather has type 2 diabetes (diagnosed at age 40 years).

Laboratory test results at hospital admission 3 weeks ago:
Hemoglobin A_{1c} = 14.0% (4.0%-5.6%) (130 mmol/mol [20-38 mmol/mol])
C-peptide = 0.6 ng/mL (0.5-2.0 ng/mL) (SI: 0.20 nmol/L [0.17-0.66 nmol/L])
Plasma glucose = 205 mg/dL (70-99 mg/dL) (SI: 11.4 mmol/L [3.9-5.5 mmol/L])

At hospital discharge, her height was 65 in (165 cm) and weight was 222.2 lb (101 kg) (BMI = 37 kg/m^2). Renal function was normal. A regimen of insulin glargine, 30 units daily, and metformin XR, 500 mg twice daily, was initiated.

At today's visit, she reports fasting blood glucose values in the range of 85 to 112 mg/dL (4.72-6.22 mmol/L), and she has significantly changed her diet and cut out sugared beverages. No antibodies for autoimmune diabetes have been assessed.

Which of the following is the best next step in this patient's management?
- A. Measure fasting glucose and insulin
- B. Measure insulin autoantibodies
- C. Measure C-peptide and glucose
- D. Add prandial insulin
- E. Add a sulfonylurea

42 A 74-year-old man with prostate cancer presents for follow-up of his bone health in the context of long-term androgen-deprivation therapy with leuprorelin, a GnRH analogue. Five years ago, at age 69.5 years, DXA revealed bone mineral density in the osteoporotic range. Metabolic bone screen at that time was normal, and denosumab was initiated (*image A*). DXA performed 3 years later (at age 72.5 years) revealed stable mineral bone density as reflected by T-scores at the lumbar spine and femoral neck of −3.2 and −1.9, respectively.

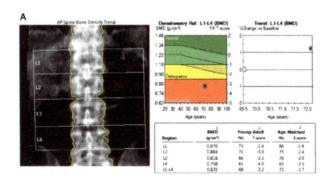

On review now, 5 years after starting denosumab, he feels well and reports adherence to his regimen of calcium and vitamin D supplementation and denosumab injections administered by his primary care physician every 6 months. He continues androgen-deprivation therapy with goserelin administered by his primary care physician, but he has not followed up with his urologist. His only additional medication is venlafaxine for hot flashes.

Current laboratory test results (sample drawn at 8 AM while fasting):
  TSH = 2.0 mIU/L (0.5-5.0 mIU/L)
  Hemoglobin = 12.4 g/dL (13.8-17.2 g/dL) (SI: 124 g/L [138-172 g/L])
  ALT = 35 U/L (10-40 U/L) (SI: 0.58 μkat/L [0.17-0.67 μkat/L])
  Alkaline phosphatase = 325 U/L (50-120 U/L) (SI: 5.43 μkat/L [0.84-2.00 μkat/L])
  Total testosterone = <50 ng/dL (300-900 ng/dL) (SI: <1.7 nmol/L [10.4-31.2 nmol/L])
  LH = 0.2 mIU/mL (1.0-9.0 mIU/mL) (SI: 0.2 IU/L [1.0-9.0 IU/L])
  C-terminal telopeptide of type 1 collagen = 2139 ng/L (100-750 ng/L)
  N-terminal propeptide of type 1 procollagen = 652 μg/L (15-115 μg/L)

Current DXA is shown (*image B*).

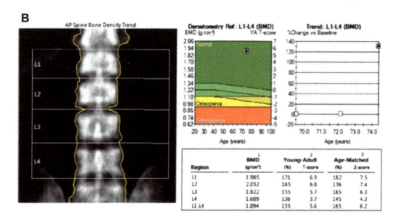

Which of the following is the most important diagnostic assessment to order now?
  A. Serum calcium measurement
  B. Serum 25-hydroxyvitamin D measurement
  C. Serum 1,25-dihydroxyvitamin D measurement
  D. Whole-body bone scintigraphy
  E. Determination of trabecular bone score

43 A 36-year-old man with classic congenital adrenal hyperplasia (21-hydroxylase deficiency) seeks evaluation for infertility. A salt-wasting crisis occurred a few days after birth, and the diagnosis of congenital adrenal hyperplasia was confirmed by documenting a very high 17-hydroxyprogesterone level. He has been treated with glucocorticoids and mineralocorticoids since that time. His growth and pubertal development were reportedly normal. He currently takes hydrocortisone, 20 mg in the morning and 5 mg in the afternoon, and fludrocortisone, 0.1 mg daily. He reports good energy and quality of life and normal libido. He has no orthostasis or salt cravings. He and his wife have been trying to conceive for more than 1 year without success. His wife is 32 years old and has undergone a complete infertility evaluation with no identified abnormality.

On physical examination, he has Tanner stage 5 pubic hair and normal hair growth on his face and chest. There are no physical signs of Cushing syndrome.

Testicular ultrasonography 2 years ago showed normal-sized testes and no evidence of rest tumors. He has not had testicular ultrasonography in the last 2 years.

The patient undergoes biochemical testing in the morning:
  17-Hydroxyprogesterone = 18,504 ng/dL (<220 ng/dL) (SI: 560.7 nmol/L [<6.67 nmol/L])

ACTH = 121 pg/mL (10-60 pg/mL) (SI: 26.6 pmol/L [2.2-13.2 pmol/L])
Androstenedione = 1390 ng/dL (65-210 ng/dL) (SI: 48.5 nmol/L [2.27-7.33 nmol/L])
Total testosterone = 171 ng/dL (300-900 ng/dL) (SI: 5.9 nmol/L [10.4-31.2 nmol/L])
Free testosterone = 3.1 ng/dL (9.0-30.0 ng/dL) (SI: 0.11 nmol/L [0.31-1.04 nmol/L])
SHBG = 9.0 μg/mL (1.1-6.7 μg/mL) (SI: 80 nmol/L [10-60 nmol/L])
LH = 0.2 mIU/L (1.0-9.0 mIU/mL) (SI: 0.2 IU/L [1.0-9.0 IU/L])
FSH = 0.9 mIU/L (1.0-13.0 mIU/mL) (SI: 0.9 IU/L [1.0-13.0 IU/L])
TSH = 2.8 mIU/L (0.5-5.0 mIU/L)

Semen analysis:
12.7 million/mL
98% sperm with abnormal morphology
38% immotile sperm

Which of the following is the most likely cause of this patient's infertility?
A. ACTH-producing pituitary adenoma
B. Adrenal hyperandrogenism
C. Klinefelter syndrome
D. Nonfunctioning pituitary tumor
E. Testicular adrenal rest tumor

44

A 60-year-old woman with gastroesophageal reflux disease, type 2 diabetes mellitus, and longstanding hypothyroidism due to Hashimoto thyroiditis presents for evaluation of worsening fatigue and forgetfulness over the past several months. Review of systems is notable for constipation, bloating, oral discomfort, and occasional falls.

Type 2 diabetes was diagnosed 6 months ago, at which time she began treatment with metformin and met with a certified diabetes educator. Dilated eye examination, bilateral foot examination, and measurements of urine albumin and serum creatinine were normal. She has subsequently lost 10 lb (4.5 kg) through changes to her diet.

Current medications are levothyroxine, 175 mcg daily; metformin, 1000 mg twice daily; and ranitidine, 150 mg daily before dinner. The patient has required increasing dosages of levothyroxine over the last year. She has been refilling her medications regularly.

On physical examination, her blood pressure is 130/88 mm Hg and pulse rate is 60 beats/min. Her height is 64 in (162.6 cm), and weight is 150 lb (68.2 kg) (BMI = 26 kg/m^2). Her tongue appears smooth and mildly swollen on oral examination. The thyroid gland is normal in size without nodules. Neurologic examination is remarkable for impaired sense of vibration and proprioception in the lower extremities, as well as delayed relaxation phase of the deep tendon reflexes. Skin examination is notable for patchy hypopigmentation.

Laboratory test results:
White blood cell count = 3800/μL (4500-11,000/μL) (SI: 3.8 × 10^9/L [4.5-11.0 × 10^9/L])
Hemoglobin = 11.0 g/dL (12.1-15.1 g/dL) (SI: 110 g/L [121-151 g/L])
Mean corpuscular volume = 100 μm^3 (80-100 μm^3) (SI: 100 fL [80-100 fL])
Platelet count = 150 × 10^3/μL (150-450 × 10^3/μL) (SI: 150 × 10^9/L [150-450 × 10^9/L])
Hemoglobin A$_{1c}$ = 6.0% (4.0%-5.6%) (42 mmol/mol [20-38 mmol/mol])
TSH = 12.0 mIU/L (0.5-5.0 mIU/L)
Free T$_4$ = 0.72 ng/dL (0.8-1.8 ng/dL) (SI: 9.27 pmol/L [10.30-23.17 pmol/L])

Which of the following is the most likely explanation for the abnormal thyroid laboratory values in this patient?
A. Medication nonadherence
B. Consumptive hypothyroidism
C. Autoimmune atrophic gastritis with pernicious anemia
D. Metformin
E. Ranitidine

45 A 23-year-old man is referred for management of hypertriglyceridemia. He was initially noted to have elevated triglycerides when he had his first episode of pancreatitis at age 19 years. At that time, his parents took him to the local emergency department because of severe abdominal pain and intolerance of oral intake. During that episode of pancreatitis, his triglyceride concentration was greater than 1000 mg/dL (>11.30 mmol/L). The patient reports a long history of recurrent episodes of abdominal pain that started when he was a teenager. Since his diagnosis of elevated triglycerides, he has tried different medications such as fenofibrate, gemfibrozil, atorvastatin, rosuvastatin, pravastatin, and high-dosage omega-3 fatty acids. However, no medication has changed his triglyceride level. His brother also has high triglycerides. The patient has no history of type 2 diabetes mellitus. He does not drink alcohol. He currently takes no medications.

On physical examination, his blood pressure is 102/76 mm Hg and pulse rate is 84 beats/min. His height is 71 in (180.3 cm), and weight is 180 lb (81.8 kg) (BMI = 25 kg/m^2). He has eruptive xanthomas on his elbows and knees. His heart sounds are regular in rate and rhythm, and his lungs are clear to auscultation bilaterally. Bowel sounds are present, and there is mild tenderness in the epigastric area.

Laboratory test results:
    Total cholesterol = 213 mg/dL (<200 mg/dL [optimal]) (SI: 5.52 mmol/L [<5.18 mmol/L])
    Triglycerides = 2784 mg/dL (<150 mg/dL [optimal]) (SI: 31.46 mmol/L [<1.70 mmol/L])
    HDL cholesterol = 30 mg/dL (>60 mg/dL [optimal]) (SI: 0.78 mmol/L [>1.55 mmol/L])
    Direct LDL cholesterol = 100 mg/dL (<100 mg/dL [optimal]) (SI: 2.59 mmol/L [<2.59 mmol/L])

Which of the following best explains this patient's clinical presentation?
    A. LDL-cholesterol receptor deficiency
    B. Lipoprotein lipase deficiency
    C. Defective apolipoprotein E
    D. Defective apolipoprotein B$_{100}$
    E. Defective apolipoprotein CIII

46 A 62-year-old woman is referred for follow-up after parathyroidectomy. On initial presentation 6 months ago, she was found to have hypercalcemia based on a serum calcium concentration (corrected for albumin) of 11.2 mg/dL (2.8 mmol/L). A concomitant intact PTH measurement was 270 pg/mL (270 ng/L). Additional laboratory results at the time of her diagnosis included normal serum creatinine and a 25-hydroxyvitamin D concentration of 10 ng/mL (25.0 nmol/L). She has no history of nephrolithiasis or fractures, and her family history is negative for hyperparathyroidism, nephrolithiasis, and endocrine tumors. She has normal bone density in the lumbar spine, proximal femur, and proximal left one-third radius.

On the basis of her clinical presentation and current guidelines, she was referred to endocrine surgery for consideration of parathyroidectomy for primary hyperparathyroidism. Preoperative imaging studies revealed a candidate parathyroid adenoma in the left lower neck region. She underwent successful parathyroidectomy of a 200-mg adenoma 3 months ago, with a greater than 50% intraoperative drop in her intact PTH level. She was prescribed supplemental calcium and vitamin D postoperatively, with dosages of 600 mg of elemental calcium twice daily and 2000 IU daily, respectively.

Since her parathyroid resection, her energy level has improved. On physical examination, she appears well. She has a healing suprasternal scar on her neck. No neck masses or adenopathy are appreciated. Findings on spine examination are normal with no evident kyphosis, and the rest of her physical examination findings are unremarkable.

Laboratory test results (ordered by her primary care physician 1 week ago):
    Calcium = 9.5 mg/dL (8.2-10.2 mg/dL) (SI: 2.4 mmol/L [2.1-2.6 mmol/L])
    Phosphate = 3.5 mg/dL (2.3-4.7 mg/dL) (SI: 1.1 mmol/L [0.7-1.5 mmol/L])
    Creatinine = 1.0 mg/dL (0.6-1.1 mg/dL) (SI: 88.4 μmol/L [53.0-97.2 μmol/L])
    Albumin = 4.0 g/dL (3.5-5.0 g/dL) (SI: 40 g/L [35-50 g/L])
    Magnesium = 2.1 mg/dL (1.5-2.3 mg/dL) (SI: 0.9 mmol/L [0.6-0.9 mmol/L])
    Intact PTH = 95 pg/mL (10-65 pg/mL) (SI: 95 ng/L [10-65 ng/L])
    25-Hydroxyvitamin D = 30 ng/mL (30-80 ng/mL [optimal]) (SI: 74.9 nmol/L [74.9-199.7 nmol/L])

On the basis of this patient's current clinical findings, which of the following is the best clinical recommendation?
- A. Refer to endocrine surgery for minimally invasive parathyroidectomy
- B. Perform 4-dimensional CT of the neck
- C. Start calcitriol
- D. Start cinacalcet
- E. Monitor calcium, albumin, and PTH levels every 6 months

47

A 29-year-old man with a history of a skull base chordoma is referred for a second opinion about his pituitary function. He underwent surgery 3 years ago and then received proton-beam radiation to the remnant tumor. He reported feeling chronically fatigued to his radiation oncologist who then referred him to an endocrinologist. After hormonal workup, he was told that his pituitary function was normal. The patient has continued to feel tired and is requesting another opinion. He is currently taking no medication.

On physical examination, his blood pressure is 129/86 mm Hg and pulse rate is 65 beats/min. His height is 72 in (183 cm), and weight is 170 lb (77.1 kg) (BMI = 23 kg/m²). He appears normally androgenized and has normal-sized testes.

Laboratory test results:
- TSH = 0.8 mIU/L (0.5-5.0 mIU/L)
- Free T_4 = 1.2 ng/dL (0.8-1.8 ng/dL) (SI: 15.4 pmol/L [10.30-23.17 pmol/L])
- Serum cortisol (9 AM) = 17.0 μg/dL (5-25 μg/dL) (SI: 469.0 nmol/L [137.9-689.7 nmol/L])
- IGF-1 = 176 ng/mL (117-321 ng/mL) (SI: 23.1 nmol/L [15.3-42.1 nmol/L])
- Testosterone = 487 ng/dL (300-900 ng/dL) (SI: 16.9 nmol/L [10.4-31.2 nmol/L])

A GH-stimulation test with oral macimorelin (0.5 mg/kg) shows a peak GH concentration of 4.0 ng/mL (4.0 μg/L). The macimorelin package insert notes that the FDA-recommended cutoff for normal response is greater than 2.8 ng/mL (>2.8 μg/L).

Which of the following is the best next step?
- A. Reassure the patient that he currently has normal pituitary function
- B. Perform a glucagon-stimulation test
- C. Repeat the GH-stimulation test with oral macimorelin (1 mg/kg)
- D. Measure IGFBP-3
- E. Perform an arginine-stimulation test

48

A 30-year-old woman with cystic fibrosis–related diabetes mellitus is interested in becoming pregnant. Cystic fibrosis–related diabetes was diagnosed when she was in college based on a 2-hour blood glucose value of 232 mg/dL (12.9 mmol/L) during a 75-g oral glucose tolerance test. Her fasting blood glucose concentration was normal at 98 mg/dL (5.4 mmol/L). She recalls being prescribed basal insulin, but she developed hypoglycemia. Currently, she takes only prandial insulin aspart at a dose of 1 unit per 15 to 20 g of carbohydrates. Fasting glucose values range from 90 to 100 mg/dL (5.0-5.6 mmol/L), and postprandial values range from 120 to 180 mg/dL (6.7-10.0 mmol/L). She is concerned about maintaining optimal glucose control over the course of her pregnancy.

Which of the following should be initiated at the time of pregnancy as the best next step to improve both glycemic and neonatal outcomes in this patient?
- A. Basal insulin
- B. Continuous glucose monitoring
- C. Continuous subcutaneous insulin infusion or insulin pump therapy
- D. Hybrid closed-loop system (combined insulin pump and continuous glucose monitoring)
- E. Increased self-monitoring of blood glucose to 7 times daily

49 A 25-year-old woman presents for follow-up of a right thyroid nodule. The patient detected the nodule herself when learning how to perform a thyroid examination as a third-year medical student. She underwent FNA biopsy of the nodule 2 weeks ago and returns today to discuss her results.

She has no anterior neck pain, dysphagia or globus sensation, hoarseness, shortness of breath, or cough. There is no personal history of head or neck radiation or family history of thyroid cancer. She takes no medications.

On physical examination, her blood pressure is 125/72 mm Hg and pulse rate is 80 beats/min. Her height is 60 in (152.4 cm), and weight is 124 lb (56.4 kg) (BMI = 24 kg/m^2). Palpation of her thyroid gland reveals a 1.5-cm firm nodule in the right lobe. There is no cervical lymphadenopathy. The rest of her examination findings are normal.

A TSH measurement 2 months ago was 2.0 mIU/L (0.5-5.0 mIU/L).

Neck ultrasonography (*see images*) performed 2 months ago demonstrated a mixed solid and cystic lesion in the right lobe of the thyroid gland measuring 1.7 × 1.5 × 1.2 cm. Punctate echogenic foci were present within the solid component of the nodule. No abnormal cervical lymph nodes were observed.

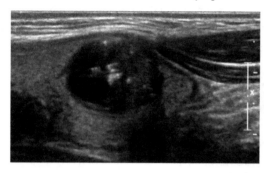
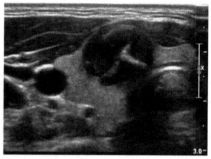

Pathology results from the FNA procedure 2 weeks ago described a benign follicular nodule with a sample that was satisfactory for evaluation.

Which of the following is the most appropriate next step in this patient's management?
- A. No further evaluation or follow-up
- B. Ultrasound-guided drainage of cyst fluid
- C. Referral for right lobectomy and isthmusectomy
- D. Repeated neck ultrasonography and ultrasound-guided FNA biopsy in 6 to 12 months
- E. CT imaging of the neck and chest

50 A 28-year-old woman is referred by dermatology for evaluation of androgenetic alopecia. The visit is conducted via real-time audio/video technology. Menses have been regular since she started puberty at age 12 years. She initiated oral contraceptives in college for birth control and continued them until 2 years ago when she and her partner tried to conceive. She had an uncomplicated pregnancy and birth. After she stopped lactating, monthly menses returned, but she developed significant hair thinning that has progressively worsened over the last year. Her primary care physician referred her to dermatology, and the dermatologist then referred her to endocrinology because of an androgenetic pattern. The dermatologist did not think that a scalp biopsy was indicated.

The patient's scalp appears to have classic male-pattern hair loss without any patches of hair loss. She has no striae, facial plethora, or dorsocervical or supraclavicular fat pads.

Laboratory test results from the dermatology visit (day 4 of the menstrual cycle):
TSH = 2.6 mIU/L (0.5-5.0 mIU/L)
Total testosterone = 48 ng/dL (8-60 ng/dL) (SI: 3.2 nmol/L [0.3-2.1 nmol/L])
DHEA-S = 410 µg/dL (44-332 µg/dL) (SI: 8.40 µmol/L [1.19-9.00 µmol/L])

Which of the following is the best next step in this patient's management?
   A. Initiate spironolactone
   B. Initiate topical minoxidil
   C. Initiate finasteride
   D. Measure androstenedione and free testosterone
   E. Perform adrenal CT

51

A 49-year-old man presents for management of type 2 diabetes mellitus that was diagnosed 12 years ago. He was initially prescribed metformin therapy but quickly required additional measures to maintain glycemic control. Comorbidities include coronary artery disease, hypothyroidism, obstructive sleep apnea, hypertension, and hyperlipidemia.

Current medications include U500 insulin, 225 units daily; metformin; metoprolol; lisinopril; fenofibrate; atorvastatin; and levothyroxine. His blood glucose concentration is usually around 200 mg/dL (11.1 mmol/L), and he says it remains near this level regardless of what he eats. He reports adherence to his medications, and pharmacy records document that refills have been dispensed consistently. His most recent hemoglobin A_{1c} measurement was 8.7% (72 mmol/mol) 6 months ago. He has no chest pain or shortness of breath, but he becomes fatigued with minimal activity. His weight has progressively increased, particularly since initiating U500 insulin. As a result of this weight gain, his ability to ambulate is reduced. He has difficulty rising from the seated position. He is frustrated that most of the weight gain is in his abdomen. While continuous positive airway pressure therapy has improved his daytime fatigue, he still feels tired most of the time.

On physical examination, his blood pressure is 142/76 mm Hg and pulse rate is 72 beats/min. His height is 70 in (177.8 cm), and weight is 330 lb (150 kg) (BMI = 47 kg/m²). He has prominent abdominal adiposity. His face is slightly rounded in appearance, but otherwise no abnormal facial features are appreciated. Dentition appears normal. Acanthosis nigricans is noted in the skin folds of his neck and over his knuckles bilaterally. His lungs are clear to auscultation bilaterally, and his heart has a regular rate and rhythm. Palpation of abdominal organs is limited as a result of his body habitus. Subtle proximal muscle weakness is appreciated in his hip flexors (+4/5). The rest of his examination findings are otherwise unremarkable.

Laboratory test results:
  TSH = 7.2 mIU/L (0.5-5.0 mIU/L)
  Total testosterone = 258 ng/dL (300-900 ng/dL) (SI: 9.0 nmol/L [10.4-31.2 nmol/L])
  Total hemoglobin A_{1c} = 9.2% (4.0%-5.6%) (77 mmol/mol [20-38 mmol/mol])

Which of the following is the best next step in this patient's evaluation and management?
   A. Add an SGLT-2 inhibitor
   B. Add a GLP-1 receptor agonist
   C. Measure serum free T_4
   D. Measure IGF-1
   E. Perform a 1-mg overnight dexamethasone-suppression test

52

A 54-year-old woman with a history of hypothyroidism and depression is concerned about fatigue, leg swelling, and a 15-lb (6.8-kg) weight gain. Over the last several months, her levothyroxine dosage has been adjusted because of persistently elevated TSH. She currently takes levothyroxine, 200 mcg daily, and bupropion, 300 mg daily. She has been referred because her most recent serum TSH concentration remains elevated. She states that she takes her levothyroxine every day on an empty stomach and waits 2 hours before eating. She does not take any multivitamins, iron tablets, or calcium supplements. She had an upper endoscopy earlier this year, and the findings were unremarkable. There is no family history of hypothyroidism or other autoimmune disease. She has no coronary artery disease.

On physical examination, her blood pressure is 135/90 mm Hg and pulse rate is 52 beats/min. Her height is 63 in (160 cm), and weight is 170 lb (77.1 kg) (BMI = 30 kg/m²). Her thyroid gland is mildly enlarged with no palpable nodules. Her pulse rate is regular, and lungs are clear to auscultation bilaterally. There is 2+ nonpitting lower-extremity edema.

Laboratory test results:

Timepoint	TSH	Free T₄	Levothyroxine dosage
4 years ago	1.8 mIU/L	1.0 ng/dL (SI: 12.87 pmol/L)	112 mcg daily
3 months ago	54 mIU/L	0.4 ng/dL (SI: 5.15 pmol/L)	Increased to 150 mcg daily
2 months ago	50 mIU/L	0.6 ng/dL (SI: 7.72 pmol/L)	Increased to 175 mcg daily
1 month ago	58 mIU/L	0.19 ng/dL (SI: 2.44 pmol/L)	Increased to 200 mcg daily

Reference ranges: TSH, 0.5-5.0 mIU/L; free T₄, 0.8-1.8 ng/dL (SI: 10.30-23.17 pmol/L).

Additional laboratory test results:
  25-Hydroxyvitamin D = 32 ng/mL (30-80 ng/mL) (SI: 79.9 nmol/L [74.9-199.7 nmol/L])
  Complete blood cell count, normal
  Celiac disease screening, negative

Her levothyroxine tablets are changed to levothyroxine oral solution and the dosage is increased to 300 mcg daily. A repeated TSH measurement 4 weeks later is 64 mIU/L. Her levothyroxine tablets have always come from the same manufacturer.

On the basis of these laboratory results, which of the following is the best next step in the management of this patient's hypothyroidism?
  A. Change to intravenous levothyroxine
  B. Change to desiccated thyroid
  C. Add liothyronine to the current levothyroxine regimen
  D. Increase the dosage of the levothyroxine oral solution to 400 mcg daily
  E. Recommend weekly oral administration of the full week's dose of levothyroxine in the clinic

53

A consultation is requested for 60-year-old man with mild intellectual disability and polycythemia associated with an elevated serum testosterone concentration. He has been admitted to the hospital's stroke unit for a left cerebellar infarction. Workup performed by the treating neurology team revealed no risk factors for stroke, with the exception of polycythemia. There is no history of sleep apnea. He does not smoke cigarettes.

Laboratory test results:
  Hemoglobin = 22.0 g/dL (13.8-17.2 g/dL) (SI: 220 g/L [138-172 g/L])
  Serum total testosterone = 1010 ng/dL (300-900 ng/dL) (SI: 35.0 nmol/L [10.4-31.2 nmol/L])
  LH = 0.2 mIU/mL (1.0-9.0 mIU/mL) (SI: 0.2 IU/L [1.0-9.0 IU/L])

He is awaiting an opinion from hematology.

Physical examination findings are notable for short stature (height 55.1 in [140 cm]), skin hyperpigmentation, and androgenetic alopecia. His blood pressure is normal. On genital examination, he has atypical genitalia. Abdominal CT, performed to evaluate self-limiting abdominal pain, shows incidental bilateral radiologic abnormalities (*see images, arrows*).

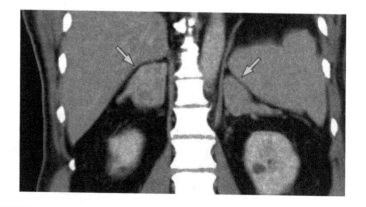

Which of the following is the most important diagnostic test to order now?
- A. Serum 17-hydroxyprogesterone measurement
- B. Whole-body fluorodeoxyglucose-PET
- C. Pituitary-directed MRI
- D. Serum estradiol measurement
- E. Serum hCG measurement

54 A 48-year-old man is concerned about fatigue, lethargy, nausea, and occasional diarrhea 4 months after undergoing surgery to remove a 14-cm left adrenal tumor. Histology confirmed a high-grade adrenocortical carcinoma. CT of the chest, abdomen, and pelvis 6 weeks after surgery revealed postoperative appearances in the left adrenal bed but no evidence of metastatic disease. His current medications are hydrocortisone, 30 mg daily in divided doses, and mitotane, 3 g twice daily.

On physical examination, his blood pressure is 120/75 mm Hg and pulse rate is 88 beats/min and regular. His height is 72 in (182.9 cm), and weight is 180 lb (81.6 kg) (BMI = 24 kg/m^2). He has a well-healed scar at the site of his recent surgery, but no other abnormalities on physical examination.

Laboratory test results:
- Hemoglobin = 10.8 g/dL (13.8-17.2 g/dL) (SI: 108 g/L [138-172 g/L])
- Mean corpuscular volume = 83 μm^3 (80-100 μm^3) (SI: 83 fL [80-100 fL])
- Platelet count = 192 × 10^3/μL (150-450 × 10^3/μL) (SI: 192 × 10^9/L [150-450 × 10^9/L])
- Serum sodium = 133 mEq/L (136-142 mEq/L) (SI: 133 mmol/L [136-142 mmol/L])
- Serum potassium = 4.0 mEq/L (3.5-5.0 mEq/L) (SI: 4.0 mmol/L [3.5-5.0 mmol/L])
- Serum creatinine = 1.0 mg/dL (0.7-1.3 mg/dL) (SI: 88.4 μmol/L [61.9-114.9 μmol/L])
- Serum urea nitrogen = 14.5 mg/dL (8-23 mg/dL) (SI: 5.2 mmol/L [2.9-8.2 mmol/L])
- Serum TSH = 1.9 mIU/L (0.5-5.0 mIU/L)
- Serum free T$_4$ = 0.7 ng/dL (0.8-1.8 ng/dL) (SI: 9.01 pmol/L [10.30-23.17 pmol/L])
- Plasma mitotane concentration = 16 μg/mL (14-20 μg/mL)

Which of the following is the most appropriate next step in this patient's management?
- A. Increase the hydrocortisone dosage
- B. Reduce the mitotane dosage
- C. Start fludrocortisone therapy
- D. Start levothyroxine therapy
- E. Stop mitotane and start streptozocin

55 A 35-year-old woman is seen in clinic to discuss weight management options. She has a lifelong history of difficulty managing her weight and has tried to lose weight multiple times over the years, including most recently with a commercial meal replacement program. Her pattern is one of initial success followed by weight regain. She has knee and back pain as a result of carrying extra weight and gastroesophageal reflux for which she takes pantoprazole. One year ago, Barrett esophagus was diagnosed, and she has periodic surveillance endoscopies.

She has met with a dietician on several occasions and is currently tracking her caloric intake. Physical activity consists of walking at a moderate pace for 20 minutes daily. She logs approximately 5000 steps per day.

On physical examination, her height is 61.5 in (156 cm) and weight is 243 lb (110 kg) (BMI = 45 kg/m^2). Examination findings are notable for symmetric weight distribution and no edema. Findings on thyroid examination are normal. Fasting glucose is normal.

She is in ongoing discussions about using assisted reproductive technology for the treatment of infertility. Her current weight is a barrier to undergoing in vitro fertilization. She has been given a goal BMI of 40 kg/m^2 or less before in vitro fertilization will be considered. Her primary goal is to have a successful pregnancy.

Which of the following is the best recommendation for this patient?
- A. Roux-en-Y gastric bypass; delay pregnancy for 1 year after surgery
- B. Laparoscopic sleeve gastrectomy; delay pregnancy for 1 year after surgery
- C. Adjustable gastric banding; delay pregnancy for 1 year after surgery
- D. Liraglutide (3 mg subcutaneously) while she undergoes in vitro fertilization
- E. Extended-release phentermine/topiramate while she undergoes in vitro fertilization

56

A 46-year-old woman with acromegaly due to a 1.6-cm pituitary adenoma underwent transsphenoidal surgery 2 years ago. Pathologic examination confirmed the diagnosis of a densely granulated GH-staining adenoma. The neurosurgeon indicated that there was tumor in the left cavernous sinus, and she was concerned that there was some residual disease. Indeed, 3 months after surgery, the patient's IGF-1 concentration was still abnormal, and a GH-suppression test showed a nadir GH concentration of 1.2 ng/mL (1.2 µg/L). Lanreotide depot, 90 mg every 28 days, was initiated, which normalized her IGF-1.

She comes to an appointment for yearly follow-up and describes persistent low back pain, hip pain, and wrist discomfort, which have continued to worsen over the past 2 years. Her IGF-1 concentration is 187 ng/mL (91-246 ng/mL [SI: 24.5 nmol/L (11.9-32.2 nmol/L)]), and a fasting GH concentration is 0.9 ng/mL (SI: 0.9 µg/L). Pituitary MRI shows a possible small residual adenoma in the left cavernous sinus. X-ray of the spine and hips shows worsening degenerative joint disease compared with an x-ray obtained 1 month after pituitary surgery.

Which of the following is the best next step in this patient's management?
- A. Refer for radiation therapy for the residual adenoma
- B. Increase the lanreotide dosage to 120 mg every 28 days
- C. Refer for a second pituitary surgery
- D. Add pegvisomant
- E. Recommend nonsteroidal antiinflammatory agents and physical therapy

57

A 34-year-old man with a 4-year history of type 2 diabetes mellitus presents for follow-up. He eats a well-balanced diet, but he has not been exercising regularly (less than 1 hour per week of activity greater than 2 metabolic equivalents). His most recent hemoglobin A_{1c} measurement is 7.4% (57 mmol/mol). He has no diabetes-related complications, including no history of atherosclerotic cardiovascular disease. He does not smoke cigarettes and drinks 1 to 2 alcoholic beverages a week. He takes metformin, 1000 mg twice daily.

On physical examination, his blood pressure is 138/94 mm Hg (repeated 144/92 mm Hg) and pulse rate is 88 beats/min. His height is 70 in (178 cm), and weight is 230 lb (104.5 kg) (BMI = 33 kg/m²). There are no carotid bruits. His heart rate and rhythm are regular. No murmurs are appreciated. Bilateral radial, dorsalis pedis, and posterior tibial pulses are palpable (2+).

Laboratory test results:
  Complete metabolic panel, normal
  LDL cholesterol = 92 mg/dL (<100 mg/dL [optimal]) (SI: 2.38 mmol/L [<2.59 mmol/L])
  Triglycerides = 165 mg/dL (<150 mg/dL [optimal]) (SI: 1.86 mmol/L [<1.70 mmol/L])
  Urine albumin-to-creatinine ratio = 22 mg/g creat (<30 mg/g creat)

The patient is counseled that consistent, moderate exercise may help to improve insulin sensitivity and reduce cardiovascular risk factors.

In addition to initiating an exercise program, which of the following should be recommended as the best next step to reduce this patient's risk of cardiovascular disease?
A. No further intervention now
B. Start atorvastatin
C. Start aspirin
D. Start icosapent ethyl
E. Start lisinopril

58

A 54-year-old woman with stage IV medullary thyroid carcinoma and postoperative hypothyroidism presents to the emergency department to evaluate chest pain. Three months ago, the patient underwent total thyroidectomy and bilateral central and lateral neck dissection.

Preoperative laboratory test results:
  Serum calcitonin = 2603 pg/mL (<8 pg/mL) (SI: 760.1 pmol/L [<2.34 pmol/L])
  Carcinoembryonic antigen = 13.5 ng/mL (<2.5 ng/mL) (SI: 13.5 µg/L [<2.5 µg/L])

Extensive imaging was completed before surgery to evaluate for metastatic disease because of the very high preoperative serum markers. Chest CT demonstrated right hilar and subcarinal lymphadenopathy, but the rest of the imaging findings, including those from bone scintigraphy and liver and brain MRI, were unremarkable. Genetic testing for germline *RET* pathogenic variants performed before surgery was negative. Subsequent testing of the patient's tumor also did not demonstrate a pathogenic variant in the *RET* gene.

Today the patient reports 6/10 substernal chest pain and dyspnea on exertion, both of which have been worsening over the past 2 weeks. Review of systems is negative for fever, cough, hemoptysis, leg swelling, abdominal pain, and diarrhea.

There is no family history of medullary thyroid cancer. The patient's only medication is levothyroxine.

On physical examination, her blood pressure is 113/74 mm Hg and pulse rate is 101 beats/min. Her height is 71 in (180.3 cm), and weight is 158 lb (71.8 kg) (BMI = 22 kg/m²). Examination of her neck reveals well-healed anterior and bilateral lateral neck scars and no mass in the thyroid bed. There is no cervical lymphadenopathy. The rest of her examination findings, including those from cardiac and respiratory examinations, are normal.

Laboratory test results:
  Complete blood cell count, normal
  Complete metabolic panel, normal
  Troponin = ≤0.05 ng/mL (<0.6 ng/mL) (SI: ≤0.05 µg/L [<0.6 µg/L])

Laboratory test results from 2 weeks ago:
  Serum TSH = 1.6 mIU/L (0.5-5.0 mIU/L)
  Calcitonin = 3916 pg/mL (<8 pg/mL) (SI: 1143.5 pmol/L [<2.34 pmol/L])
  Carcinoembryonic antigen = 10.2 ng/mL (<2.5 ng/mL) (SI: 10.2 µg/L [<2.5 µg/L])

Electrocardiography demonstrates sinus tachycardia and no acute ST- or T-wave changes. Pulmonary embolism protocol CT shows increased size of hilar lymphadenopathy, new mediastinal lymphadenopathy, and the interval development of lymphangitic spread of neoplasm in the right lung. There is no evidence of pulmonary embolism.

Which of the following is the most appropriate treatment to prescribe next?
A. Cabozantinib
B. Cyclophosphamide-vincristine-dacarbazine
C. External beam radiotherapy
D. Octreotide LAR
E. Selpercatinib

59 A 71-year-man is referred for evaluation of elevated alkaline phosphatase. At a recent annual visit, he was noted to have a slightly high alkaline phosphatase level that, in retrospect, had been borderline-high for at least the last 5 years. He was recently evaluated for lower abdominal pain. CT findings of the abdomen and pelvis were negative for obvious intraabdominal pathology, but he did have extensive cortical and trabecular thickening involving the right iliac bone and pubic bone. In light of these findings, he was referred for consultation.

His medical history is notable for hypertension and osteoarthritis involving the left knee and lower lumbar spine. Medications include hydrochlorothiazide, atenolol, and ibuprofen. His family history is negative for calcium or bone disorders, including no history of osteoporosis. Review of systems is notable for mild gastroesophageal reflux disease, for which he takes calcium carbonate on an as-needed basis. He also has intermittent low back pain that is exacerbated by excessive activity, but he has no other history of musculoskeletal pain.

On physical examination, his vital signs are unremarkable. Height is equivalent to his self-reported maximum adult height. Spine examination shows a somewhat flattened lumbar lordotic curve without elicitable tenderness to palpation. Passive range of motion of the right hip is full and painless. There is no direct tenderness to palpation over the right lateral pelvis or inguinal region.

Laboratory test results:
- Calcium = 9.5 mg/dL (8.2-10.2 mg/dL) (SI: 2.4 mmol/L [2.1-2.6 mmol/L])
- Phosphate = 3.6 mg/dL (2.3-4.7 mg/dL) (SI: 1.2 mmol/L [0.7-1.5 mmol/L])
- Creatinine = 1.0 mg/dL (0.7-1.3 mg/dL) (SI: 88.4 µmol/L [61.9-114.9 µmol/L])
- Total protein = 6.5 g/dL (6.3-7.9 g/dL) (SI: 65 g/L [63-79 g/L])
- Albumin = 4.0 g/dL (3.5-5.0 g/dL) (SI: 40 g/L [35-50 g/L])
- Alkaline phosphatase = 140 U/L (50-120 U/L) (SI: 2.3 µkat/L [0.84-2.00 µkat/L])
- γ-Glutamyltransferase = 24 U/L (2-30 U/L) (SI: 0.40 µkat/L [0.03-0.50 µkat/L])
- PSA = 1.5 ng/mL (<7.0 ng/mL) (SI: 1.5 µg/L [<7.0 µg/L])
- 25-Hydroxyvitamin D = 25 ng/mL (30-80 ng/mL [optimal]) (SI: 62.4 nmol/L [74.9-199.7 nmol/L])

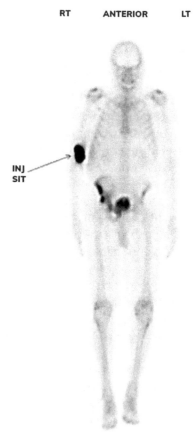

Subsequent bone-specific alkaline phosphatase measurement is abnormal at 26 µg/L (normal ≤20 µg/L). Given these results, a whole-body bone scan is ordered (*see image*).

On the basis of this patient's biochemical and radiographic results, which of the following is the best next step in the evaluation and management of his skeletal disorder?
- A. Treatment with zoledronic acid
- B. Treatment with alendronate
- C. Serum C-telopeptide measurement
- D. Serum and urine electrophoresis
- E. Reassurance and repeated alkaline phosphatase measurement in 12 months

60 A 50-year-old woman was diagnosed with Li-Fraumeni syndrome after her son was treated for leukemia 5 years ago. Her son underwent genetic testing, which documented a germline *TP53* pathogenic variant. Subsequent genetic testing of family members revealed that the patient also carries the same pathogenic variant. She was advised to undergo an imaging surveillance protocol for Li-Fraumeni syndrome, which identified a low-grade central nervous system glioma and a high-grade uterine leiomyosarcoma. Both tumors were successfully removed, and she has been in remission. She also decided to proceed with prophylactic bilateral mastectomy.

Now, on annual surveillance imaging, MRI of the abdomen reveals a new left adrenal nodule. Imaging from 1 year ago showed normal adrenal glands. The 1.2-cm nodule is described as being round, homogenous, and without signal dropout on in-phase and out-of-phase imaging.

She has no signs or symptoms of Cushing syndrome. She is normokalemic and normotensive. Biochemical testing documents a normal result from a low-dose overnight dexamethasone-suppression test, normal adrenal androgens, and normal plasma metanephrines.

Which of the following is the most likely characterization of the adrenal nodule?
- A. Adrenocortical carcinoma
- B. Adrenomedullary cyst
- C. Lipid-rich adrenocortical adenoma
- D. Lipid-poor adrenocortical adenoma
- E. Pheochromocytoma

61 A 56-year-old woman is referred for further assessment after she is found to have bitemporal hemianopia during a routine visit to her optometrist. She has hypertension and hypercholesterolemia treated with amlodipine and atorvastatin. She also has epilepsy, which has been well controlled for many years on carbamazepine.

On physical examination, her height is 67 in (170 cm) and weight is 169 lb (76.7 kg) (BMI = 26.5 kg/m^2). Her resting pulse rate is 76 beats/min and regular, and blood pressure is 125/80 mm Hg. Visual acuity is 20/40 (6/12) in the right eye and 20/80 (6/24) in the left eye.

Laboratory test results:
  Serum sodium = 129 mEq/L (136-142 mEq/L) (SI: 129 mmol/L [136-142 mmol/L])
  Serum potassium = 4.1 mEq/L (3.5-5.0 mEq/L) (SI: 4.1 mmol/L [3.5-5.0 mmol/L])
  Serum creatinine = 0.7 mg/dL (0.7-1.3 mg/dL) (SI: 61.9 µmol/L [61.9-114.9 µmol/L])
  Serum urea nitrogen = 8.4 mg/dL (8-23 mg/dL) (SI: 3.0 mmol/L [2.9-8.2 mmol/L])
  Hemoglobin A$_{1c}$ = 5.3% (4.0%-5.6%) (SI: 34 mmol/mol [20-38 mmol/mol])
  Prolactin = 80 ng/mL (4-30 ng/mL) (SI: 3.48 nmol/L [0.17-1.30 nmol/L])
  TSH = 1.3 mIU/L (0.5-5.0 mIU/L)
  Free T$_4$ = 0.7 ng/dL (0.8-1.8 ng/dL) (SI: 9.01 pmol/L [10.30-23.17 pmol/L])
  Serum cortisol (8 AM) = 16.5 µg/dL (5-25 µg/dL) (SI: 455.2 nmol/L [137.9-689.7 nmol/L])
  IGF-1 = 185 ng/mL (78-220 ng/mL) (SI: 24.2 nmol/L [10.2-28.8 nmol/L])
  FSH = 43.4 mIU/mL (>30 mIU/mL [postmenopausal]) (SI: 43.4 IU/L [>30 IU/L])
  LH = 37.2 mIU/mL (>30 mIU/mL [postmenopausal]) (SI: 37.2 IU/L [>30 IU/L])

MRI of the sella is shown (*see images*).

T1 coronal (postcontrast) T2 coronal

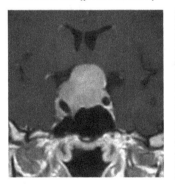
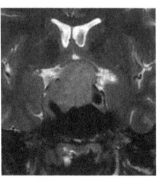

Which of the following is the most likely explanation for this patient's abnormal thyroid biochemistry?
- A. Coincidental primary hypothyroidism
- B. Cushing disease
- C. Hypopituitarism
- D. Medication
- E. Nonthyroidal illness

62 A 32-year-old woman presents for a second opinion regarding the diagnosis of nonclassic congenital adrenal hyperplasia. She initially sought evaluation from her primary care physician 8 years ago for symptoms of androgen excess. As a teenager, she had irregular menses but also developed hair growth on the chin and around the umbilicus. This led to testing, which documented an elevated DHEA-S concentration. She thinks the DHEA-S value was initially quite high but that it was lower on subsequent measurements. A gynecologist told her she did not have polycystic ovary syndrome based on ultrasonography findings and referred her to endocrinology because of the elevated DHEA-S. The endocrinologist ordered cosyntropin-stimulation testing.

Nonclassic congenital adrenal hyperplasia was diagnosed based on a stimulated 17-hydroxypregnenolone value of 1363 ng/dL (41.0 nmol/L). The patient was prescribed dexamethasone, 0.25 mg 3 times weekly; an oral contraceptive pill; and spironolactone. One year ago, she stopped the oral contraceptive pill and spironolactone and her regimen was switched to prednisone, 1 mg daily, in preparation for trying to conceive. The prednisone dosage was then increased to 2 mg daily based on elevated androgens. She began to have significant hair loss. Scalp biopsy findings were consistent with androgenetic alopecia. More recently, her prednisone dosage was increased to 3 mg daily. Genetic testing did not identify any pathogenic variants in the *CYP21A2* gene. She is now questioning her diagnosis. Menses have become irregular, every 45 to 60 days since discontinuing the oral contraceptive pill.

Her current medications are prednisone, 3 mg daily, and a daily prenatal multivitamin.

On physical examination, her blood pressure is 110/74 mm Hg. Her height is 65 in (165 cm), and weight is 145 lb (65.9 kg) (BMI = 24 kg/m^2). She has terminal hair growth on her chin and abdomen with a Ferriman-Gallwey score of 6. The rest of her examination findings are unremarkable.

Laboratory test results on day 3 of her cycle:
TSH = 2.5 mIU/L (0.5-5.0 mIU/L)
Prolactin = 12 ng/mL (4-30 ng/mL [nonlactating female]) (SI: 0.52 nmol/L [0.17-1.30 nmol/L])
LH = 4.5 mIU/mL (1.0-18.0 mIU/mL [follicular]) (SI: 4.5 IU/L [1.0-18.0 IU/L])
FSH = 6.2 mIU/mL (2.0-12.0 mIU/mL [follicular]) (SI: 6.2 IU/L [2.0-12.0 IU/L])
Estradiol = 40 pg/mL (10-180 pg/mL [follicular]) (SI: 146.8 pmol/L [36.7-660.8 pmol/L])
Total testosterone = 56.8 ng/dL (8-60 ng/dL) (SI: 2.0 nmol/L [0.3-2.1 nmol/L])
DHEA-S = 302 µg/dL (15-200 µg/dL) (SI: 8.18 µmol/L [0.41-5.42 µmol/L])
Androstenedione = 125 ng/dL (80-240 ng/dL) (SI: 4.36 nmol/L [2.79-8.38 nmol/L])
Fasting glucose = 95 mg/dL (70-99 mg/dL) (SI: 5.3 mmol/L [3.9-5.5 mmol/L])

Results from a standard 250-mcg cosyntropin-stimulation test the day of the consultation are shown in the table.

Measurement	Baseline	30 min	60 min
Cortisol	9.7 µg/dL (SI: 267.6 nmol/L)	18.0 µg/dL (SI: 496.6 nmol/L)	21.0 µg/dL (SI: 579.3 nmol/L)
17-Hydroxyprogesterone	<40 ng/dL (SI: <1.2 nmol/L)	76 ng/dL (SI: 2.3 nmol/L)	67 ng/dL (SI: 2.0 nmol/L)
17-Hydroxypregnenolone	55 ng/dL (SI: 1.7 nmol/L)	100 ng/dL (SI: 3.0 nmol/L)	84 ng/dL (SI: 2.5 nmol/L)

Which of the following is the most likely diagnosis?
A. Nonclassic congenital adrenal hyperplasia due to 21-hydroxylase deficiency
B. Nonclassic congenital adrenal hyperplasia due to 3β-hydroxysteroid dehydrogenase deficiency
C. Polycystic ovary syndrome
D. Idiopathic hirsutism
E. Cannot be determined; additional testing is needed while off prednisone

63 A 62-year-old man presents for management of type 2 diabetes mellitus, which was diagnosed 6 years ago. His hemoglobin A$_{1c}$ has been well controlled on metformin therapy. He was initially taking only 500 mg daily, but the dosage has been slowly titrated to 1000 mg twice daily. His most recent hemoglobin A$_{1c}$ measurement was 6.4% (46 mmol/mol). Coronary artery disease was diagnosed 3 years ago, and he has had 3 coronary artery bypass grafts. He has no symptoms of chest pain or shortness of breath. He recently underwent transthoracic echocardiography, and his left ventricular ejection fraction was 50%.

He has a 45 pack-year history of cigarette smoking, but he quit 3 years ago. He has hypertension controlled with atenolol, 50 mg once daily, and lisinopril/hydrochlorothiazide, 20 mg/12.5 mg once daily, and hyperlipidemia controlled with atorvastatin, 80 mg daily.

On physical examination, his blood pressure is 126/78 mm Hg and pulse rate is 66 beats/min. His height is 63 in (160 cm), and weight is 176 lb (80 kg) (BMI = 31 kg/m^2).

Laboratory test results:
Total cholesterol = 112 mg/dL (<200 mg/dL [optimal]) (SI: 2.90 mmol/L [<5.18 mmol/L])
LDL cholesterol = 45 mg/dL (<100 mg/dL [optimal]) (SI: 1.17 mmol/L [<2.59 mmol/L])
HDL cholesterol = 35 mg/dL (>60 mg/dL [optimal]) (SI: 0.91 mmol/L [>1.55 mmol/L])
Triglycerides = 105 mg/dL (<150 mg/dL [optimal]) (SI: 1.19 mmol/L [<1.70 mmol/L])
Estimated glomerular filtration rate = 63 mL/min per 1.73 m^2 (>60 mL/min per 1.73 m^2)

Which of the following is the best next step to reduce this patient's cardiovascular risk?
A. Increase the lisinopril dosage
B. Add once-weekly subcutaneous semaglutide
C. Add spironolactone
D. Add icosapent ethyl
E. Add ezetimibe

64 A 47-year-old man is referred for evaluation of elevated PTH. Nephrolithiasis was diagnosed after he presented to the emergency department with flank pain and hematuria. Abdominal CT confirmed the presence of an 8-mm stone in the right ureter. This was the patient's first episode of nephrolithiasis.

He underwent Roux-en-Y gastric bypass approximately 8 years ago. He lost 85 lb (38.5 kg) with subsequent remission of type 2 diabetes mellitus and has maintained this weight loss over the years. He currently takes a mineral-containing multivitamin twice daily; cholecalciferol, 5000 IU daily; vitamin B$_{12}$ injections monthly; and calcium citrate, 500 mg 3 times daily.

On physical examination, his height is 67 in (170 cm) and weight is 189.5 lb (86 kg) (BMI = 30 kg/m^2). He has no other notable features on examination.

Laboratory test results:
Serum calcium = 9.2 mg/dL (8.2-10.2 mg/dL) (SI: 2.3 mmol/L [2.1-2.6 mmol/L])
Serum albumin = 3.8 g/dL (3.5-5.0 g/dL) (SI: 38 g/L [35-50 g/L])
PTH = 70 pg/mL (10-65 pg/mL) (SI: 70 ng/L [10-65 ng/L])
Phosphate = 3.1 mg/dL (2.3-4.7 mg/dL) (SI: 1.0 mmol/L [0.7-1.5 mmol/L])
25-Hydroxyvitamin D = 26 ng/mL (30-80 ng/mL [optimal]) (SI: 65 nmol/L [74.9-199.7 nmol/L])
Serum creatinine = 1.0 mg/dL (0.7-1.3 mg/dL) (SI: 88.4 µmol/L [61.9-114.9 µmol/L])
Urinary calcium excretion = 90 mg/24 h (100-300 mg/24 h) (SI: 2.25 mmol/d [2.5-7.5 mmol/d])

Review of his medical record reveals that his serum calcium concentration has been as high as 10.1 mg/dL (2.5 mmol/L) in the past, with a corresponding PTH concentration of 50 pg/mL (50 ng/L).

Which of the following best explains this patient's presentation?
A. Normocalcemic primary hyperparathyroidism
B. Secondary hyperparathyroidism
C. Calcium phosphate nephropathy as a consequence of Roux-en-Y gastric bypass
D. Familial hypocalciuric hypercalcemia
E. Parathyroid carcinoma

65 A 33-year-old Black man returns for follow-up of type 1 diabetes mellitus. He has no microvascular complications, but he expresses concern about frequent hyperglycemia. His treatment regimen includes insulin aspart delivered by an external subcutaneous insulin pump. He reports no symptoms of hypoglycemia. He wears a continuous glucose monitor that shows a mean glucose value of 197 mg/dL (10.9 mmol/L) over the last 4 weeks. His glucose values are in the target range 44% of the time (70-180 mg/dL [3.9-10.0 mmol/L]), below the range 1% of the time, and above the range 55% of the time. A point-of-care hemoglobin A_{1c} measurement is 6.1% (43 mmol/mol). His medical history is notable for nephrolithiasis, iron deficiency anemia, and hypertension. Other medications include emtricitabine/tenofovir, iron sulfate, lisinopril, and acetaminophen. Emtricitabine/tenofovir is prescribed to be taken daily for HIV preexposure prophylaxis.

Laboratory test results:
    White blood cell count = 10,000/μL (4500-11,000/μL) (SI: 10 × 10⁹/L [4.5-11.0 × 10⁹/L])
    Red blood cell count = 5.31 million cells/μL (4.35-5.65 million cells/μL)
    Hemoglobin = 15.5 g/dL (13.8-17.2 g/dL) (SI: 155 g/L [138-172 g/L])
    Hematocrit = 46.5% (41%-50%) (SI: 0.465 [0.41-0.50])
    Mean corpuscular volume = 87.4 μm³ (80-100 μm³) (SI: 87.4 fL [80-100 fL])
    Mean corpuscular hemoglobin = 35.6 g/dL (31-37 g/dL)
    Red blood cell distribution width = 11.9% (11.5%-14.5%)
    Platelet count = 339 × 10³/μL (150-350 × 10³/μL) (SI: 339 × 10⁹/L [150-350 × 10⁹/L])
    Urinary albumin-to-creatinine ratio = 12 mg/g creat (<30 mg/g creat)
    Comprehensive metabolic panel, normal
    HIV-1/2 antibody screen, negative
    Fructosamine = 360 μmol/L (200-285 μmol/L)

Which of the following is the most likely explanation for the discrepancy between this patient's hemoglobin A_{1c} level and mean glucose value on continuous glucose monitoring?
    A. Race/ancestry
    B. Iron deficiency
    C. Acetaminophen
    D. Inaccuracy of continuous glucose monitoring values
    E. Emtricitabine/tenofovir

66 A 70-year-old man with urinary retention and long-term indwelling Foley catheter is referred for evaluation of Paget disease of bone after he presented to his orthopedist with left-sided hip pain. On imaging, he was found to have severe left-sided hip osteoarthritis. Total hip arthroplasty was recommended, and he plans to schedule this procedure soon. He was also found to have widespread cortical and trabecular thickening, as well as patchy sclerosis/lucency, consistent with Paget disease. His bone pain has somewhat improved by taking ibuprofen as needed. He has not had any fractures. He has no family history of Paget disease. He takes calcium and vitamin D supplementation.

Examination of his pelvis and hips does not reveal any palpable bony abnormalities, and there is no tenderness to palpation.

Laboratory test results:
    Serum calcium = 9.6 mg/dL (8.2-10.2 mg/dL) (SI: 2.4 mmol/L [2.1-2.6 mmol/L])
    Serum creatinine = 0.9 mg/dL (0.7-1.3 mg/dL) (SI: 79.6 μmol/L [61.9-114.9 μmol/L])
    Serum 25-hydroxyvitamin D = 48 ng/mL (30-80 ng/mL [optimal]) (SI: 119.8 nmol/L [74.9-199.7 nmol/L])
    Serum albumin = 4.5 g/dL (3.5-5.0 g/dL) (SI: 45 g/L [35-50 g/L])
    Serum total alkaline phosphatase = 168 U/L (50-120 U/L) (SI: 2.80 μkat/L [0.84-2.00 μkat/L])
    Serum bone-specific alkaline phosphatase = 28 μg/L (≤20 μg/L)

His imaging results are shown.

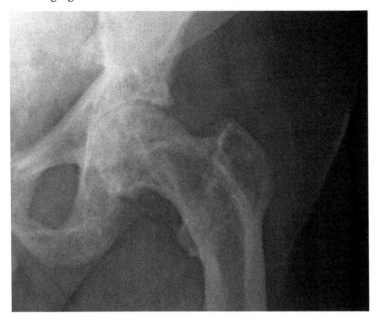

Plain x-ray of the left hip (anteroposterior view).

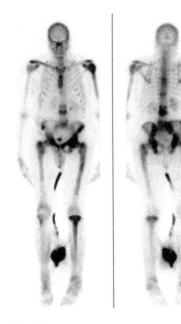

Bone scan.

Which of the following is the best treatment choice for this patient?

A. Calcitonin
B. Alendronate
C. Zoledronic acid
D. Denosumab
E. No treatment at this time

---

67 A 26-year-old woman with a history of lupus sees her primary care physician for fatigue, weight gain, and bloating. Laboratory tests document pregnancy and hypothyroidism. Gestational age is estimated to be 7 weeks. Her primary care physician prescribes levothyroxine, 100 mcg daily, but the patient would like to start desiccated thyroid. She is referred to endocrinology for the management of hypothyroidism. She currently takes no medications.

On physical examination, her blood pressure is 120/60 mm Hg and pulse rate is 60 beats/min. Her height is 66 in (167.6 cm), and weight is 124 lb (56.2 kg) (BMI = 20 kg/m^2). Her thyroid gland is palpable and visible as she swallows. There is no cervical adenopathy. Her heart rate is regular, and lungs are clear to auscultation bilaterally. Her abdomen is soft and nontender. There is no lower-extremity edema. The rest of the examination findings are normal.

Initial laboratory test results:
  Basic metabolic panel, normal
  Complete blood cell count, normal
  TSH = 15.0 mIU/L (0.5-5.0 mIU/L)
  Free T$_4$ = 0.6 ng/dL (0.8-1.8 ng/dL) (SI: 7.72 pmol/L [10.30-23.17 pmol/L])
  Pregnancy test, positive

In addition to referring her to an obstetrician-gynecologist, which of the following should be recommended to treat her hypothyroidism?

A. Levothyroxine, 100 mcg daily
B. Levothyroxine, 50 mcg daily
C. Liothyronine, 25 mcg twice daily
D. Levothyroxine, 75 mcg daily, and liothyronine, 25 mcg daily
E. Desiccated thyroid, 60 mg (1 grain) daily

68 A 56-year-old man with type 2 diabetes mellitus complicated by moderate nonproliferative diabetic retinopathy and recent myocardial infarction (but preserved ejection fraction) seeks help with diabetes management. Diabetes was diagnosed 12 years ago. His current regimen consists of basal insulin, 0.5 unit/kg at 50 units, and metformin, 1000 mg twice daily.

On physical examination, his height is 69 in (175.3 cm) and weight is 243 lb (110.5 kg) (BMI = 36 kg/m²). His blood pressure is 136/84 mm Hg, and pulse rate is 76 beats/min. He appears to be comfortable and in no acute distress. Monofilament testing is 5/5 but vibratory sensation is diminished in the lower extremities below the ankle. Distal pulses are 2+.

Laboratory test results:
    Hemoglobin A_{1c} = 9.1% (4.0%-5.6%) (80 mmol/mol [20-38 mmol/mol])
    Creatinine = 0.9 mg/dL (0.7-1.3 mg/dL) (SI: 79.6 µmol/L [61.9-114.9 µmol/L])
    Serum urea nitrogen = 24 mg/dL (8-23 mg/dL) (SI: 8.6 mmol/L [2.9-8.2 mmol/L])
    Plasma glucose = 278 mg/dL (70-99 mg/dL) (SI: 15.4 mmol/L [3.9-5.5 mmol/L])
    Sodium = 136 mEq/L (136-142 mEq/L) (SI: 136 mmol/L [136-142 mmol/L])

Last month, his primary care physician added semaglutide, 0.25 mg weekly, to his regimen.

Which of the following is the best next step in this patient's management?
    A. Titrate semaglutide to goal dosage every 4 weeks based on nausea symptoms
    B. Continue semaglutide, 0.25 mg weekly, but do not titrate because of retinopathy
    C. Continue semaglutide, 0.25 mg weekly, and add empagliflozin
    D. Stop semaglutide and start pioglitazone
    E. Stop semaglutide and increase basal insulin

69 A 66-year-old man is referred for evaluation of secondary hypogonadism. Over the past few months, he has experienced headaches, tiredness, and 10-lb (4.5-kg) weight loss. He has noticed reduced libido, erectile dysfunction, and reduced appetite. He has no history of polyuria or polydipsia, tingling, or paresthesia. His primary care physician has documented a low serum testosterone concentration and inappropriately normal gonadotropin levels:

    Total testosterone = 50 ng/dL (300-900 ng/dL) (SI: 1.7 nmol/L [10.4-31.2 nmol/L])
    LH = 2.5 mIU/L (1.0-9.0 mIU/mL) (SI: 2.5 IU/L [1.0-9.0 IU/L])
    FSH = 3.2 mIU/mL (1.0-13.0 mIU/mL) (SI: 3.2 IU/L [1.0-13.0 IU/L])

His medical history is remarkable for autoimmune pancreatitis, retroperitoneal fibrosis, and primary hypothyroidism. Findings on recent cardiac evaluation are normal, including those from echocardiography. Chest x-ray is normal. Current medications are levothyroxine, 125 mcg daily; atorvastatin, 10 mg daily; and pancreatic enzymes with meals.

On physical examination, he is a thin man in no acute distress. His blood pressure is 120/65 mm Hg, and pulse rate is 85 beats/min. His height is 64 in (162.6 cm), and weight is 148.5 lb (67.5 kg) (BMI = 26 kg/m²). He has no jaundice or skin hyperpigmentation. His thyroid is diffusely enlarged and firm. Testes are soft and testicular volume is approximately 10 mL bilaterally.

Laboratory test results:
    TSH = 0.3 mIU/L (0.5-5.0 mIU/L)
    Free T_4 = 1.2 ng/dL (0.8-1.8 ng/dL) (SI: 15.4 pmol/L [10.30-23.17 pmol/L])
    Cortisol (8 AM) = 5.2 µg/dL (5-25 µg/dL) (SI: 143.5 nmol/L [137.9-689.7 nmol/L])
    ACTH (8 AM) = 9 pg/mL (10-60 pg/mL) (SI: 2.0 pmol/L [2.2-13.2 pmol/L])

A gadolinium-enhanced pituitary MRI is shown (*see images*).

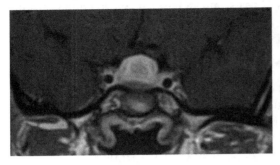
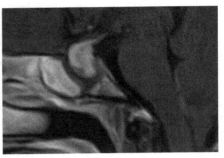

Which of the following is this patient's most likely diagnosis?
- A. Pituitary amyloidosis
- B. Pituitary sarcoidosis
- C. IgG4-related hypophysitis
- D. Granulomatous hypophysitis
- E. Lymphocytic hypophysitis

70

A 65-year-old man presents with erectile dysfunction but preserved libido. He has a 10-year history of type 2 diabetes mellitus, hypertension, and dyslipidemia. He is a former cigarette smoker, with a 30 pack-year history. He had a myocardial infarction 18 months ago, treated with a drug-eluting stent. He has no symptoms suggestive of myocardial ischemia and reports good exercise tolerance. Current medications include metformin, a sulfonylurea, a statin, aspirin, and an angiotensin 2 receptor blocker.

On physical examination, his height is 69 in (175.3 cm) and weight is 210 lb (95.5 kg) (BMI = 31 kg/m^2). His blood pressure is 132/78 mm Hg. There is no evidence of congestive cardiac failure. He has normal body hair, normal penile length, and 20-mL testes bilaterally. Visual fields are full to confrontation, and he has full range of eye movements.

Laboratory test result (sample drawn at 8 AM while fasting):
　Total testosterone = 250 ng/dL (300-900 ng/dL) (SI: 8.7 nmol/L [10.4-31.2 nmol/L])
　　(repeated measurement 1 week later = 234 ng/dL [SI: 8.1 nmol/L])
　LH = 5.0 mIU/mL (1.0-9.0 mIU/mL) (SI: 5.0 IU/L [1.0-9.0 IU/L])
　Thyroid function normal
　Iron studies, normal
　Prolactin, normal

In additional to lifestyle modification, optimization of comorbidities, and psychosexual counseling, which of the following is the best initial management to improve this patient's erectile dysfunction?
- A. Initiate a phosphodiesterase type 5 inhibitor
- B. Initiate testosterone
- C. Initiate a phosphodiesterase type 5 inhibitor plus testosterone
- D. Hold treatment for now and perform pituitary-directed MRI
- E. Advise that medical therapy is contraindicated due to underlying cardiovascular risk

71

A 63-year-old woman with recently diagnosed ectopic ACTH syndrome due to small cell lung cancer has a follow-up appointment. She reports an improvement in her general well-being since commencing medical treatment for hypercortisolism, but she has been troubled in recent days by fatigue, malaise, and nausea. Her current medications are metyrapone, 750 mg 4 times daily; spironolactone, 25 mg twice daily; and metformin, 500 mg twice daily. Her oncologist is planning to begin systemic chemotherapy within the next week.

On physical examination, her height is 68 in (172.7 cm) and weight is 152 lb (68.9 kg) (BMI = 23.1 kg/m²). Her blood pressure is 145/90 mm Hg, and pulse rate is 72 beats/min and regular. She has thin skin with several old bruises on both forearms and bilateral pedal edema.

Laboratory test results:
- Serum sodium = 143 mEq/L (136-142 mEq/L) (SI: 143 mmol/L [136-142 mmol/L])
- Serum potassium = 3.4 mEq/L (3.5-5.0 mEq/L) (SI: 3.4 mmol/L [3.5-5.0 mmol/L])
- Serum creatinine = 0.6 mg/dL (0.7-1.3 mg/dL) (SI: 53.0 µmol/L [61.9-114.9 µmol/L])
- Hemoglobin A_{1c} = 6.8% (4.0%-5.6%) (SI: 51 mmol/mol [20-38 mmol/mol])
- Serum ALT = 125 U/L (10-40 U/L) (SI: 2.09 µkat/L [0.17-0.67 µkat/L])
- Serum alkaline phosphatase = 195 U/L (50-120 U/L) (SI: 3.26 µkat/L [0.84-2.00 µkat/L])
- Serum cortisol (8 AM) = 11.1 µg/dL (5-25 µg/dL) (SI: 306.2 nmol/L [137.9-689.7 nmol/L])
- Plasma ACTH = 132 pg/mL (10-60 pg/mL) (SI: 29.0 pmol/L [2.2-13.2 pmol/L])

CT of the chest, abdomen, and pelvis at presentation documented a 2.3-cm right lung tumor with mediastinal lymphadenopathy, multiple hepatic metastases, and bilateral adrenal enlargement.

Which of the following is the most appropriate immediate next step in management?
A. Add ketoconazole
B. Add mifepristone
C. Increase the metyrapone dosage
D. Start dexamethasone
E. Start octreotide LAR

72

A 35-year-old woman is referred for recommendations regarding management of hypercalcemia. She has a history of hypercalcemia dating back at least 10 years, with reasonably stable albumin-adjusted calcium levels between 10.5 and 11.5 mg/dL (2.6-2.9 mmol/L). She has no history of fractures, nephrolithiasis, or previous head and neck irradiation. She has primary hypothyroidism, and medications include levothyroxine and a multivitamin. She does not take calcium supplements. She has no bone pain, flank pain, hematuria, depression, or anxiety. Available family history is negative for calcium disorders, nephrolithiasis, head and neck surgery, and endocrine tumors.

On physical examination, she appears well. Vital signs are unremarkable. Her height is only 0.5 in (1.3 cm) shorter than her self-reported maximum adult height. She has no thyroid enlargement or palpable nodules, and there is no supraclavicular or precervical adenopathy. Spinal curvature is normal without elicitable vertebral tenderness to palpation.

Laboratory test results:
- Serum calcium = 11.0 mg/dL (8.2-10.2 mg/dL (SI: 2.8 mmol/L [2.1-2.6 mmol/L])
- Serum phosphate = 4.0 mg/dL (2.3-4.7 mg/dL) (SI: 1.3 mmol/L [0.7-1.5 mmol/L])
- Serum magnesium = 2.3 mg/dL (1.5-2.3 mg/dL) (SI: 0.9 mmol/L [0.6-0.9 mmol/L])
- Serum albumin = 4.2 g/dL (3.5-5.0 g/dL) (SI: 42 g/L [35-50 g/L])
- Serum creatinine = 1.0 mg/dL (0.6-1.1 mg/dL) (SI: 88.4 µmol/L [53.0-97.2 µmol/L])
- Serum intact PTH = 85 pg/mL (10-65 pg/mL) (SI: 85 ng/L [10-65 ng/L])
- Serum 25-hydroxyvitamin D = 30 ng/mL (30-80 ng/mL [optimal]) (SI: 74.9 nmol/L [74.9-199.7 nmol/L])
- Serum TSH = 1.2 mIU/L (0.5-5.0 mIU/L)
- Urinary calcium = 150 mg/24 h (100-300 mg/24 h) (SI: 3.8 mmol/d [2.5-7.5 mmol/d])
- Urinary creatinine = 1.2 g/24 h (1.0-2.0 g/24 h) (SI: 10.6 mmol/d [8.8-17.7 mmol/d])
- Urinary volume = 1000 mL/24 h
- Fractional excretion of calcium = 0.015

DXA bone mineral density of the lumbar spine, proximal femur, and proximal one-third radius is within the expected range for age.

Technetium ^{99}Tc parathyroid scintigraphy does not identify a candidate parathyroid lesion, and ultrasonography of the neck is likewise negative for neck masses.

Which of the following is the best next step in the evaluation and management of this patient's hypercalcemic disorder?
- A. Refer to endocrine surgery for consideration of parathyroidectomy
- B. Start zoledronic acid
- C. Order genetic testing for pathogenic variants in the *CASR*, *AP2S1*, and *GNA11* genes
- D. Start cinacalcet
- E. Perform a thiazide challenge (hydrochlorothiazide, 25 mg twice daily for 2 weeks with repeated calcium and PTH measurement)

73

A 43-year-old Black man with a 2-year history of type 2 diabetes mellitus is seen for follow-up. He has had good glycemic control on metformin monotherapy. However, at recent clinic visits, his blood pressure measurements have been slightly elevated. Measurements taken at home are in the range of 135-145/85-95 mm Hg.

In clinic today, his blood pressure is 148/92 mm Hg and pulse rate is 88 beats/min. His height is 72.5 in (185 cm), and weight is 242 lb (110 kg) (BMI = 32 kg/m^2) He appears well. He has no carotid or renal bruits. The rest of the examination findings are normal.

Laboratory test results:
- Hemoglobin A$_{1c}$ = 6.9% (4.0%-5.6%) (52 mmol/mol [20-38 mmol/mol])
- Creatinine = 1.2 mg/dL (0.7-1.3 mg/dL) (SI: 106.1 μmol/L [61.9-114.9 μmol/L])
- Potassium = 4.1 mEq/L (3.5-5.0 mEq/L) (SI: 4.1 mmol/L [3.5-5.0 mmol/L])
- Urine albumin-to-creatinine ratio = 10 mg/g creat (<30 mg/g creat)

He is advised to start regular exercise, make improvements in dietary intake, and decrease salt intake. Despite these interventions, his blood pressure at a 3-month follow-up visit is 144/95 mm Hg.

Which of the following is the most appropriate antihypertensive agent to use as monotherapy in this patient?
- A. Amlodipine
- B. Lisinopril
- C. Hydralazine
- D. Metoprolol
- E. Clonidine

74

A 38-year-old woman presents for follow-up of recently diagnosed thyroid cancer. The patient detected a right-sided thyroid nodule while palpating her own neck. Neck ultrasonography showed a 1.6-cm right thyroid nodule, no nodules in the left lobe, and no abnormal lymph nodes. Ultrasound-guided FNA biopsy of the nodule demonstrated a follicular neoplasm (Bethesda IV cytology). Molecular testing was positive with an abnormal gene expression profile conferring a malignancy risk of approximately 60%.

The patient underwent a right lobectomy and isthmusectomy 4 weeks ago. Final pathology revealed a 2.4-cm minimally invasive follicular thyroid carcinoma. Capsular invasion was present, but there was no extrathyroidal extension or angioinvasion and the surgical margins were negative.

The patient states that she is feeling tired but is otherwise well. She has no family history of thyroid malignancy. She takes no medications. She has a copper intrauterine device for contraception.

On physical examination, her blood pressure is 95/63 mm Hg and pulse rate is 78 beats/min. Her height is 66 in (167.6 cm), and weight is 123 lb (55.8 kg) (BMI = 20 kg/m^2). There is an anterior neck scar. Palpation of her left thyroid lobe demonstrates no nodules. There is no cervical lymphadenopathy. The rest of the examination findings are normal.

Laboratory test results today:
- TSH = 1.9 mIU/L (0.5-5.0 mIU/L)
- Thyroglobulin = 15.9 ng/mL (3-42 ng/mL) (SI: 15.9 μg/L [3-42 μg/L])
- Thyroglobulin antibodies = <4.0 IU/mL (≤4.0 IU/mL) (SI: <4.0 kIU/L [≤4.0 kIU/L])

Which of the following should be recommended now as the most appropriate next step in this patient's management?
- A. No additional testing or treatment
- B. Repeated neck ultrasonography
- C. Completion thyroidectomy
- D. Completion thyroidectomy and radioactive iodine therapy
- E. Initiation of levothyroxine

75 A 45-year-old man is interested in starting a weight-loss medication for medically complicated obesity. In the last 3 years, he has had worsening symptoms of spinal stenosis, which is limiting his mobility. He can ambulate for about 10 minutes before experiencing back and leg pain, and he takes oxycodone as needed. He has gained approximately 20 lb (9.1 kg) in the last year. He has reduced his caloric intake but has difficulty sustaining his efforts because of cravings and hunger. His medical history is notable for hypertension, for which he takes hydrochlorothiazide, hydralazine, and enalapril. His blood pressure is not well controlled on this regimen, and he admits to occasionally missing doses of scheduled medication. He has stage 3 chronic kidney disease, which has been relatively stable for the last 2 years, with an estimated glomerular filtration rate of 45 mL/min per 1.73 m². He smokes cigarettes.

On physical examination, his blood pressure is 156/88 mm Hg. His height is 65 in (166 cm), and weight is 196 lb (89 kg) (BMI = 33 kg/m²). He has truncal obesity. There is mild pitting edema of the lower extremities to the shins. He has preserved muscle strength in the upper and lower extremities.

Laboratory test results:
- Hemoglobin = 12.1 g/dL (13.8-17.2 g/dL) (SI: 121 g/L [138-172 g/L])
- Serum creatinine = 1.9 mg/dL (0.7-1.3 mg/dL) (SI: 168.0 μmol/L [61.9-114.9 μmol/L])
- Fasting glucose = 105 mg/dL (70-99 mg/dL) (SI: 5.8 mmol/L [3.9-5.5 mmol/L])
- LDL cholesterol = 110 mg/dL (<100 mg/dL [optimal]) (SI: 2.85 mmol/L [<2.59 mmol/L])
- HDL cholesterol = 53 mg/dL (>60 mg/dL [optimal]) (SI: 1.37 mmol/L [>1.55 mmol/L])
- Triglycerides = 185 mg/dL (<150 mg/dL [optimal]) (SI: 2.09 mmol/L [<1.70 mmol/L])

Which of the following would be an appropriate weight-loss prescription for this patient?
- A. Extended-release phentermine/topiramate
- B. Phentermine monotherapy
- C. Naltrexone/bupropion
- D. Liraglutide
- E. Metformin

76 A 54-year-old woman with hypertension and metastatic medullary thyroid carcinoma presents for a follow-up visit. She reports excessive fatigue and weakness. She is unable to walk for more than 1 to 2 minutes due to extreme fatigue. Her blood pressure has been difficult to control lately. She currently takes levothyroxine, 125 mcg daily; losartan, 100 mg daily; amlodipine, 10 mg daily; and hydrochlorothiazide, 12.5 mg daily. *RET* genetic testing is negative.

On physical examination, her blood pressure is 176/90 mm Hg and pulse rate is 96 beats/min. Her temperature is 98.6°F (37°C). Her height is 64.5 in (164 cm), and weight is 170 lb (77 kg) (BMI = 29 kg/m²). There is a well-healed scar over her neck. Her heart rate is regular and rapid, and lungs are clear to auscultation. Her abdomen is tender in the right upper quadrant. There is bilateral lower-extremity edema. The rest of the examination findings are normal.

Laboratory test results:
- TSH = 2.1 mIU/L (0.5-5.0 mIU/L)
- Calcitonin = 1020 pg/mL (<8 pg/mL) (SI: 298 pmol/L [<2.34 mmol/L])
- Carcinoembryonic antigen = 7 ng/mL (<2.5 ng/mL) (SI: 7 μg/L [<2.5 μg/L])
- Calcium = 9.0 mg/dL (8.2-10.2 mg/dL) (SI: 2.3 mmol/L [2.1-2.6 mmol/L])
- Sodium = 140 mEq/L (136-142 mEq/L) (SI: 140 mmol/L [136-142 mmol/L])
- Potassium = 2.7 mEq/L (3.5-5.0 mEq/L) (SI: 2.7 mmol/L [3.5-5.0 mmol/L])
- Glucose = 186 mg/dL (70-99 mg/dL) (SI: 10.3 mmol/L [3.9-5.5 mmol/L])
- Creatinine = 1.4 mg/dL (0.6-1.1 mg/dL) (SI: 123.8 μmol/L [53.0-97.2 μmol/L])
- ALT = 210 U/L (10-40 U/L) (SI: 3.51 μkat/L [0.17-0.67 μkat/L])
- AST = 180 U/L (20-48 U/L) (SI: 3.00 μkat/L [0.33-0.80 μkat/L])
- Complete blood cell count, normal

Which of the following is the best next step to determine the etiology of this patient's new symptoms?

A. Perform a dedicated adrenal CT
B. Measure 24-hour urinary free cortisol
C. Perform kidney ultrasonography with Doppler
D. Measure plasma free metanephrines
E. Measure serum aldosterone and renin plasma

77 A 59-year-old man returns for continued management of type 2 diabetes mellitus, which was diagnosed 15 years ago. He was initially treated with oral agents, but he has been receiving insulin therapy for 5 years. His hemoglobin A_{1c} level has ranged from 7.0% to 9.0% (53-75 mmol/mol) over the past few years, and his most recent hemoglobin A_{1c} measurement was 8.4% (68 mmol/mol). He has a history of coronary artery disease and had 2 coronary drug-eluting stents placed 2 years ago for recurrent angina, which has since resolved. He has chronic kidney disease and macroalbuminuria. Peripheral neuropathy is well controlled with pregabalin. He also has hypertension and hyperlipidemia.

Current medications:
- Metformin, 1000 mg twice daily
- Insulin aspart, 20 units before meals (3 times daily)
- Insulin degludec, 40 units at bedtime
- Lisinopril, 20 mg daily
- Aspirin, 81 mg daily
- Clopidogrel, 75 mg daily
- Metoprolol, 25 mg twice daily
- Chlorthalidone, 25 mg once daily
- Rosuvastatin, 20 mg once daily

On physical examination, his blood pressure is 136/82 mm Hg and pulse rate is 74 beats/min. His height is 68 in (172.7 cm), and weight is 225 lb (102.3 kg) (BMI = 34 kg/m²). He has 1+ pitting edema and 2+ dorsalis pedis pulse in the bilateral lower extremities. His lungs are clear to auscultation, and his heart has a regular rate and rhythm with no audible murmur. There is decreased sensation to 10-g monofilament testing on the distal plantar aspect of his feet bilaterally.

Laboratory test results:
- Electrolytes, normal
- Creatinine = 1.5 mg/dL (0.7-1.3 mg/dL) (SI: 132.6 μmol/L [61.9-114.9 μmol/L])
- Estimated glomerular filtration rate = 50 mL/min per 1.73 m² (>60 mL/min per 1.73 m²)
- Hemoglobin A_{1c} = 8.4% (4.0%-5.6%) (68 mmol/mol [20-38 mmol/mol])
- Albumin-to-creatinine ratio = 520 mg/g creat (<30 mg/g creat)

Which of the following medications should be started as the best next step in this patient's treatment?
- A. Exenatide LAR
- B. Aliskiren
- C. Pioglitazone
- D. Canagliflozin
- E. Losartan

78

A 52-year-old woman is seen in the pituitary clinic 3 months after undergoing transsphenoidal surgery for acromegaly. At diagnosis, her IGF-1 concentration was 3.5 times the upper normal limit. She did not receive medical therapy before surgery. Her previous headaches have resolved, and she no longer has sweating episodes or greasy skin. However, she is still troubled by arthralgia affecting both hips and knees. Her current medications are atorvastatin, 20 mg daily; ramipril, 10 mg daily; and naproxen, 250 mg twice daily. She has diet-controlled type 2 diabetes.

On physical examination, her height is 70 in (177.8 cm) and weight is 192 lb (87.3 kg) (BMI = 27.5 kg/m^2). Her blood pressure is 130/75 mm Hg, and resting pulse rate is 68 beats/min and regular. Visual acuity is 20/20 (6/6) in both eyes, and her visual fields are normal. She has mild residual clinical features of acromegaly.

Laboratory test results:
- Prolactin = 32.2 ng/mL (4-30 ng/mL) (SI: 1.40 nmol/L [0.17-1.30 nmol/L])
- TSH = 2.1 mIU/L (0.5-5.0 mIU/L)
- Free T$_4$ = 1.3 ng/dL (0.8-1.8 ng/dL) (SI: 16.73 pmol/L [10.30-23.17 pmol/L])
- Cortisol (8 AM) = 17.5 µg/dL (5-25 µg/dL) (SI: 482.8 nmol/L [137.9-689.7 nmol/L])
- GH (fasting) = 0.35 ng/mL (0.01-3.61 ng/mL) (SI: 0.35 µg/L [0.01-3.61 µg/L])
- IGF-1 = 327 ng/mL (84-233 ng/mL) (SI: 42.8 nmol/L [11.0-30.5 nmol/L])
- FSH = 39.5 mIU/mL (>30.0 mIU/mL) (SI: 39.5 IU/L [>30.0 IU/L])
- LH = 25.6 mIU/mL (>30.0 mIU/mL) (SI: 25.6 IU/L [>30.0 IU/L])
- Hemoglobin A$_{1c}$ = 6.1% (4.0%-5.6%) (SI: 43 mmol/mol [20-38 mmol/mol])

MRI of the sella is shown (*see images*).

Presurgery
T1 coronal (postcontrast)
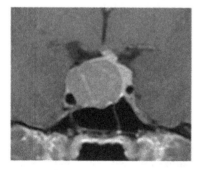

Postsurgery
T1 coronal (postcontrast)
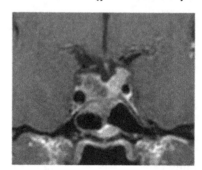

Which of the following is the most appropriate next step in this patient's management?
- A. Observation
- B. Referral for pituitary radiotherapy
- C. Repeated transsphenoidal surgery
- D. Initiation of cabergoline
- E. Initiation of depot somatostatin receptor ligand therapy

79 A 25-year-old woman with a 10-year history of type 1 diabetes mellitus complicated by severe nonproliferative retinopathy and microalbuminuria presents for outpatient follow-up. Her weight is 138 lb (62.7 kg). Kidney function is normal. Her current hemoglobin A_{1c} value is 7.5% (58 mmol/mol). In the past month, she has had 3 blood glucose measurements less than 50 mg/dL (<2.8 mmol/L) around 2 AM. She previously had been without insurance and was using NPH insulin, 12 units in the morning and 8 units with dinner; regular insulin, 6 units with meals; and a correctional dose of 1 unit for every 50 mg/dL (2.8 mmol/L) greater than 150 mg/dL (>8.3 mmol/L) at meals. She takes no correction insulin at bedtime.

She has new insurance and states that her preferred basal insulin is detemir (rDNA origin) and her preferred short-acting insulin is lispro.

Results of 3 days of 7-point glucose monitoring are shown.

Glucose	Fasting glucose	2 hours after breakfast	Prelunch	2 hours after lunch	Predinner	Bedtime
Day 1	88 mg/dL (SI: 4.9 mmol/L)	190 mg/dL (SI: 10.5 mmol/L)	81 mg/dL (SI: 4.5 mmol/L)	213 mg/dL (SI: 11.8 mmol/L)	131 mg/dL (SI: 7.3 mmol/L)	122 mg/dL (SI: 6.8 mmol/L)
Day 2	202 mg/dL (SI: 11.2 mmol/L)	170 mg/dL (SI: 9.4 mmol/L)	77 mg/dL (SI: 4.3 mmol/L)	183 mg/dL (SI: 10.2 mmol/L)	90 mg/dL (SI: 5.0 mmol/L)	188 mg/dL (SI: 10.4 mmol/L)
Day 3	93 mg/dL (SI: 5.2 mmol/L)	210 mg/dL (SI: 11.7 mmol/L)	111 mg/dL (SI: 6.2 mmol/L)	150 mg/dL (SI: 8.3 mmol/L)	78 mg/dL (SI: 4.3 mmol/L)	176 mg/dL (SI: 9.8 mmol/L)

The best recommendation for this patient regarding insulin detemir is to convert the dosing to which of the following?

A. 10 units in the morning and 10 units at bedtime
B. 16 units in the morning
C. 7 units at bedtime
D. 20 units at bedtime
E. 7 units in the morning and 7 units at bedtime

80 A 25-year-old woman presents for evaluation and management of a left-sided thyroid nodule. She presented to her local emergency department 6 weeks ago with abdominal pain and vomiting and was found to have pyelonephritis. Abdominal CT at that time demonstrated incidental pulmonary nodules, and subsequent chest CT confirmed the presence of multiple small (<1 cm) nodules in the lower lung fields bilaterally and a left thyroid mass.

Neck ultrasonography was performed to evaluate the thyroid mass and this showed a 2.9 × 2.3 × 3.0-cm mixed cystic and solid nodule in the left thyroid lobe with a hypoechoic solid component containing microcalcifications, as well as multiple enlarged lymph nodes with cystic changes and peripheral blood flow in the left central and lateral neck (neck zones 3, 4, and 6). Ultrasound-guided FNA biopsy of the left thyroid nodule demonstrated findings suspicious for a follicular neoplasm (SFN; Bethesda IV), while FNA of a left supraclavicular lymph node was nondiagnostic (no lymph node elements).

The patient presents today to discuss the next management steps. She reports no current symptoms. There is no personal history of head and neck radiation exposure, but she states that her paternal uncle had thyroid cancer. She takes no medications.

On physical examination, her blood pressure is 136/71 mm Hg and pulse rate is 90 beats/min. Her height is 65 in (165.1 cm), and weight is 169 lb (76.7 kg) (BMI = 28 kg/m^2). Palpation of her thyroid gland reveals a 3-cm firm nodule in the left lobe. There is no palpable cervical lymphadenopathy. The rest of the examination findings, including those from heart, lung, and abdominal examinations, are normal.

Her TSH concentration is 1.0 mIU/L (0.5-5.0 mIU/L).

The characteristic appearance of one of her lymph nodes is shown (*see images*).

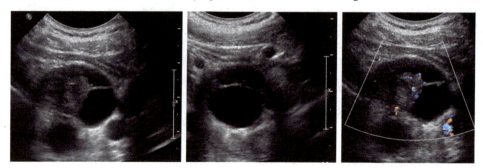

Which of the following is the most appropriate next step in this patient's management?
A. Refer for diagnostic left lobectomy
B. Refer for total thyroidectomy
C. Repeat ultrasound-guided FNA of the left thyroid nodule for cytology
D. Repeat ultrasound-guided FNA of a left lateral lymph node for cytology with thyroglobulin washout
E. Perform rhTSH-stimulated radioactive iodine (^{123}I) whole-body scanning

81 A 60-year-old woman presents for evaluation of new symptoms of anxiety, hypertension, and tremulousness. Multiple family members have had paragangliomas, including metastatic paraganglioma. Previous evaluation revealed that several family members, including the patient, have an inherited pathogenic variant in the *SDHB* gene. The patient has been followed with whole-body MRI and plasma metanephrine measurement every 2 years and has not had any known tumors or abnormal metanephrine results. Her last evaluation was 6 months ago.

Today, she describes new symptoms that started 6 weeks ago. These include unexplained headaches and palpitations. She occasionally measures her blood pressure during these symptomatic episodes and notes it to be 160-180/90-100 mm Hg. When she is asymptomatic, her blood pressure is usually 130-140/90 mm Hg. The symptoms start without provocation and resolve spontaneously within a few minutes to hours. She has had new work-related stress, as well as increased family tension in the last 2 months, but she is not sure whether these factors are contributing to her symptoms.

Measurements of plasma metanephrines and 24-hour urinary metanephrines are normal.

Which of the following is the most likely contributor to this patient's symptoms?
A. Anxiety unrelated to a functional pheochromocytoma or paraganglioma
B. Epinephrine-producing pheochromocytoma
C. Norepinephrine-producing pheochromocytoma
D. Norepinephrine-producing paraganglioma
E. Nonfunctional paraganglioma

82 A 62-year-old woman seeks consultation for diabetes mellitus that was diagnosed 2 weeks ago based on a random blood glucose value of 250 mg/dL (13.9 mmol/L) that was included as part of routine laboratory testing.

Her medical history is notable for Lynch syndrome with rectosigmoid malignancy, concurrent cervical and endometrial cancer, and gastric adenocarcinoma with signet ring features. She has had multiple surgeries, including hysterectomy, gastrectomy, and colectomy. There is a history of metastases to the right-sided posterior thoracic rib and right paravertebral region for which she has received radiation therapy and chemotherapy.

Medications are notable for pembrolizumab, which was initiated 6 months ago for rising levels of carcinoembryonic antigen. Insulin lispro was prescribed on a correctional scale of 1 unit per 30 mg/dL.

In retrospect, she endorses polyuria and polydipsia for the last 10 to 14 days. For many years, she notes that she has often felt thirsty, and she has always attributed this to her gastrointestinal issues. Her weight has declined from 117 lb (53.2 kg) to 108 lb (49.1 kg), but her weight often fluctuates in this range. Her son has type 1 diabetes mellitus.

Physical examination findings are unremarkable.

Laboratory test results:
Basic metabolic panel, normal except for a glucose value of 220 mg/dL (SI: 12.2 mmol/L)
Hemoglobin A_{1c} = 7.4% (4.0%-5.6%) (57 mmol/mol [20-38 mmol/mol])
Glutamic acid decarboxylase 65 antibodies = ≤0.02 nmol/L (≤0.02 nmol/L)
Islet-cell antibodies = ≤0.02 nmol/L (≤0.02 nmol/L)
Insulinoma-associated 2 antibodies = ≤0.02 nmol/L (≤0.02 nmol/L)
Zinc transporter 8 antibodies = <15 U/L (<15 U/L)
Lipase = 356 U/L (0-160 U/L) (SI: 5.95 μkat/L [0.17-1.22 μkat/L])

Which of the following should be prescribed as the best next step in this patient's treatment?
A. Metformin
B. Basal insulin
C. Sulfonylurea
D. SGLT-2 inhibitor
E. GLP-1 receptor agonist

83 A 56-year-old man with a history of gastric bypass surgery is referred for evaluation of recurrent nephrolithiasis. He has had multiple episodes of calcium oxalate kidney stones over the past 5 years, some of which required lithotripsy. He has very good dietary calcium intake (~900 mg daily). Osteoporosis was diagnosed based on a screening bone density test done 6 months ago (lowest T-score of –3.0 at the left femoral neck [Z-score –2.4]). Due to malabsorption, he has been maintained on calcium citrate supplementation, 3000 mg (600 mg elemental) 4 times daily; ergocalciferol, 50,000 units daily; and calcitriol, 0.25 mcg daily. He has no history of fragility fractures.

On physical examination, he has an intact gait and no spine tenderness to palpation.

Laboratory test results:
Serum calcium = 9.6 mg/dL (8.2-10.2 mg/dL) (SI: 2.4 mmol/L [2.1-2.6 mmol/L])
Serum phosphate = 4.0 mg/dL (2.3-4.7 mg/dL) (SI: 1.3 mmol/L [0.7-1.5 mmol/L])
Serum creatinine = 0.9 mg/dL (0.7-1.3 mg/dL) (SI: 79.6 μmol/L [61.9-114.9 μmol/L])
Serum intact PTH = 70 pg/mL (10-65 pg/mL) (SI: 70 ng/L [10-65 ng/L])
Serum 25-hydroxyvitamin D = 56 ng/mL (30-80 ng/mL [optimal]) (SI: 139.8 nmol/L [74.9-199.7 nmol/L])
Serum 1,25-dihydroxyvitamin D = 50 pg/mL (16-65 pg/mL) (SI: 130 pmol/L [41.6-169.0 pmol/L])
Serum albumin = 3.7 g/dL (3.5-5.0 g/dL) (SI: 37 g/L [35-50 g/L])
Urinary calcium = 40 mg/24 h (100-300 mg/24 h) (SI: 1.0 mmol/d [2.5-7.5 mmol/d])
Urinary sodium = 190 mEq/24 h (40-217 mEq/24 h) (SI: 190 mmol/d [40-217 mmol/d])
Urinary oxalate = 140 mg/24 h (<40 mg/24 h) (SI: 1596 mmol/d [<456 mmol/d])
Urinary uric acid = 600 mg/24 h (<800 mg/24 h) (SI: 3.5 mmol/d [<4.7 mmol/d])
Urinary citrate = 300 mg/24 h (320-1240 mg/24 h) (SI: 15.6 mmol/d [16.7-64.5 mmol/d])
Urinary creatinine = 1.8 g/24 h (1.0-2.0 g/24 h) (SI: 15.9 mmol/d [8.8-17.7 mmol/d])
Urine total volume = 2200 mL/24 h

Which of the following should be recommended now to decrease this patient's future risk of developing kidney stones?
A. Discontinue calcitriol
B. Discontinue calcium supplementation
C. Decrease ergocalciferol to weekly dosing
D. Decrease dietary oxalate intake
E. Increase orange juice intake

84

A 25-year-old woman is referred by reproductive endocrinology for secondary amenorrhea, infertility, and a significantly elevated total testosterone concentration (>200 ng/dL [>6.9 nmol/L]). DHEA-S levels as high as 800 μg/dL (21.7 μmol/L) have also been documented. Thelarche was at age 14 years, but she still did not have spontaneous menstrual cycles by age 15 years. Therefore, oral contraceptives were initiated at that time. On birth control pills, the patient had regular menstrual cycles for approximately 1 year. She discontinued birth control pills a year ago but never had a spontaneous period. At age 15 years, she noted terminal hair growth on her face. This has slowly worsened over the years and is also present on her arms and legs. She has had laser treatment to remove hair from her face and neck but not from her body.

On physical examination, her height is 62.2 in (158.0 cm) and weight is 151 lb (68.5 kg) (BMI = 27.4 kg/m^2). Her blood pressure is 114/63 mm Hg. There is evidence of significant terminal hair growth over her arms and upper abdomen, but in other areas it has been mechanically removed. In the areas where hair has not been removed, the Ferriman-Gallwey score is 4. Taking into account her description of treated areas, the Ferriman-Gallwey score exceeds 12. Examination of external genitalia reveals a slightly enlarged clitoris.

Laboratory test results:
    TSH = 1.9 mIU/L (0.5-5.0 mIU/L)
    Total testosterone = 190 ng/dL (8-60 ng/dL) (SI: 6.6 nmol/L [0.3-2.1 nmol/L])
    Prolactin = 8.2 ng/mL (4-30 ng/mL) (SI: 0.36 nmol/L [0.17-1.30 nmol/L])
    FSH = 2.4 mIU/mL (1.0-9.0 mIU/mL [luteal]) (SI: 2.4 IU/L [1.0-9.0 IU/L])
    DHEA-S = 447 μg/dL (44-332 μg/dL) (SI: 12.11 μmol/L [1.19-9.00 μmol/L])
    Androstenedione = 601 ng/dL (30-200 ng/dL) (SI: 21.0 nmol/L [1.05-6.98 nmol/L])
    Antimullerian hormone = 13 ng/mL (0.9-9.5 ng/mL) (SI: 92.9 pmol/L [6.4-67.9 pmol/L])
    17-Hydroxyprogesterone = 268 ng/dL (SI: 8.1 nmol/L)

Dexamethasone is prescribed, 0.5 mg every 6 hours for 2 days, and laboratory tests are then repeated:
    Total testosterone = 206 ng/dL (8-60 ng/dL) (SI: 7.1 nmol/L [0.3-2.1 nmol/L])
    DHEA-S = 106 μg/dL (44-332 μg/dL) (SI: 2.87 μmol/L [1.19-9.00 μmol/L])
    Androstenedione = 352 ng/dL (30-200 ng/dL) (SI: 12.3 nmol/L
        [1.05-6.98 nmol/L])

Pelvic ultrasonography reveals more than 25 follicles (2-9 mm) in the left ovary (31 cc) and more than 25 follicles (2-9 mm) in the right ovary (27 cc).

Subsequent pelvic MRI (*see image*) reveals numerous (>25) subcentimeter follicles in each ovary consistent with polycystic ovary morphology. The right ovary measures 3.0 × 2.5 × 5.3 cm (16.6 cc), and the left ovary measures 3.1 × 2.7 × 4.2 cm (14.7 cc). No ovarian tumors are seen.

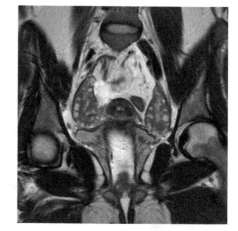

Results from ovarian/adrenal venous sampling.

Measurement	Right ovarian vein	Left ovarian vein	Right adrenal	Left adrenal	Inferior vena cava
Total testosterone	6180 ng/dL (SI: 214.4 nmol/L)	8750 ng/dL (SI: 303.6 nmol/L)	253 ng/dL (SI: 8.8 nmol/L)	224 ng/dL (SI: 7.8 nmol/L)	271 ng/dL (SI: 9.4 nmol/L)
Androstenedione	33,100 μg/dL (SI: 1155.2 μmol/L)	38,700 μg/dL (SI: 1350.6 μmol/L)	1622 μg/dL (SI: 56.6 μmol/L)	1570 μg/dL (SI: 54.8 μmol/L)	498 μg/dL (SI: 17.4 μmol/L)

The right ovarian vein-to-inferior vena cava ratio is 22.8, and the left ovarian vein-to-inferior vena cava ratio is 32.3.

Which of the following is the best next step in this patient's management to help her conceive?
A. Combined oral contraceptives
B. Left oophorectomy
C. Ovarian drilling
D. Letrozole
E. Dexamethasone

85

A 46-year-old woman presents for a general examination. She is particularly concerned about her risk of developing type 2 diabetes mellitus and wishes to be screened. She developed gestational diabetes with her last pregnancy 10 years ago, which was managed with diet alone. Her father and paternal aunt have type 2 diabetes.

She is otherwise in good health and takes no medications on a regular basis. She uses a rescue inhaler intermittently for exercise-induced asthma. She does not smoke cigarettes. She runs for 20 minutes 5 days a week.

On physical examination, her height is 61 in (155 cm) and weight is 128 lb (58 kg) (BMI = 24 kg/m^2). There is no thyroid enlargement. She has no stigmata of hypercortisolism.

Laboratory test results:
  Fasting glucose = 99 mg/dL (70-99 mg/dL) (SI: 5.5 mmol/L [3.9-5.5 mmol/L])
  Hemoglobin A$_{1c}$ = 5.3% (4.0%-5.6%) (34 mmol/mol [20-38 mmol/mol])

In addition to maintaining a healthy body weight, which of the following strategies would be most appropriate to reduce this patient's risk of developing type 2 diabetes?
A. Limiting carbohydrate intake to less than 30 g daily
B. Following a healthy dietary pattern (emphasizing high-quality foods primarily derived from plant sources)
C. Prescribing acarbose
D. Following an intermittent fasting program 2 days a week (<500 kcal daily) with ad libitum intake the other 5 days a week
E. Increasing physical activity to ensure at least 20 minutes of moderate-intensity activity daily

86

A 56-year-old man with Graves disease and hypertension presents to the emergency department with shortness of breath and tachycardia. Community-acquired pneumonia was recently diagnosed. While waiting for initial laboratory results, his condition deteriorates. He becomes lethargic and requires intubation. Electrocardiography shows atrial fibrillation with a heart rate of 160 beats/min. Chest x-ray shows right lower-lobe pneumonia.

Initial laboratory test results:
  TSH = <0.01 mIU/L (0.5-5.0 mIU/L)
  Free T$_4$ = 6.2 ng/dL (0.8-1.8 ng/dL) (SI: 79.8 pmol/L [10.30-23.17 pmol/L])
  Free T$_3$ = 8.4 pg/mL (2.3-4.2 pg/mL) (SI: 12.9 pmol/L [3.53-6.45 pmol/L])
  Sodium = 142 mEq/L (136-142 mEq/L) (SI: 142 mmol/L [136-142 mmol/L])
  Potassium = 5.6 mEq/L (3.5-5.0 mEq/L) (SI: 5.6 mmol/L [3.5-5.0 mmol/L])
  Glucose = 102 mg/dL (70-99 mg/dL) (SI: 5.7 mmol/L [3.9-5.5 mmol/L])
  Calcium = 10.1 mg/dL (8.2-10.2 mg/dL) (SI: 2.53 mmol/L [2.1-2.6 mmol/L])
  Creatinine = 2.9 mg/dL (0.7-1.3 mg/dL) (SI: 256.4 µmol/L [61.9-114.9 µmol/L])
  ALT = 78 U/L (10-40 U/L) (SI: 1.30 µkat/L [0.17-0.67 µkat/L])
  AST = 80 U/L (20-48 U/L) (SI: 1.34 µkat/L [0.33-0.80 µkat/L])

On physical examination, his blood pressure is 90/60 mm Hg, pulse rate is 158 beats/min, and temperature is 101°F (38.3°C). His height is 67 in (170 cm), and weight is 164 lb (74.5 kg) (BMI = 26 kg/m^2). He is sedated and intubated. There is bilateral proptosis. His thyroid gland is approximately 60 g, and there is a bruit over his thyroid. His heart has an irregularly irregular rate and rhythm. Lungs are clear to auscultation bilaterally except for rales in the right lower lobe. The abdomen is soft to palpation. There is 1+ lower-extremity edema.

The endocrinology team is consulted in the intensive care unit, and thyroid storm is diagnosed. The patient is immediately started on propylthiouracil, 200 mg every 4 hours; propranolol, 80 mg every 4 hours; and hydrocortisone, 100 mg intravenously every 8 hours. He is also started on ceftriaxone intravenously. Several hours later, SSKI, 5 drops 3 times daily, is also initiated. On day 2, repeated thyroid function tests yield the same results and his clinical status remains critical. Cholestyramine, 4 g twice daily, is added to his regimen. On day 3, free thyroid hormones remain elevated with slight improvement in free T_3, and his hepatic function test values remain elevated as on admission. His renal function worsens without the need for dialysis. The cholestyramine dosage is increased to 4 g 3 times daily.

In addition to intensive care, which of the following is the best next step in the management of this patient's thyroid storm?
- A. Start lithium
- B. Perform plasma exchange
- C. Change propylthiouracil to methimazole
- D. Perform thyroidectomy
- E. Increase the propranolol dosage

87

A 30-year-old woman with type 2 diabetes mellitus requests a refill of her sulfonylurea prescription. Diabetes was diagnosed at age 13 years when workup for polyuria documented fasting blood glucose values of 140 to 160 mg/dL (7.9-8.9 mmol/L). At the time, she was overweight and recalls being treated with metformin and then with glyburide for about 10 years. Gliclazide was also prescribed at one point. Four weeks ago, she decided to stop all medications because of occasional episodes of hypoglycemia. She began monitoring her blood glucose and has documented fasting values ranging from 91 to 140 mg/dL (5.1-7.8 mmol/L) and postprandial values ranging from 140 to 200 mg/dL (7.8-11.1 mmol/L). Values as high as 253 mg/dL (14.0 mmol/L) occur on rare occasions.

Her family history is notable for her mother being diagnosed with diabetes mellitus in her 20s (she now takes multiple oral medications). Her father was diagnosed with diabetes mellitus in his 60s. Her brother does not have diabetes.

On physical examination, her blood pressure is 114/61 mm Hg and pulse rate is 81 beats/min. Her height is 63 in (160 cm), weight is 132 lb (60 kg) (BMI = 23.4 kg/m^2). She has no acanthosis nigricans or any other notable findings.

Laboratory test results:
   Hemoglobin A_{1c} = 7.0% (4.0%-5.6%) (53 mmol/mol [20-38 mmol/mol])
   Fasting glucose = 167 mg/dL (70-99 mg/dL) (SI: 9.3 mmol/L [3.9-5.5 mmol/L])
   Concurrent C-peptide = 1.03 ng/mL (0.5-2.0 ng/mL) (SI: 0.34 nmol/L [0.17-0.66 nmol/L])

She expresses frustration about her current glucose levels.

In addition to emphasizing appropriate lifestyle interventions, which of the following is the best recommendation for this patient?
- A. Acarbose
- B. GLP-1 receptor agonist
- C. Metformin
- D. Sulfonylurea
- E. Basal insulin

88

A 62-year-old man with stage 3 chronic kidney disease is admitted to the hospital for parathyroidectomy. Hypercalcemia and osteoporosis were diagnosed due to severe primary hyperparathyroidism 6 months before the current admission. He underwent a 3-gland parathyroidectomy 5 days ago, complicated by postoperative hypocalcemia. He reports paresthesias in his extremities, as well as muscle cramping. Despite treatment with intravenous and oral calcium and vitamin D supplements, he remains hypocalcemic. He is currently receiving calcium citrate, 3000 mg (600 mg elemental) by mouth 4 times daily, and cholecalciferol, 2000 IU daily. He also takes a proton-pump inhibitor.

The Chvostek sign is elicited on physical examination.

Laboratory test results:
- Serum calcium = 6.5 mg/dL (8.2-10.2 mg/dL) (SI: 1.6 mmol/L [2.1-2.6 mmol/L])
- Serum phosphate = 2.2 mg/dL (2.3-4.7 mg/dL) (SI: 0.7 mmol/L [0.7-1.5 mmol/L])
- Serum creatinine = 1.4 mg/dL (0.7-1.3 mg/dL) (SI: 123.8 μmol/L [61.9-114.9 μmol/L])
- Glomerular filtration rate (estimated) = 52 mL/min per 1.73 m^2 (>60 mL/min per 1.73 m^2)
- Serum intact PTH = 50 pg/mL (10-65 pg/mL) (SI: 50 ng/L [10-65 ng/L])
- Serum 25-hydroxyvitamin D = 30 ng/mL (30-80 ng/mL [optimal]) (SI: 74.9 nmol/L [74.9-199.7 nmol/L])
- Serum albumin = 4.0 g/dL (3.5-5.0 g/dL) (SI: 40 g/L [35-50 g/L])
- Serum magnesium = 1.4 mg/dL (1.5-2.3 mg/dL) (SI: 0.6 mmol/L [0.6-0.9 mmol/L])

In addition to repleting his magnesium, which of the following is the most appropriate next step in the management of this patient's hypocalcemia?
- A. Increase oral elemental calcium intake to 900 mg 4 times daily
- B. Increase oral cholecalciferol intake to 4000 IU daily
- C. Start intravenous phosphate therapy
- D. Start oral calcitriol therapy
- E. Start rhPTH (1-84) subcutaneous injections once daily

89

A 27-year-old woman is referred for evaluation of hyperprolactinemia, which was diagnosed during the workup of galactorrhea and oligomenorrhea. She would like to conceive. Her prolactin concentration was found to be elevated at 104 ng/mL (4.5 nmol/L). A repeated measurement documents a similar value (97 ng/mL [4.2 nmol/L], 90% monomeric). Brain MRI shows a left-sided microadenoma (*see image, white arrow*).

Cabergoline is initiated at a dosage of 0.5 mg twice weekly. After 1 month, her prolactin concentration decreases to 25 ng/mL (1.1 nmol/L). Cabergoline is continued at the same dosage. Four months later, she calls the office because she has just learned that she is pregnant after missing her period last week.

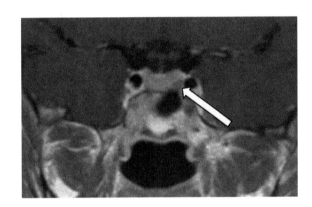

Which of the following is the best next step in this patient's management?
- A. Continue the current cabergoline dosage
- B. Reduce the cabergoline dosage to 0.25 mg twice weekly
- C. Stop cabergoline
- D. Stop cabergoline and obtain periodic visual field testing during pregnancy
- E. Switch cabergoline to bromocriptine

90

A 64-year-old man presents with low libido, fatigue, and muscle weakness that has gradually worsened over the last few years. At his request, his primary care physician measured serum testosterone, drawn in the morning in the fasted state, and the value was 144 ng/dL (300-900 ng/dL) (SI: 5.0 nmol/L [10.4-31.2 nmol/L]). He reports a history of mumps as a teenager and recalls a painful left testis at that time. He is otherwise healthy and takes no regular medications. He has no lower urinary tract symptoms. There is no family history of prostate cancer.

On physical examination, his height is 70 in (177.8 cm) and weight is 190 lb (86.4 kg) (BMI = 27 kg/m^2). He has reduced body hair, mild muscle wasting, and mild palpable gynecomastia bilaterally. On rectal examination, there is no palpable prostate irregularity. His left testis is 5 mL, and his right testis is 15 mL.

Initial laboratory test results (sample drawn at 8 AM while fasting):
    Repeated total testosterone = 164 ng/dL (300-900 ng/dL) (SI: 5.7 nmol/L [10.4-31.2 nmol/L])
    LH = 25.0 mIU/mL (1.0-9.0 mIU/mL) (SI: 25.0 IU/L [1.0-9.0 IU/L])
    FSH = 28.0 mIU/mL (1.0-13.0 mIU/mL) (SI: 28.0 IU/L [1.0-13.0 IU/L])

Testosterone replacement therapy is recommended. He elects to do PSA monitoring. His baseline PSA concentration before commencing testosterone replacement is 0.8 ng/mL (<5.3 ng/mL) (SI: 0.8 µg/L [<5.3 µg/L]). He starts topical testosterone replacement at the standard replacement dosage with marked clinical improvement. Six months later, he continues to feel well.

Current laboratory test results (sample drawn at 8 AM while fasting):
    Serum testosterone = 432 ng/dL (300-900 ng/dL) (SI: 15.0 nmol/L [10.4-31.2 nmol/L])
    LH = 7.0 mIU/mL (1.0-9.0 mIU/mL) (SI: 7.0 IU/L [1.0-9.0 IU/L])
    PSA = 1.8 ng/mL (<5.3 ng/mL) (SI: 1.8 µg/L [<5.3 µg/L]) (repeated 3 weeks later = 1.9 ng/mL [SI: 1.9 µg/L])

He reports no new lower urinary tract symptoms, and findings on rectal examination are unchanged.

Which of the following is the best next step in this patient's management?
    A. Refer to a urologist for prostate biopsy
    B. Stop testosterone replacement therapy and measure PSA in 3 months
    C. Reduce current testosterone dosage by 50% and measure PSA in 3 months
    D. Perform prostate ultrasonography
    E. Continue testosterone treatment and measure PSA in 3 months

91

A 63-year-old woman with hypertension, mixed hyperlipidemia, rheumatoid arthritis, and fibromyalgia returns for follow-up. She was initially referred because of statin intolerance. She had tried lovastatin, simvastatin, and atorvastatin and developed severe myalgias with each medication. At her initial visit (when she was off statins), her 10-year atherosclerotic cardiovascular disease risk was calculated to be 16%. Given her risk, it was recommended that she try rosuvastatin. She developed myalgias despite different dosages and administration frequencies. Three months ago, her regimen was switched to pravastatin, 40 mg at bedtime, and she reports no adverse effects.

The patient has been limiting her fat intake; however, she has been having difficulty limiting her carbohydrate intake. For exercise, she walks 30 minutes 4 to 5 days a week. Despite trying to quit cigarette smoking, she still smokes one-half pack daily. She has a family history of premature heart disease.

On physical examination, her blood pressure is 107/69 mm Hg and pulse rate is 80 beats/min. Her height is 64 in (162.5 cm), and weight is 139 lb (63.2 kg) (BMI = 24 kg/m^2). She is alert, oriented, and in no distress. Her lungs are clear to auscultation bilaterally, and heart sounds are regular in rate and rhythm. She has swelling and decreased range of motion of all her fingers. Findings on abdominal examination are unremarkable.

Laboratory test results:
    Total cholesterol = 240 mg/dL (<200 mg/dL [optimal]) (SI: 6.22 mmol/L [<5.18 mmol/L])
    Triglycerides = 320 mg/dL (<150 mg/dL [optimal]) (SI: 3.62 mmol/L [<1.70 mmol/L])
    HDL cholesterol = 45 mg/dL (>60 mg/dL [optimal]) (SI: 1.17 mmol/L [>1.55 mmol/L])
    LDL cholesterol = 131 mg/dL (<100 mg/dL [optimal]) (SI: 3.39 mmol/L [<2.59 mmol/L])

Which of the following medications should be added next to the patient's cholesterol-lowering regimen?
    A. Evolocumab
    B. Bempedoic acid
    C. Colestipol
    D. Icosapent ethyl
    E. Ezetimibe

92

A 31-year-old pregnant woman (G1P0) with a history of asthma presents for evaluation and management of a thyroid nodule. She is currently 10 weeks' gestation. At an appointment with her obstetrician at 8 weeks' gestation, a right-sided thyroid nodule was detected on clinical neck examination. The patient's pregnancy has otherwise been uncomplicated. She plans to breastfeed after delivery.

Over the past month, she has been experiencing intermittent headaches relieved with acetaminophen and daily nausea without vomiting. She reports no history of head or neck radiation and no family history of thyroid malignancy.

On physical examination, her blood pressure is 115/73 mm Hg and pulse rate is 78 beats/min. Her height is 62 in (157.5 cm), and weight is 135 lb (61.4 kg) (BMI = 25 kg/m²). Thyroid examination is notable for a 3-cm firm right thyroid mass that is well-circumscribed and mobile. There is no palpable cervical lymphadenopathy. The rest of the examination findings are normal.

Laboratory test results:
TSH = 0.091 mIU/L (0.5-5.0 mIU/L)
Free T_4 = 1.39 ng/dL (0.8-1.8 ng/dL) (SI: 17.9 pmol/L [10.30-23.17 pmol/L])

Neck ultrasonography demonstrates a 3.5 × 1.8 × 2.4-cm hypoechoic nodule in the right thyroid lobe with irregular margins. There are abnormal-appearing lymph nodes in the right lateral neck.

Ultrasonography images are shown.

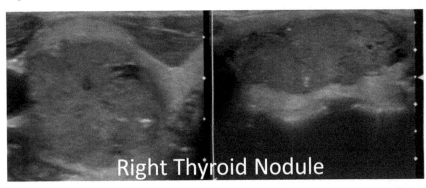

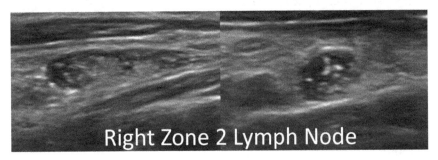

The patient undergoes ultrasound-guided FNA biopsy of the right thyroid nodule and a right zone 2 lymph node, both of which demonstrate findings consistent with papillary thyroid carcinoma.

Which of the following is the most appropriate management to recommend next?
A. Order neck and chest MRI
B. Prescribe levothyroxine
C. Proceed with surgery now
D. Proceed with surgery during the second trimester of pregnancy
E. Proceed with surgery and radioactive iodine therapy 4 weeks after delivery

93 A 21-year-old man with type 1 diabetes mellitus is seen for preoperative evaluation. He has no known diabetes-related complications, and a recent creatinine measurement was normal. Surgery is scheduled to correct a deviated septum. The procedure will be performed under general anesthesia and is likely to last about 1.5 hours. He uses an insulin pump and a continuous glucose monitor (nonhybrid closed loop). His total basal insulin dose is 20 units daily, with an insulin-to-carbohydrate ratio of 1:10, a sensitivity factor of 40 mg/dL (2.2 mmol/L), and a target glucose value of 120 mg/dL (6.7 mmol/L).

Review of the sensor data shows infrequent nocturnal hypoglycemia about once a month. A hemoglobin A_{1c} measurement 4 weeks ago was 6.6% (49 mmol/mol). He would like assistance in adjusting insulin therapy preoperatively.

Which of the following would be the most reasonable approach to insulin delivery perioperatively?
- A. Continue pump use throughout the procedure
- B. Continue pump use, but start a temporary basal rate at 75% of the usual rate the morning of the procedure
- C. Discontinue pump use the morning of the procedure and inject insulin glargine, 10 units; use correction dosing 1:40 as needed
- D. Discontinue pump use the morning of the procedure and initiate an intravenous insulin drip
- E. Discontinue pump use the evening before the procedure and inject insulin glargine, 20 units; use an insulin-to-carbohydrate ratio of 1:15 for the evening meal with 1:40 correction dosing

94 A 65-year-old man presents with fatigue and low mood. He recently had a normal sleep study. He has a 3-year history of type 2 diabetes mellitus treated with metformin. He sustained an acute myocardial infarction 2 years ago. At that time, he had coronary angiography, and a cardiologist recommended medical management. Findings on recent stress echocardiography were reported to be normal. He also has stable stage 2 chronic kidney disease. His medications include metformin, a statin, aspirin, and an ACE inhibitor.

On physical examination, his height is 69 in (175 cm) and weight is 252 lb (114.5 kg) (BMI = 37 kg/m²). His blood pressure is 134/72 mm Hg. He has prominent lipomastia and mildly reduced muscle bulk. Testes are 20 mL bilaterally. Eye movements are full, and there is no clinical visual field defect.

Current laboratory test results (sample drawn at 8 AM while fasting):
- Total testosterone = 225 ng/dL (300-900 ng/dL) (SI: 7.8 nmol/L [10.4-31.2 nmol/L]) (repeated total testosterone [sample drawn 1 week later at 8 AM while fasting] = 207 ng/dL [SI: 7.2 nmol/L])
- LH = 4.8 mIU/mL (1.0-9.0 mIU/mL) (SI: 4.8 IU/L [1.0-9.0 IU/L])
- SHBG = 1.1 µg/mL (1.1-6.7 µg/mL) (SI: 9.8 nmol/L [10-60 nmol/L])
- Hemoglobin = 15.4 g/dL (13.8-17.2 g/dL) (SI: 154 g/L [138-172 g/L])
- ALT = 68 U/L (10-40 U/L) (SI: 1.14 µkat/L [0.17-0.67 µkat/L])
- Hemoglobin A_{1c} = 8.1% (4.0%-5.6%) (65 mmol/mol [20-38 mmol/mol])
- Thyroid function, normal
- Prolactin, normal

In addition to lifestyle modification, which of the following is the most appropriate next step in this patient's management?
- A. Initiate liraglutide
- B. Initiate testosterone
- C. Initiate a selective estrogen receptor modulator
- D. Perform pituitary-directed MRI
- E. Measure serum estradiol

95 A 64-year-old man with prostate cancer is referred for evaluation of low bone density, which was diagnosed based on results of DXA done 4 months ago (lowest T-score of −1.9 at the left femoral neck). He recently started androgen-deprivation therapy, which he will continue long-term. The FRAX calculator reveals a 10-year probability for major fracture and hip fracture of 8.2% and 2.8%, respectively. He smokes cigarettes but has no personal history of fractures. He has good dietary calcium intake and takes vitamin D supplementation. He has no family history of osteoporosis or fractures.

His physical examination findings are unremarkable.

Laboratory test results:
Serum calcium = 9.6 mg/dL (8.2-10.2 mg/dL) (SI: 2.4 mmol/L [2.1-2.6 mmol/L])
Serum creatinine = 1.6 mg/dL (0.7-1.3 mg/dL) (SI: 141.4 µmol/L [61.9-114.9 µmol/L])
Glomerular filtration rate (estimated) = 35 mL/min per 1.73 m^2 (>60 mL/min per 1.73 m^2)
Serum 25-hydroxyvitamin D = 48 ng/mL (30-80 ng/mL [optimal]) (SI: 119.8 nmol/L [74.9-199.7 nmol/L])
Serum albumin = 4.5 g/dL (3.5-5.0 g/dL) (SI: 45 g/L [35-50 g/L])
Serum total alkaline phosphatase = 140 U/L (50-120 U/L) (SI: 2.34 µkat/L [0.84-2.00 µkat/L])

A whole-body bone scan shows no evidence of skeletal metastatic disease.

Which of the following is the most appropriate next step in the management of this patient's low bone density?
- A. No additional therapy
- B. Alendronate
- C. Zoledronic acid
- D. Teriparatide
- E. Denosumab

96 A 36-year-old woman is referred for evaluation of positive TPO antibodies. Her mother and sister have hypothyroidism and take levothyroxine. Her brother has celiac disease. She has had fatigue for the past 6 months and reports an 8-lb (3.6-kg) weight gain during the same period. She has no plans for pregnancy. Her primary care physician ordered laboratory measurement of TPO antibodies and TSH:

TSH = 2.5 mIU/L (0.5-5.0 mIU/L)
TPO antibodies = 140 IU/mL (<2.0 IU/mL) (SI: 140 kIU/L [<2.0 kIU/L])

On physical examination, her blood pressure is 120/68 mm Hg and pulse rate is 60 beats/min. Her height is 65 in (165 cm), and weight is 176.5 lb (80.2 kg) (BMI = 29 kg/m^2). She has a small, palpable thyroid gland with no nodules. The rest of the examination findings are normal.

Which of the following is the best next step in this patient's evaluation and management?
- A. Start levothyroxine
- B. Recommend no treatment now; measure TSH in 12 months
- C. Start desiccated thyroid
- D. Recommend no treatment now; measure TPO antibodies in 12 months
- E. Perform thyroid ultrasonography

97 A 68-year-old man presents for management of type 2 diabetes mellitus, which was diagnosed 10 years ago. His hemoglobin A$_{1c}$ level has hovered around 7.0% (53 mmol/mol) for the past few years. He takes metformin, 500 mg twice daily; glimepiride, 4 mg daily; and insulin glargine, 28 units daily. He has a history of coronary artery disease, 2 myocardial infarctions, and placement of 2 drug-eluting stents. Congestive heart failure was diagnosed after the second myocardial infarction. An ejection fraction of 35% was noted on recent echocardiography. He reports some shortness of breath, particularly with prolonged exertion. He also has swelling in his lower extremities that is usually worse at the end of the day. He has had no cardiac events since his second drug-eluting stent was placed 3 years ago.

His most recent hemoglobin A_{1c} value was 7.3% (56 mmol/mol). He has a 30 pack-year history of cigarette smoking, but he quit 8 years ago. He has hypertension and hyperlipidemia controlled with metoprolol; losartan; furosemide; and rosuvastatin, 20 mg daily.

On physical examination, his blood pressure is 136/62 mm Hg, and pulse rate is 58 beats/min. His height is 71 in (180.3 cm), and weight is 228 lb (103.6 kg) (BMI = 32 kg/m²).

Laboratory test results:
  Hemoglobin A_{1c} = 7.3% (4.0%-5.6%) (56 mmol/mol [20-38 mmol/mol])
  Total cholesterol = 139 mg/dL (<200 mg/dL [optimal]) (SI: 3.60 mmol/L [<5.18 mmol/L])
  HDL cholesterol = 28 mg/dL (>60 mg/dL [optimal]) (SI: 0.73 mmol/L [>1.55 mmol/L])
  LDL cholesterol = 55 mg/dL (<100 mg/dL [optimal]) (SI: 1.42 mmol/L [<2.59 mmol/L])
  Triglycerides = 110 mg/dL (<150 mg/dL [optimal]) (SI: 1.24 mmol/L [<1.70 mmol/L])
  Serum creatinine = 1.4 mg/dL (0.7-1.3 mg/dL) (SI: 123.8 µmol/L [61.9-114.9 µmol/L])
  Estimated glomerular filtration rate = 54 mL/min per 1.73 m² (>60 mL/min per 1.73 m²)
  Potassium = 5.2 mEq/L (3.5-5.0 mEq/L) (SI: 5.2 mmol/L [3.5-5.0 mmol/L])

Which of the following should be added as the best next step in this patient's management?
  A. Dapagliflozin
  B. Alogliptin
  C. Eplerenone
  D. Icosapent ethyl
  E. Exenatide LAR

98

A 33-year-old woman with polycystic ovary syndrome presents via telemedicine consultation for progressive hirsutism and virilization that began during pregnancy. Immediately after delivery, a significantly elevated testosterone level was documented. Her gynecologist is very concerned and is recommending ovarian venous sampling to identify the source, which she suspects is related to a large hemorrhagic ovarian cyst. The patient is now 7 weeks postpartum.

Polycystic ovary syndrome was diagnosed 2 years ago while she was undergoing workup for planned ovulation induction and intrauterine insemination with donor sperm. Polycystic ovarian morphology was documented on ultrasonography by report. She had normal testosterone and DHEA-S concentrations at that time. She had a history of difficulty losing weight and mild hirsutism during her teenage years, but menstruation had always been regular. Fertility status was not clear, as her spouse is a woman, and she had not tried to conceive spontaneously. Letrozole was administered with monitoring by reproductive endocrinology for ovulation induction, and pregnancy was achieved with the first cycle of intrauterine insemination.

During pregnancy, she developed excessive facial hair growth, expanding across her jaw, sides of her face, and abdomen. She developed cystic acne along the lower half of her face and noticed deepening of her voice during the third trimester. Her baby was born via cesarean delivery 7 weeks ago at full term. At the time, her obstetrician noted that her ovaries were large. When she experienced difficulty with lactation and mentioned her recent symptoms, laboratory tests were ordered. Her only medication is a prenatal vitamin.

Laboratory test results:
  Total testosterone = 1034 ng/dL (8-60 ng/dL) (SI: 35.9 nmol/L [0.3-2.1 nmol/L])
  Free testosterone = 44 ng/dL (0.3-1.9 ng/dL) (SI: 1.5 nmol/L [0.01-0.07 nmol/L])
  SHBG = 125 µg/mL (2.2-14.6 µg/mL) (SI: 1112 nmol/L [20-130 nmol/L])
  TSH = 1.48 mIU/L (0.5-5.0 mIU/L)
  Prolactin = 125 ng/mL (10-200 ng/mL [lactating]) (SI: 5.4 nmol/L [0.43-8.70 nmol/L])

Laboratory test results 1 week later:
  Total testosterone = 333 ng/dL (8-60 ng/dL) (SI: 11.6 nmol/L [0.3-2.1 nmol/L])
  Free testosterone = 17 ng/dL (0.3-1.9 ng/dL) (SI: 0.59 nmol/L [0.01-0.07 nmol/L])
  SHBG = 182 µg/mL (2.2-14.6 µg/mL) (SI: 1619 nmol/L [20-130 nmol/L])

No adrenal masses are observed on abdominal CT. On pelvic ultrasonography, the left ovary is normal and measures 3.6 × 3.7 × 2.4 cm with a volume of 16.7 cc. The right ovary is enlarged and measures 6.1 × 6.3 × 3.1 cm with a volume of 62.3 cc. It is polycystic in appearance with a 6-cm complex cystic mass.

Six weeks later, her total testosterone concentration is 25 ng/dL (0.9 nmol/L). She has started to lactate successfully, and her acne has improved. Hair growth is still present in the same distribution.

Which of the following is this patient's most likely diagnosis?
A. Polycystic ovary syndrome
B. Theca-cell tumor
C. Extraovarian/extraadrenal tumor
D. Luteoma of pregnancy
E. Idiopathic hirsutism

99

A 45-year-old woman is diagnosed with breast cancer following screening mammography. A mastectomy is planned. She is referred for routine genetic testing for breast cancer at a tertiary care genetics clinic, and an 83-gene panel study is ordered. No pathogenic variants known to increase breast cancer risk are found; however, a pathogenic variant in the *RET* gene is identified.

She has no personal or family history of medullary thyroid cancer, hyperparathyroidism, or pheochromocytoma. She has no neck masses, neck pain, or difficulty swallowing. She has longstanding anxiety, but no palpitations, high blood pressure, or episodes of sweating. Her medications include venlafaxine, 175 mg daily, and lorazepam, 0.5 mg as needed (both for anxiety).

Thyroid ultrasonography reveals a normal thyroid gland without nodules. Abdominal CT documents a 9-mm nodularity in the left adrenal gland with an unenhanced attenuation of 2 Hounsfield units. The right adrenal gland is normal.

Laboratory test results:
    Calcitonin, normal
    Plasma normetanephrine = 220 pg/mL (<165 pg/mL) (SI: 1.20 nmol/L [<0.90 nmol/L])
    Plasma metanephrine = 90 pg/mL (<99 pg/mL) (SI: 0.46 nmol/L [<0.50 nmol/L])

Which of the following is the most appropriate next step in this patient's management?
A. Proceed with planned mastectomy
B. Perform left laparoscopic adrenalectomy after preoperative α-adrenergic blockade
C. Perform an MIBG scan
D. Perform a ^{68}Ga-DOTATATE PET-CT
E. Perform abdominal MRI

100

A 30-year-old premenopausal woman is referred for evaluation of low bone density. She recently sustained a Colles fracture of her right wrist after falling. DXA documents a Z-score of −3.1 in the lumbar spine. Her dietary calcium intake is approximately 400 mg daily. She does not take any calcium or vitamin D supplements. She has been using depot medroxyprogesterone for the past 5 years. She has no history of thyroid disease or parathyroid disease. She has no family history of bone disease. Her mother has breast cancer.

Her physical examination findings, including vital signs, are unremarkable.

Laboratory test results:
    Serum 25-hydroxyvitamin D = 26 ng/mL (30-80 ng/mL [optimal]) (SI: 64.9 nmol/L [74.9-199.7 nmol/L])
    Complete blood cell count, normal
    Complete metabolic panel, normal
    TSH, normal

Which of the following should be recommended in addition to adequate calcium and vitamin D supplementation?
  A. Measure tissue transglutaminase antibodies
  B. Measure 24-hour urinary calcium excretion
  C. Discontinue depot medroxyprogesterone
  D. Start raloxifene
  E. Start alendronate

101

A 44-year-old man with hypertension, stomatocytosis, and macrothrombocytopenia is referred after a myocardial infarction. His primary care provider would like a recommendation regarding the best therapy. The patient has no history of a cholesterol problem. His older brother underwent coronary artery bypass surgery at age 45 years. His other 4 siblings do not have a personal history of premature heart disease. The patient does not drink alcohol or smoke cigarettes. His medications include lisinopril, aspirin, metoprolol, and clopidogrel.

On physical examination, his blood pressure is 121/66 mm Hg, pulse rate is 84 beats/min, and respiratory rate is 14 breaths/min. His height is 72 in (183 cm), and weight is 215 lb (97.7 kg) (BMI = 29 kg/m²). His lungs are clear to auscultation bilaterally and heart sounds are regular without a murmur. His abdomen is soft and nontender and bowel sounds are normal. His spleen is not palpable. His skin is nonicteric. He does not have xanthelasmas; however, he has bilateral Achilles tendon xanthomas.

Laboratory test results:
  White blood cell count = 6600/μL (4500-11,000/μL) (SI: 6.6×10^9/L [4.5-11.0×10^9/L])
  Hemoglobin = 11.3 g/dL (13.8-17.2 g/dL) (SI: 113 g/L [138-172 g/L])
  Platelet count = 39×10^3/μL (150-450×10^3/μL) (SI: 39×10^9/L [150-450×10^9/L])
  Total cholesterol = 158 mg/dL (<200 mg/dL [optimal]) (SI: 4.09 mmol/L [<5.18 mmol/L])
  Triglycerides = 162 mg/dL (<150 mg/dL [optimal]) (SI: 1.83 mmol/L [<1.70 mmol/L])
  HDL cholesterol = 42 mg/dL (>60 mg/dL [optimal]) (SI: 1.09 mmol/L [>1.55 mmol/L])
  LDL cholesterol = 84 mg/dL (<100 mg/dL [optimal]) (SI: 2.18 mmol/L [<2.59 mmol/L])
  Campesterol = 84.9 μg/mL (0-7 μg/mL)

Which of the following is this patient's most likely diagnosis?
  A. Familial combined hyperlipidemia
  B. Familial hypobetalipoproteinemia
  C. Familial dysbetalipoproteinemia
  D. Sitosterolemia
  E. Familial hypercholesterolemia

102

A 64-year-old man is seen for consultation regarding postoperative glycemic management. He had an emergent exploratory laparotomy yesterday for small-bowel obstruction not responsive to conservative measures.

His medical history is notable for type 2 diabetes mellitus of 7 years' duration, coronary artery disease, and hypertension. He has a 30 pack-year history of cigarette smoking, although he quit 7 years ago. At the time diabetes was diagnosed, his hemoglobin A_{1c} level was 8.3% (67 mmol/mol), and he was prescribed metformin and lifestyle management. After 1 year of treatment, his hemoglobin A_{1c} level remained above 7.0% (>53 mmol/mol) and glipizide was started. His hemoglobin A_{1c} level subsequently decreased to 6.7% (50 mmol/mol). Four years ago, glipizide was changed to empagliflozin.

Outpatient medications are metformin, empagliflozin, lisinopril, aspirin, hydrochlorothiazide, and metoprolol. He reports good adherence. At the time of surgery, all oral antidiabetes medications were stopped, and diabetes is currently being managed with an intravenous insulin drip alone, on a protocol that targets a glucose concentration of 110 to 140 mg/dL (6.1-7.8 mmol/L). His glycemic control has been stable on about 3 units per hour. The team plans to convert the regimen to subcutaneous insulin today.

On physical examination, his blood pressure is 134/78 mm Hg and pulse rate is 72 beats/min. His height is 68 in (173 cm), and weight is 184 lb (83.5 kg) (BMI = 28 kg/m²). Achilles deep tendon reflexes are absent. His surgical incisions are clean. There is no evidence of heart failure.

Recent laboratory test results:
- Sodium = 134 mEq/L (136-142 mEq/L) (SI: 134 mmol/L [136-142 mmol/L])
- Potassium = 5.2 mEq/L (3.5-5.0 mEq/L) (SI: 5.2 mmol/L [3.5-5.0 mmol/L])
- Chloride = 106 mEq/L (96-106 mEq/L) (SI: 106 mmol/L [96-106 mmol/L])
- Bicarbonate = 17 mEq/L (21-28 mEq/L) (SI: 17 mmol/L [21-28 mmol/L])
- Glucose = 130 mg/dL (70-99 mg/dL) (SI: 7.2 mmol/L [3.9-5.5 mmol/L])
- Serum urea nitrogen = 24 mg/dL (8-23 mg/dL) (SI: 8.6 mmol/L [2.9-8.2 mmol/L])
- Creatinine = 1.1 mg/dL (0.7-1.3 mg/dL) (SI: 97.2 µmol/L [61.9-114.9 µmol/L])
- Hemoglobin A_{1c} = 8.1% (4.0%-5.6%) (65 mmol/mol [20-38 mmol/mol])

Which of the following additional recommendations would be most reasonable to help avoid postoperative complications?
- A. Measure blood lactic acid
- B. Measure serum β-hydroxybutyrate
- C. Check urine for ketones
- D. Continue insulin drip (rather than switch to subcutaneous insulin)
- E. Start a GLP-1 receptor agonist

103

A 67-year-old woman is referred for evaluation following recent multiple fractures. She has a history of orthotopic liver transplant for hepatitis B 15 years ago, although she has been off prednisone therapy for more than 10 years. A bone density study done 5 years ago showed osteopenia in the lumbar spine with T-scores of −2.3, −1.3, −2.4, and −2.1 in the lumbar spine, right femoral neck, total hip, and left proximal one-third radius, respectively. She was prescribed alendronate, 70 mg weekly. However, because of worsening renal function, alendronate was discontinued after 1 year and raloxifene was started, which she continues to take.

Approximately 9 months ago, she fell after rising from a chair and incurred a left proximal humeral fracture and a right intertrochanteric proximal femoral fracture. She underwent operative repair of her femoral fracture, with initial conservative therapy of her proximal humeral fracture. Due to poor healing, she still had left hip pain with limited weightbearing and also eventually had plate fixation of her proximal humeral fracture 3 months ago.

Additional medical history includes persistent hepatitis B infection and chronic renal insufficiency secondary to calcineurin inhibitor therapy. Current medications include mycophenolate, tacrolimus, tenofovir, famotidine, calcium with vitamin D, and raloxifene. She does not smoke cigarettes or drink alcohol. Her family history is negative for osteoporosis or hip fracture.

On physical examination, she is in mild distress because of hip pain. Vital signs are unremarkable, including her height, which is only 1.0 in (2.5 cm) shorter than her self-stated maximum adult height. She has no thyromegaly or neck masses. Spine examination shows normal curvature without kyphosis. She has tenderness over the right groin and lateral hip. The rest of her examination findings are unremarkable.

Laboratory test results:
- Calcium = 9.4 mg/dL (8.2-10.2 mg/dL) (SI: 2.4 mmol/L [2.1-2.6 mmol/L])
- Phosphate = 1.9 mg/dL (2.3-4.7 mg/dL) (SI: 0.6 mmol/L [0.7-1.5 mmol/L])
- Creatinine = 2.0 mg/dL (0.6-1.1 mg/dL) (SI: 176.8 µmol/L [53.0-97.2 µmol/L])
- Albumin = 4.0 g/dL (3.5-5.0 g/dL) (SI: 40 g/L [35-50 g/L])
- Magnesium = 2.0 mg/dL (1.5-2.3 mg/dL) (SI: 0.8 mmol/L [0.6-0.9 mmol/L])
- Alkaline phosphatase = 154 U/L (50-120 U/L) (SI: 2.57 µkat/L [0.84-2.00 µkat/L])
- Intact PTH = 95 pg/mL (10-65 pg/mL) (SI: 95 ng/L [10-65 ng/L])
- 25-Hydroxyvitamin D = 25 ng/mL (30-80 ng/mL [optimal]) (SI: 62.4 nmol/L [74.9-199.7 nmol/L])

A DXA scan performed at this visit on the same instrument as her previous assessment shows the following (contralateral hip measured due to interval right femoral fracture):
   Lumbar spine T-score = –3.2 (decreased 12.8% compared with previous)
   Femoral neck T-score = –3.8
   Total hip T-score = –4.3
   Proximal one-third radius T-score = –4.4

On the basis of this patient's presentation, which of the following is the best next step in the management of her metabolic bone disorder?
   A. Start ergocalciferol, 50,000 IU weekly
   B. Start zoledronic acid
   C. Start cinacalcet
   D. Discontinue tenofovir
   E. Discontinue tacrolimus

104

A 51-year-old man seeks a second opinion for androgen deficiency-like symptoms and low testosterone, which his primary care physician has attributed to overweight/metabolic syndrome. The patient reports lethargy, muscle weakness, low mood, and low libido. He describes stressful work and marital difficulties with his wife that include her being "demanding sexually." He has been advised to lose weight and engage in regular exercise, but he has lacked motivation to be adherent to these recommendations.

On physical examination, his height is 71 in (180.3 cm) and weight is 206 lb (93.6 kg) (BMI = 29.0 kg/m²). He has mild gynecomastia bilaterally. Testes are 15 mL bilaterally. Visual fields are full to confrontation, and he has a full range of eye movements.

Current laboratory test results (sample drawn at 8 AM while fasting):
   Total testosterone = 176 ng/dL (300-900 ng/dL) (SI: 6.1 nmol/L [10.4-31.2 nmol/L])
   SHBG = 1.7 µg/mL (1.1-6.7 µg/mL) (SI: 15 nmol/L [10-60 nmol/L])
   LH = 1.8 mIU/mL (1.0-9.0 mIU/mL) (SI: 1.8 IU/L [1.0-9.0 IU/L])
   TSH = 2.0 mIU/L (0.5-5.0 mIU/L)
   Free T$_4$ = 0.9 ng/dL (0.8-1.8 ng/dL) (SI: 11.6 pmol/L [10.30-23.17 pmol/L])
   Prolactin = 39 ng/mL (4-23 ng/mL) (SI: 1.70 nmol/L [0.17-1.00 nmol/L])
   Hemoglobin = 12.8 g/dL (13.8-17.2 g/dL) (SI: 128 g/L [138-172 g/L])
   ALT = 55 U/L (10-40 U/L) (SI: 0.91 µkat/L [0.17-0.67 µkat/L])
   Hemoglobin A$_{1c}$ = 6.2% (4.0%-5.6%) (44 mmol/mol [20-38 mmol/mol])

Serum electrolytes and renal function are normal. Repeated total testosterone (sample drawn 1 week later at 8 AM while fasting) is 167 ng/dL (5.8 nmol/L).

Which of the following is the best next step in this patient's management?
   A. Measure serum free testosterone
   B. Prescribe a phosphodiesterase type 5 inhibitor
   C. Perform pituitary-directed MRI
   D. Commence testosterone treatment
   E. Refer to a dietician and exercise physiologist for lifestyle measures

105

A 53-year-old man with hypertension and a 10-year history of HIV is taking bictegravir/tenofovir alafenamide/emtricitabine. Diabetes mellitus was diagnosed 6 months ago, at which time his hemoglobin A$_{1c}$ level was 8.7% (69 mmol/mol). He was prescribed metformin, 500 mg twice daily. Point-of-care hemoglobin A$_{1c}$ in the clinic today is 7.9% (63 mmol/mol). His current estimated glomerular filtration rate is 62 mL/min per 1.73 m². His height is 69 in (175.3 cm), and weight is 205 lb (93.2 kg) (BMI = 30 kg/m²).

Which of the following is the best next step in this patient's management?
  A. Continue current therapy
  B. Add dulaglutide
  C. Increase the metformin dosage to 1000 mg twice daily
  D. Stop metformin and start dulaglutide
  E. Stop metformin and start sitagliptin

106 A 36-year-old man with a 4-cm right thyroid nodule undergoes FNA biopsy, which documents papillary thyroid carcinoma. Subsequently, he undergoes total thyroidectomy with bilateral central neck dissection. He has no difficulty swallowing and no tingling or numbness around his lips the day after surgery. He is discharged home. The following day, he starts noticing hoarseness. At a follow-up visit 10 days after surgery, he is concerned about hoarseness and intermittent cough. He has been taking levothyroxine daily, the same dosage he was taking before his thyroid surgery.

His medical history is notable for hypothyroidism diagnosed 8 years ago, which has been treated with levothyroxine, 125 mcg daily. He has no other relevant medical or surgical history.

On physical examination, his blood pressure is 118/64 mm Hg and pulse rate is 68 beats/min. His height is 72 in (183 cm), and weight is 185 lb (83.9 kg) (BMI = 25 kg/m²). His voice is hoarse. He has a well-healed scar at the base of his neck with no palpable neck masses. His lungs are clear to auscultation. There is no lower-extremity edema. The rest of the examination findings are normal.

Laboratory test results:
  TSH = 6.50 mIU/L (0.5-5.0 mIU/L)
  Free T$_4$ = 1.1 ng/dL (0.8-1.8 ng/dL) (SI: 14.2 pmol/L [10.30-23.17 pmol/L])
  Calcium = 8.6 mg/dL (8.2-10.2 mg/dL) (SI: 2.2 mmol/L [2.1-2.6 mmol/L])

In addition to adjusting his levothyroxine dosage, which of the following is the best next step in this patient's management?
  A. Measure TSH in 6 months
  B. Reassess his hoarseness in 3 months
  C. Refer to an otolaryngologist
  D. Refer to a pulmonologist
  E. No immediate intervention is needed

107 A 52-year-old woman presents with several months of epigastric discomfort after eating. She describes a burning sensation that is worse after consuming high-fat foods and carbonated beverages. She has been intermittently taking over-the-counter chewable calcium supplementation with relief, but these episodes are becoming more frequent and she is concerned. Her bowel movements are normal in frequency and consistency.

Approximately 2 years ago, she underwent laparoscopic sleeve gastrectomy for the primary indication of medically complicated obesity. She weighed 243 lb (110 kg) at the time of surgery and currently weighs 192 lb (87 kg), representing a 21% total body weight loss. She has successfully maintained her weight.

She takes a mineral-containing multivitamin twice daily; cholecalciferol, 5000 IU daily; and vitamin B$_{12}$ injections monthly.

On physical examination, her height is 61.5 in (156 cm) and weight is 192 lb (87 kg) (BMI = 36 kg/m²). Findings on thyroid examination are normal. Her abdomen is soft, and the laparoscopic scars are well healed. She has mild tenderness to palpation of the epigastrium.

In addition to arranging a dietician review, which of the following is the best next step in this patient's management?
- A. Pantoprazole, 40 mg daily
- B. Upper gastrointestinal endoscopy with biopsies
- C. Barium esophagography
- D. Ursodeoxycholic acid (ursodiol)
- E. Abdominal ultrasonography to screen for gallstones

108 A 45-year-old man is referred for evaluation of right hip pain and low bone density. He was in his usual state of health until 3 months ago, when he noted abrupt onset of right groin pain. The pain is worse with ambulation and flexion of the hip. He had no antecedent injury or falls. Progression of his pain prompted him to see his primary care physician who referred him to physical therapy without benefit. Subsequent plain x-ray of the right hip was normal. Bone density assessment documented low bone density for age, based on a right femoral neck Z-score of –2.2. Lumbar spine and total hip bone densities were within normal range for age with Z-scores of –1.4 and –1.6, respectively. He has no history of fractures as an adult. His medical history is notable for asthma treated with an albuterol inhaler and montelukast. Family history is negative for osteoporosis or hip fracture. He smokes 1 pack of cigarettes per day and drinks 1 to 2 beers daily. He does not exercise on a regular basis.

On physical examination, he is lying on the examination table in mild distress because of right groin pain. He has scattered expiratory wheezes. Findings on spine examination are normal, with normal curvature and no elicitable tenderness. There is tenderness to palpation over the right medial inguinal region, as well as pain elicited with both internal and external rotation of the hip.

In addition to a normal complete blood cell count, laboratory testing reveals the following:
Calcium = 9.7 mg/dL (8.2-10.2 mg/dL) (SI: 2.4 mmol/L [2.1-2.6 mmol/L])
Phosphate = 3.2 mg/dL (2.3-4.7 mg/dL) (SI: 1.0 mmol/L [0.7-1.5 mmol/L])
Creatinine = 1.0 mg/dL (0.7-1.3 mg/dL) (SI: 88.4 μmol/L [61.9-114.9 μmol/L])
Albumin = 4.4 g/dL (3.5-5.0 g/dL) (SI: 44 g/L [35-50 g/L])
Alkaline phosphatase = 85 U/L (50-120 U/L) (SI: 1.42 μkat/L [0.84-2.00 μkat/L])
Intact PTH = 42 pg/mL (10-65 pg/mL) (SI: 42 ng/L [10-65 ng/L])
25-Hydroxyvitamin D = 28 ng/mL (30-80 ng/mL [optimal]) (SI: 69.9 nmol/L [74.9-199.7 nmol/L])

MRI of the right hip is performed (*see image*).

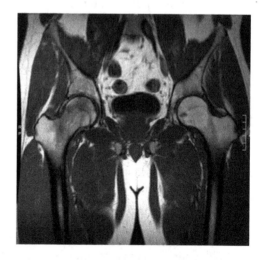

Coronal T1-weighted MRI of the right hip shows extensive bone marrow edema in the right femoral head and neck and mild joint effusion without apparent crescent sign or signs of fracture.

Which of the following is this patient's most likely diagnosis?
- A. Transient osteoporosis
- B. Trochanteric bursitis
- C. Septic arthritis
- D. Avascular necrosis
- E. Rheumatoid arthritis

109 A 51-year-old woman with type 2 diabetes mellitus is currently hospitalized for evaluation and management of abdominal pain. During this admission, numerous low fingerstick point-of-care blood glucose values have been recorded. A fingerstick point-of-care blood glucose value of 30 mg/dL (1.7 mmol/L) was documented earlier this morning. The nurse administered oral dextrose, but a repeated point-of-care measurement was only 22 mg/dL (1.2 mmol/L). The patient was reported to be conversant at the time. Intravenous dextrose and intramuscular glucagon were subsequently administered, but the patient's fingerstick blood glucose concentration remained critically low at 28 mg/dL (1.6 mmol/L). The primary service has consulted endocrinology for recurrent and refractory hypoglycemia.

She has a 10-year-history of type 2 diabetes complicated by nonproliferative retinopathy and microalbuminuria. She currently takes metformin, 850 mg twice daily, and glimepiride, 2 mg once daily. Her last hemoglobin A_{1c} measurement was 7.7% (61 mmol/mol). She has a 40 pack-year history of cigarette smoking. She has hypertension and hyperlipidemia controlled with lisinopril/hydrochlorothiazide and atorvastatin. She has a history of peripheral arterial disease and has undergone a below-the-knee amputation of her left leg.

She has no palpitations, shortness of breath, sweating, confusion, tremor, or hunger. Her only concerns at this time are weight loss, lack of appetite, and abdominal pain that worsens with prandial intake, which is what prompted the current hospital admission. She rarely checks blood glucose at home. She has no regular signs or symptoms suggestive of hypoglycemia.

On physical examination, her blood pressure is 136/78 mm Hg and pulse rate is 78 beats/min. Her height is 63 in (160 cm), and weight is 176 lb (80 kg) (BMI = 31 kg/m²). Her right lower-extremity dorsalis pedis and posterior tibial pulses are only faintly palpable. Her abdomen is diffusely tender to palpation.

Laboratory test results:
Serum creatinine = 1.1 mg/dL (0.6-1.1 mg/dL) (SI: 97.2 μmol/L [53.0-97.2 μmol/L])
Estimated glomerular filtration rate = 65 mL/min per 1.73 m² (>60 mL/min per 1.73 m²)

Which of the following is the best next step in this patient's evaluation and management?
A. Measure venous plasma glucose
B. Administer octreotide
C. Order a sulfonylurea panel
D. Initiate intravenous infusion of dextrose-containing fluids
E. Measure C-peptide

110 An 18-year-old girl is evaluated for fatigue and poor concentration in school. Laboratory testing reveals a TSH concentration of 26.0 mIU/L (0.5-5.0 mIU/L) and markedly elevated TPO antibodies. Hashimoto thyroiditis is diagnosed, and levothyroxine therapy is started. Ten days later, she reports an improved energy level.

During routine follow-up 3 weeks later, she is feeling tired again. She has lost 10 lb (4.5 kg) since her last visit. Her mother reports that it is unclear whether she has been taking her levothyroxine daily, and on some days, she has been taking a double or triple dose to "make up" for missed doses. Her appetite is significantly decreased.

Six weeks later, while at a concert with friends, the patient faints and is taken to the emergency department. Her blood pressure is 89/51 mm Hg, and pulse rate is 120 beats/min.

Laboratory test results:
Sodium = 120 mEq/L (136-142 mEq/L) (SI: 120 mmol/L [136-142 mmol/L])
Potassium = 6.9 mEq/L (3.5-5.0 mEq/L) (SI: 6.9 mmol/L [3.5-5.0 mmol/L])
Glucose = 63 mg/dL (70-99 mg/dL) (SI: 3.5 mmol/L [3.9-5.5 mmol/L])

Which of the following laboratory findings is most likely to be observed in this patient?
A. Very high free T_4
B. Very high TSH
C. Very low renin
D. Very high ACTH
E. Very high thyroid-stimulating immunoglobulins

111 Polycystic ovary syndrome was diagnosed in a 24-year-old woman based on an elevated total testosterone concentration and irregular menses since adolescence with an average intermenstrual interval of 60 days. The patient's local gynecologist ordered appropriate endocrine testing, which revealed normal thyroid function and normal levels of prolactin and 17-hydroxyprogesterone. The gynecologist referred her to endocrinology.

After reviewing her treatment priorities, she is interested in more regular menses. She does not have any unwanted hair growth. An oral contraceptive is recommended. She has concerns about adverse effects, so she is started on a lower-dosage estrogen pill. Three months later, she contacts the clinic because she is having spotting throughout the month and no withdrawal period in the expected time of the placebo week.

Laboratory test results:
  FSH, undetectable
  Estradiol, undetectable

Which of the following is the best next step in this patient's evaluation and management?
  A. Order pituitary MRI
  B. Order pelvic ultrasonography
  C. Switch to a combined oral contraceptive with a different progestin
  D. Switch to a combined oral contraceptive with a higher dose of estrogen
  E. Switch to a progestin-only oral contraceptive

112

A 30-year-old woman with a 2-year history of diabetes mellitus and no complications presents for a follow-up appointment. Schizophrenia was recently diagnosed after hospitalization. Three weeks ago, during her hospitalization, her psychiatrist started olanzapine and aripiprazole. Her diabetes has been well controlled on metformin, 1000 mg twice daily, and her hemoglobin A_{1c} value 3 months ago was 6.3% (45 mmol/mol). Her point-of-care hemoglobin A_{1c} value at today's visit is 6.7% (50 mmol/mol). She infrequently checks her blood glucose, but in preparation for this appointment she obtained 3 fasting blood glucose measurements over the past week (range, 165-193 mg/dL [9.2-10.7 mmol/L]).

Her height is 63 in (160 cm), and weight is 185 lb (84.1 kg) (BMI = 33 kg/m²).

Which of the following is the best next step in this patient's management in addition to arranging nutritional counseling?
  A. Make no changes and follow-up in 3 months
  B. Add basal insulin
  C. Add phentermine/topiramate
  D. Add semaglutide
  E. Add glimepiride

113

A 53-year-old man with type 2 diabetes mellitus, hypertension, cirrhosis secondary to alcohol use, and gastroesophageal reflux disease is referred for management of mixed hyperlipidemia. Type 2 diabetes was diagnosed 2 years ago. At that time, metformin was prescribed and shortly after he started atorvastatin. One year ago, he was evaluated for elevated liver enzymes; cirrhosis secondary to alcohol use was diagnosed. During evaluation for liver disease, statin therapy was discontinued. He has not consumed any alcohol since cirrhosis was diagnosed, and he reports this condition is stable. His medications include insulin glargine, insulin aspart, lisinopril, furosemide, and pantoprazole.

On physical examination, his blood pressure is 94/65 mm Hg, pulse rate is 86 beats/min, and respiratory rate is 16 breaths/min. His skin is pale and he has no jaundice. A few facial telangiectasias are visible. His lungs are clear to auscultation bilaterally. He has gynecomastia bilaterally. On abdominal examination, bowel sounds are present, he has no ascites, and there is no tenderness to palpation. He does not have asterixis or peripheral edema.

Laboratory test results:
  Hemoglobin A_{1c} = 6.5% (4.0%-5.6%) (48 mmol/mol [20-38 mmol/mol])
  Total bilirubin = 0.4 mg/dL (0.3-1.2 mg/dL) (SI: 6.8 μmol/L [5.1-20.5 μmol/L])
  Direct bilirubin = 0.1 mg/dL (0-0.3 mg/dL) (SI: 1.7 μmol/L [0-5.1 μmol/L])
  Alkaline phosphatase = 86 U/L (50-120 U/L) (SI: 1.44 μkat/L [0.84-2.00 μkat/L])

AST = 71 U/L (20-48 U/L) (SI: 1.19 µkat/L [0.33-0.80 µkat/L])
ALT = 89 U/L (10-40 U/L) (SI: 1.49 µkat/L [0.17-0.67 µkat/L])
Total cholesterol = 247 mg/dL (<200 mg/dL [optimal]) (SI: 6.40 mmol/L [<5.18 mmol/L])
Triglycerides = 274 mg/dL (<150 mg/dL [optimal]) (SI: 3.10 mmol/L [<1.70 mmol/L])
HDL cholesterol = 52 mg/dL (>60 mg/dL [optimal]) (SI: 1.35 mmol/L [>1.55 mmol/L])
LDL cholesterol = 140 mg/dL (<100 mg/dL [optimal]) (SI: 3.63 mmol/L [<2.59 mmol/L])

Which of the following is the best medication to recommend for this patient?
- A. Atorvastatin
- B. Ezetimibe
- C. Bempedoic acid
- D. Colesevelam
- E. Alirocumab

114 A 32-year-old woman with type 1 diabetes mellitus comes to clinic because of upper abdominal discomfort, nausea, and vomiting that have been gradually worsening over the last 3 to 4 months. She sometimes has a feeling of fullness after meals, although this is not consistent. A gastric-emptying study demonstrates gastric retention of 15% after 4 hours, described as a mild to moderate delay in gastric emptying. Upper endoscopy reveals no evidence of outlet obstruction. Her hemoglobin A_{1c} level is 8.5% (69 mmol/mol). At the time of her gastric-emptying study, her blood glucose was elevated (200-260 mg/dL [11.1-14.4 mmol/L]) based on readings from her continuous glucose monitor.

Her medical history is notable for type 1 diabetes of 18 years' duration and hypothyroidism. Medications include insulin aspart delivered via an insulin pump and levothyroxine. Recent laboratory test results are unremarkable, including a normal TSH level.

She asks what she can do to improve her symptoms.

Which of the following is the most appropriate next step in this patient's management?
- A. Repeat the gastric-emptying study and ensure glucose levels are normal at the time of the study
- B. Recommend a nutrition consult for low-fat, low-fiber, small particle size foods
- C. Intensify glucose control, targeting hemoglobin A_{1c} <7.0% (<53 mmol/mol)
- D. Initiate metoclopramide
- E. Initiate erythromycin

115 A 40-year-old premenopausal woman is referred for low bone density. She recently fell on a concrete floor and sustained a right hip fracture. DXA documents a Z-score of –2.5 in the left femoral neck. She reports numerous long-bone fractures since early childhood. She has good dietary calcium intake and takes a vitamin D supplement daily. She has no hearing loss. Her mother and maternal grandmother are being treated for osteoporosis.

On physical examination, she has short stature, moderate scoliosis, and several bone deformities in her upper and lower extremities. She has normal sclerae and normal hearing.

Laboratory test results, including a basic metabolic panel, alkaline phosphatase level, and serum 25-hydroxyvitamin D level, are unremarkable.

Which of the following is this patient's most likely diagnosis?
- A. Type V osteogenesis imperfecta
- B. Idiopathic juvenile osteoporosis
- C. Juvenile Paget disease
- D. Hereditary resistance to vitamin D
- E. Hypophosphatasia

116 A 22-year-old man is referred for evaluation of recently diagnosed diabetes insipidus. He first noticed polyuria and polydipsia about 3 months ago. His primary care physician ruled out diabetes mellitus and hypercalcemia and measured a 24-hour urine output of 13 L (urine was dilute). The patient responded well to desmopressin therapy (0.2 mg orally twice daily), with normalization of urination. His anterior pituitary function is normal, with the exception of central hypogonadism as demonstrated by the following laboratory test results:

Total testosterone = 137 ng/dL (300-900 ng/dL) (SI: 4.8 nmol/L [10.4-31.2 nmol/L])
LH = 2.5 mIU/mL (1.0-9.0 mIU/mL) (SI: 2.5 IU/L [1.0-9.0 IU/L])
FSH = 3.2 mIU/mL (1.0-13.0 mIU/mL) (SI: 3.2 IU/L [1.0-13.0 IU/L])

On physical examination, he is normally androgenized. He has a full beard. His blood pressure is 115/78 mm Hg, and pulse rate is 72 beats/min. His height is 67.5 in (171.5 cm), and weight is 195 lb (88.5 kg) (BMI = 30 kg/m^2). Examination findings are normal, with the exception of small, soft testes, about 8 mL in volume bilaterally.

A gadolinium-enhanced pituitary MRI is shown (*see images*).

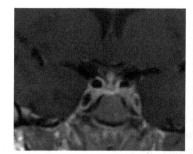
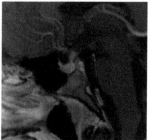

Which of the following is the best next step in this patient's evaluation?
- A. Pituitary stalk biopsy
- B. PET-CT of the brain
- C. Lumbar puncture
- D. Skeletal survey
- E. ^{68}Ga DOTATATE scan

117 A 61-year-old man with a 6-year history of type 2 diabetes mellitus returns for follow-up. He has not been seen in clinic for more than a year. Point-of-care hemoglobin A_{1c} measurement today is 6.8% (51 mmol/mol). He has no known diabetes-related complications although he has not had laboratory evaluation or eye examination in more than a year. His blood pressure is 128/72 mm Hg. Current medications are metformin, 1000 mg twice daily, and rosuvastatin, 10 mg daily.

His immunization record documents that he received tetanus-diphtheria and pneumococcal polysaccharide (PPSV23) vaccinations at the time of his diabetes diagnosis 6 years ago.

In addition to recommending an eye examination and ordering appropriate laboratory studies to screen for complications, which of the following immunizations should this patient receive?
- A. Second dose of pneumococcal polysaccharide (PPSV23)
- B. Tetanus-diphtheria booster
- C. Live attenuated influenza
- D. Hepatitis A
- E. Hepatitis B series

118 A 23-year-old man with a history of celiac disease presents for evaluation and management of subclinical hypothyroidism that was diagnosed after he completed a battery of laboratory tests while visiting his local health fair.

His initial serum TSH measurement was 34.0 mIU/L, and it was confirmed to be elevated on repeated testing. His free T_4 concentration was normal. At a visit with his primary care physician, the patient described some fatigue, as well as intermittent bloating and diarrhea when not strictly adherent to a gluten-free diet. His primary care physician diagnosed subclinical hypothyroidism and prescribed weight-based oral levothyroxine therapy, which the patient has been taking for approximately 2 months with good adherence and appropriate administration.

Today the patient reports ongoing fatigue, new heat intolerance and sweating overnight, and unchanged gastrointestinal symptoms.

On physical examination, his blood pressure is 130/82 mm Hg and pulse rate is 90 beats/min. His height is 72 in (182.9 cm), and weight is 170 lb (77.3 kg) (BMI = 23 kg/m²). Findings on thyroid examination are normal without enlargement or nodules. There is no palpable cervical lymphadenopathy. Deep tendon reflexes are brisk. There is a slight tremor of his upper extremities. The rest of the examination findings are normal.

Laboratory test results:

Analyte	Health fair	2 weeks later	After taking levothyroxine for 8 weeks
TSH	34.0 mIU/L	26.0 mIU/L	40.0 mIU/L (repeated in heterophile-blocking tube = 36.0 mIU/L)
Free T_4	...	1.1 ng/dL (SI: 14.2 pmol/L)	1.8 ng/dL (SI: 23.2 pmol/L)
TPO antibodies	...	<2.0 IU/mL (SI: <2.0 kIU/L)	...
LDL cholesterol	76 mg/dL (SI: 1.97 mmol/L)	...	...
Complete blood cell count	Normal	...	...
Complete metabolic panel	Normal	...	...

Reference ranges: TSH, 0.5-5.0 mIU/L; free T_4, 0.8-1.8 ng/dL (10.30-23.17 pmol/L); TPO antibodies, <2.0 IU/mL (SI: <2.0 kIU/L); LDL cholesterol, <100 mg/dL (optimal) (SI: <2.59 mmol/L).

Which of the following is the most appropriate next step in this patient's evaluation and management?
- A. Calculate polyethylene glycol (PEG)-precipitable TSH
- B. Measure free T_4 by equilibrium dialysis
- C. Perform pituitary MRI with and without contrast
- D. Increase the levothyroxine dosage
- E. Change the levothyroxine from tablets to oral solution

119 A 30-year-old man has multiple endocrine neoplasia type 2A. Several family members are also affected. The patient underwent prophylactic total thyroidectomy at age 13 years. He has had normal calcitonin levels since that time. He has been monitored annually for symptoms, and plasma metanephrines have been normal.

At his most recent evaluation, while entirely asymptomatic, he is found to have new-onset hypertension with a blood pressure of 141/82 mm Hg. He has no episodic palpitations, sweating, or anxiety. Plasma metanephrines are elevated:

Plasma metanephrine = 191 pg/mL (<99 pg/mL) (SI: 0.97 nmol/L [<0.50 nmol/L])
Plasma normetanephrine = 169 pg/mL (<165 pg/mL) (SI: 0.92 nmol/L [<0.90 nmol/L])
Urinary metanephrine = 898 µg/24 h (<261 µg/24 h) (SI: 4553 nmol/d [<1323 nmol/d])
Urinary normetanephrine = 586 µg/24 h (<482 µg/24 h) (SI: 3200 nmol/d [<2632 nmol/d])

Abdominal CT reveals a new left adrenal mass measuring 27 × 17 mm with an unenhanced attenuation of 41 Hounsfield units. The right adrenal gland is unremarkable. Pheochromocytoma is diagnosed and surgery is recommended.

Which of the following is the most appropriate next step in this patient's surgical management?
- A. Left cortical-sparing laparoscopic adrenalectomy
- B. Bilateral cortical-sparing laparoscopic adrenalectomy
- C. Left total laparoscopic adrenalectomy
- D. Left open adrenalectomy
- E. Bilateral total laparoscopic adrenalectomy

120

A 57-year-old man with a history of hypertension and nephrolithiasis is referred for evaluation of possible hypercortisolism. He has been experiencing weight gain, and his blood pressure has been more difficult to control than in the past. His primary care physician has considered the diagnosis of Cushing syndrome and ordered the following laboratory tests:

Serum cortisol after 1 mg of dexamethasone = 3.9 µg/dL (SI: 107.6 nmol/L)
Simultaneous ACTH = 15 pg/mL (10-60 pg/mL) (SI: 3.3 pmol/L [2.2-13.2 pmol/L])
Urinary free cortisol = 63 µg/24 h (4-50 µg/24 h) (SI: 173.9 nmol/d [11-138 nmol/d]) (volume = 1.7 L)

His medical history is remarkable for a seizure disorder since childhood and depression. His current medications include aspirin, 81 mg daily; alfuzosin, 10 mg daily; amlodipine, 10 mg daily; carbamazepine, 200 mg 3 times daily; fluoxetine, 20 mg daily; and an over-the-counter "prostate health supplement."

On physical examination, he is in no apparent distress. His blood pressure is 121/85 mm Hg, and pulse rate is 79 beats/min. His height is 69.5 in (176.5 cm), and weight is 304 lb (138 kg) (BMI = 44.2 kg/m²). His abdomen is protuberant, with some stretch marks.

Which of the following is the best next step in this patient's evaluation?
- A. Pituitary-directed MRI
- B. Two bedtime salivary cortisol measurements
- C. Adrenal-directed CT
- D. Another dexamethasone-suppression test after stopping the prostate supplement
- E. Low-dose dexamethasone-suppression test with measurement of 24-hour urinary cortisol excretion

ENDOCRINE SELF-ASSESSMENT PROGRAM 2022

Part II

1   **ANSWER: A) *HNF1A* (HNF1 homeobox A)**

In 2020, the American Diabetes Association and the European Association for the Study of Diabetes published a joint consensus statement that describes a roadmap to increasing precision in diabetes diagnosis and management. The consensus statement highlights the need to combine risk factor assessment, biomarker evaluation, and genomic assessment to develop an individualized description of a patient's diabetes. This approach is particularly important when considering monogenic causes of diabetes, as the etiology may affect management. In this patient with low BMI, multigenerational incidence of diabetes, and diagnosis of diabetes at a young age, a monogenic cause, such as maturity-onset diabetes of the young (MODY), should be considered. MODY is estimated to account for 2% to 3% of diabetes cases in children and young adults. Most cases of MODY (99%) involve pathogenic variants in 1 of the following 3 genes: *HNF1A*, *HNF4A*, and *GCK*. Of the pathogenic variants, 52% to 65% are in *HNF1A*, 15% to 32% are in *GCK*, and 10% are in *HNF4A*. It is difficult to identify the gene involved based solely on clinical characteristics. In the SEARCH for Diabetes in Youth study, patients who had diabetes diagnosed at an age younger than 20 years, negative antibody testing, and C-peptide levels greater than 0.8 ng/mL (>0.26 nmol/L) underwent DNA sequencing to look for pathogenic variants in these genes. Of the 47 cases of MODY identified this way, only 3 had been identified as having MODY based on clinical features.

Patients with MODY develop hyperglycemia due to abnormalities in β-cell development, function, and regulation. Insulin action in these individuals is normal. The clinical presentation can be variable, although some features may be seen with specific gene variants. For example, with *GCK* pathogenic variants, β-cell glucose sensing is affected, and there is a higher glucose threshold for insulin release. Individuals with *GCK* pathogenic variants do not have vascular complications. Patients with variants in *HNF1A* and *HNF4A* present in similar ways, with hyperglycemia and glucosuria. Pathogenic variants in *HNF1A* might be considered if an oral glucose load results in glucosuria. Patients with these variants can be treated with sulfonylureas early on, but they may require insulin over time and can develop diabetes-related complications.

In this vignette, the patient most likely has a pathogenic variant in the *HNF1A* gene (Answer A) because it is the most common etiology of MODY. In addition, his family members probably had MODY that was misdiagnosed as type 2 diabetes. His father has developed diabetic nephropathy, which is less likely to be associated with a *GCK* pathogenic variant (Answer C).

Pathogenic variants in *HNF1B* (Answer D), *PDX1* (Answer E), and *NEUROD1* (Answer B) are rare and much less likely to be the etiology in this patient. In addition, although the presentation can be variable, a person with an *HNF1B* pathogenic variant might present with evidence of abnormal kidney development or pancreatic atrophy, which is not the case in this vignette.

Educational Objective
Classify diabetes mellitus in a young patient with a low BMI.

Reference(s)
Pihoker C, Gilliam LK, Ellard S, et al; SEARCH for Diabetes in Youth Study Group. Prevalence, characteristics and clinical diagnosis of maturity onset diabetes of the young due to mutations in HNF1A, HNF4A, and glucokinase: results from the SEARCH for Diabetes in Youth. *J Clin Endocrinol Metab*. 2013;98(10):4055-4062. PMID: 23771925

Hattersley AT, Patel KA. Precision diabetes: learning from monogenic diabetes. *Diabetologia*. 2017;60(5):769-777. PMID: 28314945

2   **ANSWER: A) ACTH**

This patient has a pituitary macroadenoma with significant right parasellar extension, completely enveloping the intracavernous segment of the right carotid artery (*see image, yellow arrow*) (Knosp grade 4). The tumor also extends superiorly into the suprasellar cistern, but without compressing the optic chiasm (*see image, white dashed arrows*). The infundibulum is deviated to the left (*see image, white dotted arrow*), and the remaining normal pituitary gland is seen compressed against the medial wall of the left cavernous sinus (*see image, white solid arrows*).

T1 coronal (postcontrast)	T1 sagittal (postcontrast)	T2 sagittal
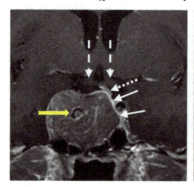	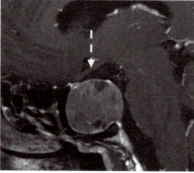	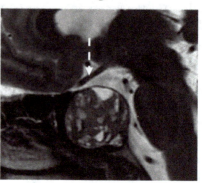

Although the pituitary adenoma is likely to have been an unexpected finding on the original CT, which was performed for investigation of headache, it is possible that the headache is related to the tumor. Several factors have been associated with a predisposition to headaches in patients with pituitary adenomas, including highly proliferative tumors, those exhibiting cavernous sinus invasion, and somatotroph adenomas. Pituitary adenoma–associated headache can mimic primary headache disorders, making recognition of an underlying secondary cause challenging. Migraine-like symptoms are the most common presentation. Unilateral headaches are usually ipsilateral to the side of cavernous sinus invasion.

Although this patient has a history of diabetes and hypertension, there are no other reported features to suggest an underlying diagnosis of acromegaly and her serum IGF-1 level is not elevated (in fact it is within the lower half of the reference range). Thus, the tumor is unlikely to be of somatotroph origin (Answer C).

The prolactin level is raised, but it is less than 3-fold the upper normal limit. Laboratory dilution studies confirm there is no evidence of the "hook effect." Therefore, given the size of the adenoma, this is very unlikely to be a lactotroph tumor (Answer D).

The thyroid biochemistry shows mild central hypothyroidism and is not therefore consistent with a TSH-secreting pituitary adenoma (Answer E).

Most clinically nonfunctioning pituitary adenomas are of gonadotrope origin, and they frequently demonstrate immunohistochemical positivity for FSH and/or LH (using staining for their respective β-subunits). Following changes to the recommendations for pathologic characterization of these tumors in the 2017 World Health Organization criteria, additional histochemical markers to define the lineage of the tumor based on transcription factor expression is recommended, and gonadotrope tumors express SF-1 (steroidogenic factor 1).

This patient has inappropriate postmenopausal gonadotropin levels and central hypothyroidism and is also likely to be GH deficient (although dynamic testing would be required to confirm the latter). The modest hyperprolactinemia is consistent with pituitary stalk compression. However, the laboratory results are unusual in that there appears to be good preservation of hypothalamic-pituitary-adrenal axis function (with very robust ACTH and cortisol levels). In addition, the T2 MRI appearances show multiple microcysts and macrocysts. Together, these findings point to a corticotrope tumor, which would be anticipated to demonstrate positive staining for ACTH (Answer A) and not FSH β-subunit (Answer B).

Silent corticotrope tumors present clinically as nonfunctional pituitary adenomas. However, subclinical ACTH-dependent hypercortisolism and/or subtle changes in cortisol dynamics (eg, loss of normal diurnal variation, failure to suppress serum cortisol following 1 mg dexamethasone) may be observed. Indeed, in the case reported here, the patient exhibited several clinical features that could be consistent with overt Cushing syndrome (type 2 diabetes, hypertension, obesity), and the surprisingly well-preserved serum cortisol in the face of anterior hypopituitarism should raise clinical suspicion.

Educational Objective

Explain that corticotrope pituitary macroadenomas may present with features related to local mass effect rather than overt hypercortisolism, and that preservation of hypothalamic-pituitary-adrenal axis function despite widespread anterior pituitary dysfunction is a clue to the diagnosis.

Reference(s)

Suri H, Dougherty C. Clinical presentation and management of headache in pituitary tumors. *Curr Pain Headache Rep.* 2018;22(8):55. PMID: 29904889

Vilar L, Vilar CF, Lyra R, Freitas MDC. Pitfalls in the diagnostic evaluation of hyperprolactinemia. *Neuroendocrinology.* 2019;109(1):7-19. PMID: 30889571

Mete O, Lopes BM. Overview of the 2017 WHO classification of pituitary tumors. *Endocr Pathol.* 2017;28(3):228-243. PMID: 28766057

Guttenberg KB, Mayson SE, Sawan C, et al. Prevalence of clinically silent corticotroph macroadenomas. *Clin Endocrinol (Oxf).* 2016;85(6):874-880. PMID: 27346850

Cazabat L, Dupuy M, Boulin A, et al. Silent, but not seen: multi microcystic aspect on T2-weighted MRI in silent corticotropin adenomas. *Clin Endocrinol (Oxf).* 2014;81(4):566-572. PMID: 24601912

3. ANSWER: E) Nonfunctioning adrenal adenoma

Adrenal incidentalomas are common and are identified on 4% to 7% of abdominal CT or MRI scans in patients older than 40 years. Most of these are truly incidental and not associated with endocrine dysfunction. However, it is important to adopt a systematic approach to assessment, and the clinician must answer 2 important questions: (1) could this be a primary (eg, adrenocortical carcinoma) or secondary (eg, metastasis) malignant tumor? and (2) is the lesion functioning?

With modern imaging techniques (triple-phase CT, in-phase and out-of-phase MRI), most adrenal incidentalomas are readily classified as benign adrenal adenomas. In this case, the identification of a 2.8-cm homogeneous adrenal mass does not raise concerns on the basis of size alone, and the Hounsfield unit measurement of 8 is consistent with a lipid-rich adrenocortical adenoma. Therefore, an adrenocortical carcinoma (Answer A) is very unlikely. The radiologic findings are also not suggestive of adrenal metastasis (Answer D).

While some clinicians recommend measurement of plasma free metanephrines or 24-hour urinary fractionated metanephrines to exclude a pheochromocytoma in all cases of adrenal incidentalomas, recent case series suggest that if the imaging assessment clearly demonstrates features of an adrenocortical adenoma, then this assessment is not necessary unless other clinical concerns dictate.

In the setting of adrenal incidentaloma, primary aldosteronism is important to exclude in any patient with hypertension and/or hypokalemia (provoked or unprovoked). This is conventionally undertaken through measurement of paired plasma aldosterone concentration and plasma renin activity or direct renin concentration. Ideally, these measurements should be conducted in the absence of confounding medications. Recently, 24-hour urinary aldosterone measurement with appropriate oral salt loading has been proposed as a more sensitive test for the detection of primary aldosteronism.

A 1-mg overnight dexamethasone-suppression test is typically used to screen for hypercortisolism in patients with adrenal incidentalomas. In this vignette, the postdexamethasone cortisol value is above the traditional threshold for excluding autonomous hypercortisolism (<1.8 µg/dL [<50 nmol/L]) and merits further investigation. Clinical features of hypercortisolism may be subtle or even absent in the presence of a cortisol-secreting adrenal adenoma (Answer B). However, in this case, both plasma ACTH and serum DHEA-S are clearly measurable and not suggestive of hypothalamic-pituitary-adrenal axis suppression, making a cortisol-secreting adrenal adenoma less likely. Indeed, if there were clinical concern of possible Cushing syndrome, then an ACTH-dependent cause would need to be considered (Answers C or D) (provided that laboratory assay interference has been excluded and plasma ACTH is not suppressed).

In this context, and before embarking on a more extensive investigation, it is important to pause and consider conditions that can be associated with a false-positive result on dexamethasone-suppression testing, including obesity, depression, alcohol excess, oral estrogen therapy (which raises cortisol-binding globulin and hence total serum cortisol levels), and enzyme-inducing agents (eg, carbamazepine, which increases dexamethasone clearance). None of these were relevant in this patient. However, it is increasingly recognized that some individuals are naturally fast metabolizers of dexamethasone. Ueland and colleagues recently demonstrated abnormal serum cortisol in study participants without Cushing syndrome in whom serum dexamethasone levels at 8 AM were low following 1 mg of dexamethasone given the previous evening at 11 PM. Accordingly, measurement of serum dexamethasone on the same sample can aid interpretation of the postdexamethasone serum cortisol value, with a serum dexamethasone concentration greater than 3.3 nmol/L deemed sufficient for the suppression of serum cortisol.

On repeat testing, this patient was found to have a detectable, but suboptimal, serum dexamethasone concentration, rendering the test invalid for the purpose of excluding hypercortisolism. This finding was also consistent with the nonsuppressed plasma ACTH and DHEA-S (DHEA-S synthesis is ACTH dependent, and if serum DHEA-S had been subnormal/suppressed, then this would have been a possible pointer to autonomous ACTH-independent cortisol secretion). Subsequent testing with 24-hour urinary free cortisol and late-night salivary cortisol measurements also excluded hypercortisolism, and the patient was therefore deemed to have a nonfunctioning adrenal adenoma (Answer E). Nonfunctioning adenomas account for most adrenal incidentalomas in published series.

Educational Objective
List potential limitations of first-line screening tests for adrenal autonomy in cases of adrenal incidentaloma.

Reference(s)
Fassnacht M, Arlt W, Bancos I, et al. Management of adrenal incidentalomas: European Society of Endocrinology clinical practice guideline in collaboration with the European Network for the Study of Adrenal Tumors. *Eur J Endocrinol.* 2016;175(2):G1-G34. PMID: 27390021

Ueland GA, Methlie P, Kellman R, et al. Simultaneous assay of cortisol and dexamethasone improved diagnostic accuracy of the dexamethasone suppression test. *Eur J Endocrinol.* 2017;176(6):705-713. PMID: 28298353

Dennedy MC, Annamalai AK, Prankerd-Smith O, et al. Low DHEAS: a sensitive and specific test for the detection of subclinical hypercortisolism in adrenal incidentalomas. *J Clin Endocrinol Metab.* 2017;102(3):786-792. PMID: 27797672

4 ANSWER: C) Bempedoic acid

Bempedoic acid (Answer C) is a new cholesterol-lowering agent that reduces cholesterol synthesis through inhibition of adenosine triphosphate citrate lyase, an enzyme upstream of HMG-CoA reductase in the cholesterol synthesis pathway. Bempedoic acid is a prodrug that is converted to its CoA-activated form by the very long-chain acyl-CoA synthetase 1. In the United States, this nonstatin LDL cholesterol–lowering agent is approved for use as an adjunct to diet in patients with atherosclerotic cardiovascular disease or heterozygous familial hypercholesterolemia who, despite taking maximally tolerated statin dosages, do not achieve the desired LDL-cholesterol target concentration. Bempedoic acid has been approved as monotherapy (180 mg tablet once daily) and as a fixed-dose combination with ezetimibe (bempedoic acid, 180 mg/ezetimibe, 10 mg once daily).

The Clear Harmony Trial was a phase 3 randomized, placebo-controlled trial that included patients with atherosclerotic cardiovascular disease, heterozygous familial hypercholesterolemia, or both who were already on maximally tolerated statin therapy. A 12.6% reduction in LDL cholesterol was observed in the bempedoic acid group compared with a 1% increase in the placebo group. Another phase 3 randomized controlled clinical trial compared the LDL-cholesterol lowering of the fixed-dose combination of bempedoic acid and ezetimibe with that of bempedoic acid, ezetimibe, or placebo in patients with high risk of cardiovascular disease who were receiving maximally tolerated statin therapy after 12 weeks of therapy. This study showed a 36% decrease in LDL cholesterol in the group taking the fixed-dose combination of bempedoic acid and ezetimibe, 17% decrease in the bempedoic acid group, 23% decrease in the ezetimibe group, and 2% increase in the placebo group. The most frequently reported adverse effects for bempedoic acid monotherapy included hyperuricemia, gout, thrombocytopenia, leukopenia, and upper respiratory tract infections.

The patient in this vignette is a candidate for a nonstatin LDL-cholesterol–lowering medication to decrease his risk of another cardiovascular event, as he has atherosclerotic cardiovascular disease and his LDL-cholesterol concentration is not at goal on the maximum tolerated statin dosage. LDL-cholesterol goals vary according to which guideline is followed. In this case, the patient's goal is less than 70 mg/dL (<1.81 mmol/L) (following the American Heart Association/American College of Cardiology recommendations), as he has atherosclerotic cardiovascular disease. Given the options provided, bempedoic acid is the best choice. Another option for this patient could be a PCSK9 inhibitor such as evolocumab or alirocumab.

Colesevelam (Answer B) is a bile acid sequestrant. It lowers LDL cholesterol by decreasing the hepatic bile acid pool, which leads to an increase in hepatic bile acid synthesis from cholesterol. The usual dosage is three 625-mg tablets twice daily. In combination with statins, it can decrease LDL cholesterol by 10% to 16%. The most frequent adverse effects are constipation, dyspepsia, nausea, and increasing triglycerides. This patient has irritable bowel syndrome, so colesevelam would not be the first choice, as it could affect his gastrointestinal disease.

Niacin (Answer A) is also known as vitamin B_3. It decreases LDL cholesterol by decreasing release of fatty acids from adipose tissue, which leads to a decrease in VLDL secretion and therefore a decrease in LDL cholesterol. The recommended dosage is 1500 mg at bedtime. The most frequent adverse effects are flushing, increased values on liver function tests, hyperglycemia, hyperuricemia, and gastrointestinal discomfort. This patient has prediabetes, and adding niacin could worsen his glycemic control. Also, niacin is no longer approved in the United States as an adjunct to statins due to the lack of evidence that it reduces the risk of cardiovascular disease.

Fenofibrate (Answer D) and icosapent ethyl (Answer E) are triglyceride-lowering agents, not LDL-cholesterol–lowering agents. This patient needs further LDL-cholesterol reduction and neither of these medications would achieve this. A randomized controlled trial that included patients with cardiovascular disease or diabetes with other risk factors who were on statin therapy and had elevated triglycerides (135-499 mg/dL [1.52-5.64 mmol/L]) showed that high dosages of icosapent ethyl reduced the primary endpoint, which was a composite of cardiovascular death, nonfatal myocardial infarction, nonfatal stroke, coronary revascularization, or unstable angina. The patient in this vignette is not a candidate for icosapent ethyl for this indication (cardiovascular event risk reduction) because his triglycerides are normal.

Educational Objective
List the indications for prescribing bempedoic acid.

Reference(s)
Markham A. Bempedoic acid: first approval. *Drugs.* 2020;80(7):747-753. PMID: 32314225

Ray KK, Bays HE, Catapano AL, et al. Safety and efficacy of bempedoic acid to reduce LDL cholesterol. *N Engl J Med.* 2019;380(11):1022-1032. PMID: 30865796

Ballantyne CM, Laufs U, Ray KK, et al. Bempedoic acid plus ezetimibe fixed-dose combination in patients with hypercholesterolemia and high CVD risk treated with maximally tolerated statin therapy. *Eur J Prev Cardiol.* 2020;27(6):593-603. PMID: 31357887

Grundy SM, Stone NJ, Bailey AL, et al. 2018 AHA/ACC/AACVPR/AAPA/ABC/ACPM/ADA/AGS/APhA/ASPC/NLA/PCNA Guideline on the management of blood cholesterol: a report of the American College of Cardiology/American Heart Association Task Force on Clinical Practice Guidelines. *Circulation.* 2019;139(25):e1082-e1143. PMID: 30586774

Bhatt DL, Steg PG, Miller M, et al; REDUCE-IT Investigators. Cardiovascular risk reduction with icosapent ethyl for hypertriglyceridemia. *N Engl J Med.* 2019;380(1):11-22. PMID: 30415628

5 ANSWER: E) Continue denosumab

Osteonecrosis of the jaw (ONJ) is defined as exposed necrotic bone in the maxillofacial region that does not heal after 8 weeks in patients with no history of craniofacial radiation. It appears as areas of exposed yellow or white hard bone with smooth or ragged borders. Risk factors for developing ONJ include dosage and duration of exposure to bisphosphonate therapy, intravenous administration of bisphosphonate therapy, glucocorticoids, cancer and anticancer therapy, cigarette smoking, poorly fitting dentures, invasive dental procedures, and preexisting dental disease. A revised ONJ staging system was recommended in the 2014 guidelines published by the American Association of Oral and Maxillofacial Surgeons (*see table*). ONJ is extremely uncommon with osteoporosis therapy and can be treated if it occurs.

Table. Staging System for ONJ

Stage of ONJ	Findings
Stage 0	Nonspecific clinical findings with no exposed bone
Stage 1 (mild)	Exposed bone with no symptoms and no infection
Stage 2 (moderate)	Exposed bone with infection
Stage 3 (severe)	Exposed bone with infection and ≥1 of the following: • Exposed and necrotic bone extending beyond the region of alveolar bone resulting in pathologic fracture • Extraoral fistula • Oral antral or oral nasal communication • Osteolysis extending to inferior border of the mandible or sinus floor

Adapted from Ruggiero SL, Dodson TB, Fantasia J, et al; American Association of Oral and Maxillofacial Surgeons. American Association of Oral and Maxillofacial Surgeons position paper on medication-related osteonecrosis of the jaw--2014 update. J Oral Maxillofac Surg. 2014;72(10):1938-1956.

This postmenopausal woman has osteoporosis in the setting of stage 1 (mild) ONJ after 2 years of zoledronic acid treatment and 1 year of denosumab treatment. She has had an improvement in her bone mineral density after 1 year of denosumab with no fragility fractures, indicating a good response to her current therapy. Denosumab, which is a fully human monoclonal antibody to the receptor activator of nuclear factor kappaB ligand (RANKL), reduces osteoclast formation, function, and survival, resulting in decreased bone resorption and increased bone density. The Fracture Reduction Evaluation of Denosumab in Osteoporosis Every 6 Months (FREEDOM) trial reported no cases of ONJ in either the denosumab or placebo group over 3 years. There were 13 adjudicated cases of ONJ in the 7-year open-label FREEDOM extension trial, most of which occurred after a reported invasive oral procedure and healed with appropriate dental treatment, despite ongoing denosumab therapy in most cases. Therefore, continuing denosumab (Answer E) would be the most appropriate option at this time. Simply discontinuing denosumab (Answer A) or delaying the dose would not be a good choice, since data have raised concern that this would result in rapid bone loss and a subsequent increase in vertebral fracture risk.

Raloxifene is a selective estrogen receptor modulator approved for the treatment of postmenopausal osteoporosis. However, it is considered a second-line agent because it only decreases the risk of vertebral fractures and has no effect on hip or other nonvertebral fracture risk. Although there has been no link between ONJ and raloxifene, switching to this agent (Answer B) would not be the best choice in this patient who is at high risk of future fracture, especially given her low T-scores at the hips. Similar to estrogen, safety concerns with raloxifene include an increased risk of venous thromboembolism.

Switching to abaloparatide (Answer C), a PTHrP analogue used as an osteoanabolic agent in the treatment of osteoporosis, would also not be appropriate in this case since the patient has already been treated with teriparatide for 2 years in the past. Both teriparatide and abaloparatide have a black box warning for potential risk of osteosarcoma, and their cumulative use is limited to 2 years in a lifetime. Contraindications to their use include history of skeletal irradiation, Paget disease of bone, or unexplained elevation in alkaline phosphatase. Of note, teriparatide may promote ONJ healing (off-label use), but limited data support its efficacy. It is important to also mention the DATA-Switch study, which showed that switching from denosumab to teriparatide in postmenopausal women with osteoporosis resulted in transient or progressive bone loss; therefore, this sequence of therapies is generally not advised.

Romosozumab is a monoclonal antibody to sclerostin, an endogenous inhibitor of bone formation. In 2019, the US FDA approved romosozumab for the treatment of postmenopausal osteoporosis. ONJ has also been reported with the use of romosozumab. Thus, there is limited advantage in switching from denosumab to romosozumab (Answer D) in such a case. Furthermore, romosozumab has a black box warning of the potential risk of myocardial infarction, stroke, and cardiovascular death and should not be initiated in patients who have had a myocardial infarction or stroke within the preceding year. Since this patient had a myocardial infarction 6 months ago, switching to romosozumab would not be appropriate at this time.

Educational Objective
Recommend the most appropriate intervention in a patient who develops osteonecrosis of the jaw while on denosumab therapy.

Reference(s)
Watts NB, Grbic JT, Binkley N, et al. Invasive oral procedures and events in postmenopausal women with osteoporosis treated with denosumab for up to 10 years. *J Clin Endocrinol Metab.* 2019;104(6):2443-2452. PMID: 30759221

Ruggiero SL, Dodson TB, Fantasia J, et al; American Association of Oral and Maxillofacial Surgeons. American Association of Oral and Maxillofacial Surgeons position paper on medication-related osteonecrosis of the jaw--2014 update. *J Oral Maxillofac Surg.* 2014;72(10):1938-1956. PMID: 25234529

Khan AA, Morrison A, Hanley DA, et al; International Task Force on Osteonecrosis of the Jaw. Diagnosis and management of osteonecrosis of the jaw: a systematic review and international consensus. *J Bone Miner Res.* 2015;30(1):3-23. PMID: 25414052

Tymlos (abaloparatide) prescribing information. Available at: https://www.accessdata.fda.gov/drugsatfda_docs/label/2017/208743lbl.pdf

Forteo (teriparatide) prescribing information. Available at: https://www.accessdata.fda.gov/drugsatfda_docs/label/2020/021318s053lbl.pdf

Leder BZ, Tsai JN, Uihlein AV, et al. Denosumab and teriparatide transitions in postmenopausal osteoporosis (the DATA-Switch study): extension of a randomised controlled trial. *Lancet.* 2015;386(9999):1147-1155. PMID: 26144908

6
ANSWER: D) Increase metformin dosage to 1000 mg twice daily and add basal insulin

Hyperglycemia and diabetes-related emergency department encounters are common and account for approximately 1% of emergency department visits. Unless a patient has diabetic ketoacidosis or hyperosmolar coma, the benefits of sending a patient to the emergency department have not been shown. Acute lowering of hyperglycemia in the emergency setting does not improve outcomes without a long-term glycemic management plan in place. Thus, sending this patient to the emergency department for fluids and acute glucose management (Answer A) would be a common clinical decision, but it is incorrect.

This patient would be better served by initiating outpatient medication therapy to combat his severe hyperglycemia. In the setting of symptomatic hyperglycemia, insulin initiation is recommended (thus, Answer D is correct and Answers B, C, and E are incorrect). Hyperglycemia causing polyuria, polydipsia, and especially weight loss should be treated with insulin. Although increasing the metformin dosage or adding sitagliptin or glimepiride may decrease glucose levels, use of these agents will not reverse the catabolic state. Basal insulin should be initiated to suppress hepatic glucose production, stimulate glucose uptake by muscle and fat, and reduce ketogenesis and risk for diabetic ketoacidosis. This patient has multiple indications for initiating insulin, including a glucose concentration greater than 300 mg/dL (>16.7 mmol/L), a hemoglobin A_{1c} value greater than 10.0% (>86 mmol/mol), and evidence of an ongoing catabolic state (weight loss).

The next decision is what dosage of insulin to introduce. The goal is to improve hyperglycemia but not significantly increase the risk of hypoglycemia. The American Diabetes Association guidelines recommend 0.1 to 0.2 units/kg, which is a conservative starting dosage. However, given this patient's hemoglobin A_{1c} value greater than 10.0% (>86 mmol/mol), obesity, normal renal function, and significant hyperglycemia, he would be better served with a higher starting dosage. The American Association of Clinical Endocrinology recommends a starting dosage of 0.2 to 0.3 units/kg in the setting of a hemoglobin A_{1c} value greater than 8.0% (>64 mmol/mol). Thus, a starting dosage of 0.3 units/kg would be appropriate for this patient.

The final caveat of this case is that once evidence of catabolism has resolved and glycemia has improved, one must consider minimizing or replacing insulin with an insulin-sparing agent such as a GLP-1 receptor agonist or an SGLT-2 inhibitor given the associated lower risk for hypoglycemia, greater potential for weight loss, and potential for cardiovascular benefit. Revaluation of the management plan at every visit is an important component of diabetes management and patient partnership.

Educational Objective
Recommend initiation of insulin therapy for a patient with symptomatic hyperglycemia.

Reference(s)

Driver BE, Klein LR, Cole JB, Prekker ME, Fagerstrom ET, Miner JR. Comparison of two glycemic discharge goals in ED patients with hyperglycemia, a randomized trial. *Am J Emerg Med.* 2019;37(7):1295-1300. PMID: 30316635

Wang Z, Hedrington MS, Gogitidze Joy N, et al. Dose-response effects of insulin glargine in type 2 diabetes. *Diabetes Care.* 2010;33(7):1555-1560. PMID: 20357371

American Diabetes Association. 9. Pharmacologic approaches to glycemic treatment: standards of medical care in diabetes-2020. *Diabetes Care.* 2020;43(Suppl 1):S98-S110. PMID: 31862752

Garber AJ, Handelsman Y, Grunberger G, et al. Consensus statement by the American Association of Clinical Endocrinologists and American College of Endocrinology on the Comprehensive type 2 diabetes management algorithm-2020 executive summary. *Endocr Pract.* 2020;26(1):107-139. PMID: 32022600

7 ANSWER: B) Take a careful drug and supplement history

This patient presents with typical features of anabolic steroid abuse, which is often not readily disclosed by patients. Even close partners may not be aware of this habit. Therefore, taking a careful drug history (Answer B) that includes direct questioning in a nonjudgmental manner, and, if appropriate, in the absence of the patient's partner, is the best next step. Many commercial laboratories offer urine anabolic steroid testing, but the ethics of ordering such testing without informing the patient are highly debatable. Moreover, anabolic steroid testing is not standardized across laboratories, and diagnostic precision is uncertain. Patients can easily avoid detection by temporarily pausing anabolic steroid use or by providing someone else's urine sample. In addition, these individuals often take multiple drugs, sometimes in an effort to prevent adverse effects of others, and this can confound laboratory testing and make the biochemical diagnosis challenging. Therefore, in clinical practice, the best "diagnostic test" remains to ask the patient directly.

While precise epidemiologic data are difficult to establish, the lifetime prevalence of anabolic steroid use among men in the general population is approximately 1% to 5%. Users often pursue a muscular physique to improve body image, and they may have underlying psychiatric disease, including muscle dysmorphia (or reverse anorexia nervosa), a condition now recognized in the *Diagnostic and Statistical Manual of Mental Disorders* (*DSM-5*). Men who abuse anabolic steroids may take other performance-enhancing drugs (eg, GH, T_4, hCG, or insulin) or classic drugs of abuse such as opioids.

Men who abuse anabolic steroids are typically in their 20s to 30s, appear muscular, and, with long-term use, have small, atrophic testes due to the suppressive effect of exogenous anabolic steroids on spermatogenesis. Of note, a normal testicular volume does not rule out anabolic steroid use. For example, testicular volume could be normal if anabolic steroid use has commenced recently and/or if hCG is coadministered. Men taking anabolic steroids may have azoospermia when evaluated for infertility. Acne involving the upper back and midline chest is virtually pathognomonic. Other adverse effects include painful gynecomastia (often mitigated by concomitant use of antiestrogens, such as aromatase inhibitors), male-pattern hair loss, and tendon injuries, especially upper-extremity tendinous ruptures. Exogenous anabolic steroids have also been associated with cardiovascular toxicity and a variety of neuropsychiatric effects. While testosterone itself is not hepatotoxic, alkylated testosterone derivatives, especially when taken orally, have been associated with liver injury, including cholestasis, hepatic peliosis, and liver tumors.

If synthetic nontestosterone anabolic steroids (eg, nandrolone, danazol) are abused, typical biochemical abnormalities include suppressed gonadotropins and serum testosterone because these synthetic anabolic steroids are not detected by standard testosterone assays. If exogenous testosterone is abused, measured serum testosterone will be high (unless a testosterone formulation with a short half-life has been stopped prior to the blood draw) and gonadotropins will be suppressed. Due to the erythropoietic actions of anabolic steroids, other typical biochemical features include polycythemia and a low SHBG level because they suppress SHBG production—these features are evident in the presented vignette. HDL cholesterol is typically low.

Given that this patient presented with classic features of anabolic steroid abuse, which explains the suppressed gonadotropins, performing a pituitary-directed MRI (Answer A) is not the best next step. The small testicular size is explained by the drug abuse, so there is no need to pursue testicular ultrasonography (Answer C) unless a testicular tumor is suspected clinically. There is no suspicion of an hCG-producing tumor, which would be associated with normal or increased serum testosterone, so measurement of hCG (Answer D) is incorrect. Of note, some men who use anabolic steroids may abuse hCG, but random hCG measurement to diagnose potential hCG abuse is not recommended. DHEA-S is an adrenal androgenic precursor with weak androgen receptor–stimulating properties; there is no suspicion of endogenous adrenal androgen excess and DHEA-S measurement (Answer E) is therefore not indicated.

While high-level data in this field are lacking, some users of anabolic steroids appear to develop an "androgen dependence syndrome," and dependency becomes a motivator for continued abuse despite adverse medical or psychosocial effects. If steroid use is stopped, some men experience a variety of neuropsychiatric withdrawal symptoms, leading to recidivism. Especially with long-term abuse, even if anabolic steroids are stopped successfully, gonadal axis suppression may persist for months or longer. A recent cross-sectional case-control study comparing current and past anabolic steroid abusers with healthy control participants reported that current abusers had suppressed reproductive function and impaired cardiac systolic function and lipoprotein parameters (lower HDL cholesterol, higher triglycerides, and reduced cholesterol efflux capacity) compared with healthy control participants or past users. For past users, the mean time to recovery was 11 months for LH and 14 months for sperm variables. Longer duration of androgen abuse was associated with slower recovery of sperm output.

Management of men who use anabolic steroids but are willing to stop is complex and controversial. Some authorities recommend a supportive approach, providing education and reassurance that reactivation of the endogenous gonadal axis should occur eventually, with regular biochemical monitoring, and not prescribing hormonal treatment. If fertility is not desired, some experts prescribe testosterone with a clearly defined "taper and no refill without follow-up visits" approach to mitigate withdrawal symptoms. If fertility is desired and there is some urgency (eg, female partner aged 30 to 35 years or older), some authorities prescribe selective estrogen modulators such as clomiphene or hCG in an attempt to hasten endogenous gonadal axis recovery (and hence spermatogenesis). However, with the exception of anecdotal case reports, there is no firm evidence to support such an approach. Of note, clomiphene may increase the risk of venous thrombosis. If clomiphene is considered, patients should be advised regarding this risk.

Educational Objective
Identify and manage anabolic steroid abuse.

Reference(s)
Shankara-Narayana N, Yu C, Savkovic S, et al. Rate and extent of recovery from reproductive and cardiac dysfunction due to androgen abuse in men. *J Clin Endocrinol Metab.* 2020;105(6):dgz324. PMID: 32030409

Anawalt BD. Diagnosis and management of anabolic androgenic steroid use. *J Clin Endocrinol Metab.* 2019;104(7):2490-2500. PMID: 30753550

8
ANSWER: D) Referral to physical therapy for acute fracture management

Osteoporosis is a significant public health problem that results in considerable morbidity and mortality. Indeed, fractures due to osteoporosis number approximately 2 million each year within the United States alone, resulting in roughly 2.5 million visits to health care professionals. Although not conferring the same degree of mortality as hip fractures, vertebral fractures are the most common osteoporotic fracture (~700,000 per year). While approximately two-thirds of vertebral fractures are identified incidentally by radiograph, approximately one-third present with acute pain that is often severe and debilitating. Vertebral fractures are classified as mild, moderate, or severe (20%-25%, 25%-40%, or >40% height loss, respectively, of the anterior, mid, or posterior vertebral body), with evidence that a greater degree of compression predicts a higher risk of subsequent fracture. Severe back pain due to vertebral fractures, which generally lasts 4 to 6 weeks followed by gradual improvement over time, can usually be treated with antiinflammatory medications such as ibuprofen or naproxen. Patients with more severe pain may be candidates for the brief use of short-acting narcotics, although extended-release narcotics should be avoided due to the limited duration of severe pain and the potential for tolerance and addiction. Thus, prescribing oxycodone (Answer C) is incorrect. Calcitonin nasal spray (Answer E) may have some analgesic benefit in patients with vertebral fractures based on limited evidence, although it is not appropriate for this patient with a history of fish allergy.

In patients who experience acute vertebral fractures, individualized physical therapy (Answer D) can be beneficial to their postfracture care. Specifically, exercises that address thoracolumbar extensor muscle strengthening can reduce the amount of axial loading to the vertebral body by increasing the cross-sectional area of the paraspinal muscles. Physical therapy following a vertebral fracture can also improve physical function (measured by the metric Timed Up and Go) and may also improve quality of life, although the overall effect of exercise on pain and physical function is less certain. Spinal bracing with orthotics such as lumbosacral or thoracolumbosacral orthoses, which was not offered as a choice in this vignette, may provide some short-term benefit to patients, although extensive and/or prolonged use may induce paraspinal muscle weakness and therefore paradoxically increase the risk for additional vertebral fractures. In addition, patients should not become completely inactive or adopt extended bed rest (Answer B) because of concerns over both paraspinal and global weakness or an attendant increase in risk for falls and fracture.

Finally, although intuitively attractive, vertebral augmentation with or without concomitant balloon inflation (kyphoplasty and vertebroplasty, respectively) (Answer A), may acutely attenuate pain in patients with a painful vertebral fracture. Importantly, however, existing evidence does not support the routine use of this procedure. A recent Cochrane review showed no clinically demonstrable benefit vs a placebo sham procedure. This lack of clear benefit was also independent of the duration of pain (less than or greater than 6 weeks). Additionally, the risk of serious complications due to epidural cement leak (nerve root compression, osteomyelitis, cement pulmonary embolism), as well as a possible risk for fractures of adjacent vertebrae, necessarily limits its clinical utility to those patients with persistent, refractory back pain and MRI evidence of lack of healing for greater than 8 to 10 weeks. Give the paucity of high-level evidence to date, however, the American Society for Bone and Mineral Research has recommended cessation of the procedures until randomized controlled trials confirm a true benefit.

Educational Objective
Recommend appropriate management for a patient with an acute osteoporotic vertebral fracture.

Reference(s)
Gibbs JC, MacIntyre NJ, Ponzano M, et al. Exercise for improving outcomes after osteoporotic vertebral fracture. *Cochrane Database Syst Rev.* 2019;7(7):CD008618. PMID: 31273764

Buchbinder R, Johnston RV, Rischin KJ, et al. Percutaneous vertebroplasty for osteoporotic vertebral compression fracture. *Cochrane Database Syst Rev.* 2018;11(11):CD006349. PMID: 30399208

Brown DB, Glaiberman CB, Gilula LA, Shimony JS. Correlation between preprocedural MRI findings and clinical outcomes in the treatment of chronic symptomatic vertebral compression fractures with percutaneous vertebroplasty. *AJR Am J Roentgenol.* 2005;184(6):1951-1955. PMID: 15908560

9 ANSWER: B) Thyroid ultrasonography again in 12 months
Thyroid nodules are very common and most are benign. Thyroid nodules can be palpable during physical examination or found incidentally on imaging studies such as neck ultrasonography, CT, MRI, PET, or carotid ultrasonography. Serum TSH should be measured during the initial evaluation of a patient with a thyroid nodule to assess the patient's thyroid status. Risk factors, including radiation exposure to the head and neck and family history of thyroid cancer, increase the risk of thyroid cancer in a patient with a known thyroid nodule. Despite increased incidence of a thyroid cancer diagnosis, mortality remains low. The presence of suspicious sonographic features is more predictive of malignancy than is thyroid nodule size. FNA biopsy should be performed if a thyroid nodule is larger than 1 cm and has 1 or more of the following suspicious sonographic features: solid composition, hypoechogenicity, irregular margins, taller-than-wide shape, extrathyroidal extension, and microcalcifications. Certain sonographic features, such as a cystic or spongiform appearance, suggest a benign condition that does not require FNA biopsy until a certain size is achieved. The risk of malignancy based on sonographic features is detailed in the 2015 American Thyroid Association management guidelines for adult patients with thyroid nodules and differentiated thyroid cancer (*see table 1*).

Table 1. Risk of Thyroid Malignancy Based on Sonographic Features

Nodules	Sonographic features	FNA biopsy	Estimated risk for malignancy
Benign	Purely cystic nodule	Not indicated	<1%
Very low suspicion	Spongiform or partially cystic nodules with no suspicious sonographic features	≥2 cm	<3%
Low suspicion	Isoechoic nodule, hyperechoic solid nodule, or partially cystic nodule with eccentric solid areas, with no suspicious sonographic features	≥1.5 cm	5%-10%
Intermediate suspicion	Hypoechoic solid nodule with no suspicious sonographic features	≥1 cm	10%-20%
High suspicion	Solid hypoechoic nodule or solid hypoechoic component of a partially cystic nodule with 1 or more suspicious sonographic features	≥1 cm	>70%-90%

Adapted from Haugen BR, Alexander EK, Bible KC, et al. 2015 American Thyroid Association management guidelines for adult patients with thyroid nodules and differentiated thyroid cancer: the American Thyroid Association Guidelines Task Force on Thyroid Nodules and Differentiated Thyroid Cancer. Thyroid. 2016;26(1):1-133.

Spongiform and other mixed cystic solid nodules may exhibit bright reflectors on ultrasonography. This is caused by colloid crystals or posterior acoustic enhancement of the back wall of a microcystic area. Less experienced sonographers and endocrinologists may interpret these findings as microcalcifications. It is well established that operator experience is correlated with accurate evaluation of internal calcifications.

In addition to the 2015 American Thyroid Association management guidelines for adult patients with thyroid nodules and differentiated thyroid cancer, the American College of Radiology has developed the Thyroid Imaging, Reporting, and Data System (TI-RADS), which also provides guidance regarding management of thyroid nodules on the basis of their sonographic appearance. The TI-RADS calculator is available online, and it requires information about composition, echogenicity, shape, margin, and echogenic foci of each nodule. Each category is assigned points (0 to 3) depending on the answer provided, and the total point value correlates to a TI-RADS score. Based on the TI-RADS score, FNA biopsy may be recommended. The introduction of TI-RADS score has been a helpful tool in the management of thyroid nodules. The 5 TI-RADS scores (TR 1, TR 2, TR 3, TR 4, and TR 5) are shown in table 2.

Table 2. Thyroid Imaging, Reporting, and Data System Scoring

TI-RADS score	Nodule	FNA biopsy
TR 1	Benign	Not indicated
TR 2	Not suspicious	Not indicated
TR 3	Mildly suspicious	If nodule ≥2.5 cm
TR 4	Moderately suspicious	If nodule ≥1.5 cm
TR 5	Highly suspicious	If nodule ≥1 cm

The patient in this vignette has a cystic nodule with comet tail artifact (*see image, arrow*), which is a benign finding. This is a colloid nodule. According to the 2015 American Thyroid Association management guidelines for adult patients with thyroid nodules and differentiated thyroid cancer and the TI-RADS calculator (TR 1), FNA biopsy (Answer A) is not recommended. This nodule can be monitored with repeated thyroid ultrasonography in 12 months (Answer B). FNA biopsy would only be indicated if there is sonographic evidence of growth (more than a 50% change in volume or 20% increase in at least 2 nodule dimensions with a minimal increase of 2 mm) or development of new suspicious sonographic features. Diagnostic FNA biopsy is not required for purely cystic thyroid nodules, but aspiration may be necessary if a cyst is large and symptomatic. Cytology should be obtained if aspiration is performed.

There is no indication for alcohol ablation now (Answer E). Alcohol ablation (ethanol ablation) is indicated in the management of benign recurrent purely cystic or predominantly cystic nodules causing pressure symptoms, hyperfunctioning thyroid nodules, and local recurrent thyroid cancer. However, alcohol ablation is not widely used in the United States.

This patient's dysphagia cannot be explained by her thyroid nodule based on its size and location. Therefore, there is no need to order neck CT (Answer C) or barium esophagography (Answer D) to evaluate her dysphagia at this time. Her difficulty swallowing happens when she takes calcium and metformin, both of which are large tablets that can affect swallowing in many individuals. In addition, she has had no weight loss. However, if her difficulty swallowing continues and she experiences problems swallowing solid food and/or liquid, further evaluation is warranted.

Educational Objective
Identify the sonographic characteristics of a colloid nodule, including recognition of the comet tail.

Reference(s)
Haugen BR, Alexander EK, Bible KC, et al. 2015 American Thyroid Association management guidelines for adult patients with thyroid nodules and differentiated thyroid cancer: the American Thyroid Association Guidelines Task Force on Thyroid Nodules and Differentiated Thyroid Cancer. *Thyroid.* 2016;26(1):1-133. PMID: 26462967

Tessler FN, Middleton WD, Grant EG, et al. ACR Thyroid Imaging, Reporting and Data System (TI-RADS): white paper of the ACR TI-RADS Committee. *J Am Coll Radiol.* 2017;14(5):587-595. PMID: 28372962

10 ANSWER: E) Pioglitazone

Nonalcoholic fatty liver disease (NAFLD) is estimated to be present in 10% to 56% of persons with type 2 diabetes. The condition can range from steatosis alone to steatosis with hepatic inflammation, hepatocyte injury, and fibrosis. When changes beyond simple steatosis are noted, the condition is termed nonalcoholic steatohepatitis (NASH). NAFLD/NASH are the leading causes of chronic liver disease in developed countries and are associated with an increased risk of cirrhosis and hepatocellular carcinoma. Individuals with NAFLD are also at increased risk for cardiovascular disease. Although increasing attention has been given to addressing NAFLD in patients with type 2 diabetes, a number of issues in diagnosis and management remain.

Transaminase levels can be normal in patients with NAFLD. Ultrasonography, CT, and MR spectroscopy may be needed to identify steatosis. Noninvasive algorithms (such as the Fibrosis-4 [FIB-4] index score) based on metabolic characteristics can also help identify patients at risk for fibrosis, although these algorithms are not very sensitive. Vibration-controlled transient elastography and MR spectroscopy are more sensitive noninvasive ways to identify patients at risk for fibrosis. Liver biopsy is currently considered the gold standard for assessment of NAFLD/NASH.

Based on current expert opinion, when NAFLD/NASH is identified by noninvasive methods, lifestyle intervention to facilitate weight loss is the first therapeutic intervention. Weight loss can reduce liver steatosis and patients should be encouraged to engage in lifestyle modification efforts to lose weight. Cardiovascular risk reduction is also an important component of care. If the patient has biopsy-proven NASH, other therapeutic interventions can be considered; however, none of the pharmacologic therapies are FDA approved for this disorder.

The patient in this vignette would benefit from an intervention that could lower blood glucose and improve hepatic inflammation and fibrosis. Obeticholic acid (Answer A) has been shown to reduce inflammation and fibrosis related to NASH in phase 3 trials, but it would not address glycemic control. Although SGLT-2 inhibitors (Answer B) have shown promising results, no prospective trial to date has demonstrated improvement in components of NASH. Similarly, DPP-4 inhibitors (Answer D) do not reduce hepatic fibrosis in NASH. Vitamin E (Answer C) improves inflammation and fibrosis in patients without diabetes, although the effect is not as clear in patients with diabetes. In addition, vitamin E would have no effect on glycemic control.

Pioglitazone (Answer E) has been shown in more than one study to improve hepatic inflammation and fibrosis in NASH, and it would also lower blood glucose. The only concern with pioglitazone is weight gain. Therefore, this patient should be counseled on continuing healthy nutrition and exercise practices.

In recent years, the use of GLP-1 receptor agonists has become increasingly common as a means to assist patients with weight loss. In this scenario, liraglutide could certainly be considered as an alternative to pioglitazone. In a prospective placebo-controlled trial, liraglutide also improved hepatic histologic findings. It is unclear whether the changes are related to the medication or due to weight loss. Another GLP-1 receptor agonist, semaglutide, was studied in the management of steatohepatitis. Semaglutide (at dosages of 0.1 mg, 0.2 mg, and 0.4 mg weekly) was compared with placebo. Weight loss was achieved with all dosages of semaglutide (about 5% weight loss in patients receiving 0.1 mg weekly to 13% weight loss in patients receiving 0.4 mg weekly). Although there appeared to be improvement in NASH, there was not significant improvement in the degree of fibrosis. Further study is required to elucidate the role of GLP-1 receptor agonists in improving liver fibrosis.

Educational Objective
Diagnose and manage nonalcoholic fatty liver disease in patients with type 2 diabetes mellitus.

Reference(s)
Stefan N, Haring H-U, Cusi K. Non-alcoholic fatty liver disease: causes, diagnosis, cardiometabolic consequences, and treatment strategies. *Lancet Diabetes Endocrinol.* 2019;7(4):313-324. PMID: 30174213

Sanyal AJ, Chalasani N, Kowdley KV, et al. Pioglitazone, vitamin E, or placebo for nonalcoholic steatohepatitis. *N Engl J Med.* 2010;362(18):1675-1685. PMID: 20427778

Newsome PN, Buchholtz K, Cusi P, et al; NN9931-4296 Investigators. A placebo-controlled trial of subcutaneous semaglutide in nonalcoholic steatohepatitis *N Engl J Med.* 2021;384(12):1113-1124. PMID: 33185364

Armstrong MJ, Gaunt P, Aithal GP, et al. Liraglutide safety and efficacy in patients with non-alcoholic steatohepatitis (LEAN): a multicenter, double-blind, randomised, placebo-controlled phase 2 study. *Lancet.* 2016;387(10019):679-690. PMID: 26608256

11 ANSWER: B) Starting gabapentin

Weight gain can be a distressing adverse effect of some medications. Certain drug classes are more frequently associated with weight gain; however, within-class differences exist that influence prescribing practices.

The anticonvulsant drug gabapentin (Answer B) is often associated with weight gain, as are other anticonvulsant agents such as pregabalin and carbamazepine, and this is the most likely cause of weight gain in this patient. Weight gain with gabapentin tends to occur within the first 3 months of therapy and is related to the dosage and duration of treatment. In this vignette, the patient's paresthesias were an adverse effect of topiramate therapy and would have most likely resolved spontaneously when the drug was discontinued.

Tricyclic antidepressants such amitriptyline, imipramine, clomipramine, and doxepin are recognized to increase appetite and cause sedation and are thus weight-promoting. Members of the selective serotonin receptor reuptake inhibitor class can be associated with weight neutrality (fluoxetine and sertraline, especially with long-term use), weight loss (bupropion), or weight gain (paroxetine). Based on data from meta-analyses, within these 2 classes of antidepressant agents, amitriptyline and paroxetine carry the greatest risk for weight gain. It is important to note that even when the drug is recognized to be associated with weight change, the average impact of these drugs on weight is modest (+4.0 lb to –2.9 lb [+1.8 kg to –1.3 kg], or approximately 2% body weight). The propensity to cause weight gain has been postulated to be related to the drug's affinity for the H1 histamine receptor and interference with the appetite regulation circuitry at the level of the hypothalamus.

Bupropion suppresses appetite and reduces food cravings. In 2014, the US FDA approved its use as a long-term weight management medication when used in combination with naltrexone. Combination therapy with bupropion and fluoxetine (Answer E) is therefore not a cause of this patient's weight gain.

Second-generation (atypical) antipsychotic drugs such as olanzapine, clozapine, and risperidone are associated with weight gain. However, with long-term use, even traditionally weight-neutral options may lead to changes in body weight. Other drug classes commonly associated with weight gain include certain antihypertensive agents such β-adrenergic blockers (eg, atenolol, metoprolol, and propranolol) and antihyperglycemic medications such as sulfonylureas, thiazolidinediones, and insulin.

When the offending medication can be substituted or withdrawn, this should be the first line of management. However, particularly with antidepressant and antipsychotic medications, it can be clinically challenging to do so without sacrificing efficacy. In these situations, the dosage and duration of therapy may be targeted instead. As with any weight-management strategy, counseling should still be directed at emphasizing caloric restriction and increased physical activity.

The oral contraceptive pill (Answer C) does not lead to significant weight changes and is therefore not the culprit in this case.

This patient has no biochemical evidence for a hormonal cause of weight gain. Thus, neither hypothyroidism (Answer A) nor hypercortisolism (Answer D) is the cause of this patient's weight gain. While weight gain can be associated with hypothyroidism, the patient has subclinical hypothyroidism that is not associated with weight gain. The patient's high-normal 8-AM serum cortisol concentration is due to the oral estrogen (oral contraceptive pill).

Educational Objective
Identify medications that are associated with weight gain, weight neutrality, and weight loss.

Reference(s)
Serretti A, Mandelli L. Antidepressants and body weight: a comprehensive review and meta-analysis. *J Clin Psychiatry*. 2010;71(10):1259-1272. PMID: 21062615

Blumenthal SR, Castro VM, Clements CC, et al. An electronic health records study of long-term weight gain following antidepressant use. *JAMA Psychiatry*. 2014;71(8):889-896. PMID: 24898363

DeToledo JC, Toledo C, DeCerce J, Ramsay RE. Changes in body weight with chronic, high-dose gabapentin therapy. *Ther Drug Monit*. 1997;19(4):394-396. PMID: 9263379

12 ANSWER: D) Consult neurology

Not all peripheral neuropathy in patients with diabetes mellitus is related to the microvascular complications associated with hyperglycemia. Furthermore, appreciating when polyneuropathy in patients with diabetes may be more than typical diabetes-related polyneuropathy is important, as some cases may be amenable to treatment beyond simple pain control with gabapentin, pregabalin, or duloxetine. Diabetes can cause several patterns of neuropathy; the most common is a distal, symmetric, axonal sensorimotor neuropathy. The second most common presentation is a small-fiber, painful neuropathy. Involvement of autonomic fibers is also common in diabetes. This patient has symmetric and significant motor deficiencies that are not typically observed in patients with classic peripheral neuropathy related to diabetes. Diabetes infrequently causes multifocal neuropathies, including the cranial nerves, asymmetric proximal motor neuropathy (diabetic amyotrophy), or symmetric proximal motor neuropathy. Accordingly, the presence of signs and symptoms of these types of presentations should raise suspicion for other etiologies. This patient's progressive symmetric proximal motor neuropathy warrants further investigation, particularly since his blood glucose has been very well controlled.

He has no signs or symptoms suggestive of an inflammatory arthropathy. Thus, measuring rheumatoid factor (Answer C) is incorrect.

The laboratory profile (normal calcium, hemoglobin/hematocrit, total protein levels, and lack of reported bone pain) make multiple myeloma an unlikely etiology. Thus, obtaining serum protein electrophoresis/urine protein electrophoresis (Answer E) is incorrect.

The patient reports only a mild worsening of painful neuropathy; thus, increasing his current gabapentin dosage (Answer A) or changing from gabapentin to duloxetine (Answer B) is not the best answer. Also, these adjustments would not address his motor symptoms.

Serum vitamin B_{12} was assessed to evaluate the patient for vitamin B_{12} deficiency, a known cause of polyneuropathy. Glutamic acid decarboxylase (GAD) 65 antibodies were assessed because of the patient's history of an autoimmune condition (Crohn disease) and some of his motor symptoms were concerning for a potential diagnosis of stiff-person syndrome. Stiff-person syndrome is a disabling autoimmune central nervous system disorder characterized by progressive muscle rigidity and gait impairment with superimposed painful spasms that involve axial and limb musculature, triggered by heightened sensitivity to external stimuli. Stiff-person syndrome is commonly associated with high GAD 65 antibody titers and a variety of other organ-specific autoantibodies and has a wide spectrum of clinical presentation.

Of the options listed, consulting neurology (Answer D) is the best answer. A neurologic evaluation will likely lead to electromyography/nerve conduction study being performed, as well as additional forms of testing. This patient was eventually diagnosed with chronic inflammatory demyelinating polyneuropathy that responded rather dramatically to immunotherapy. Chronic inflammatory demyelinating polyneuropathy has an estimated incidence of 0.7 to 1.6 cases per 100,000 persons per year. The overall prevalence is estimated at 4.8 to 8.9 cases per 100,000 persons. Typical chronic inflammatory demyelinating polyneuropathy is a fairly symmetric sensorimotor polyneuropathy in which motor involvement exceeds sensory involvement. Peripheral neuropathy syndromes are summarized in the *Box*.

Box. Peripheral Neuropathy Syndromes

Acute-subacute generalized polyneuropathies

Sensorimotor
    Acute motor and sensory axonal neuropathy syndrome
    Alcohol or nutritional deficiencies
    Toxins (metals)
Motor more than sensory
    Acute motor axonal neuropathy syndrome
    Diphtheria
    Guillain-Barre syndrome
    Porphyria
    Toxins (dapsone, vincristine)
Sensory
    Human immunodeficiency virus
    Paraneoplastic/autoimmune (anti-Hu-associated)
    Toxins (cisplatin)
    Vitamin B_6 toxicity

Chronic generalized symmetric polyneuropathies

Sensorimotor
    Alcohol or nutritional deficiencies
    Connective tissue disease
    Diabetes
    Dysproteinemias
    Uremia
Motor more than sensory
    Chronic inflammatory demyelinating polyradiculoneuropathy
    Dysproteinemias
    Hypothyroidism
    Toxins (amiodarone, cytosine arabinoside, metals, tacrolimus)
Sensory
    Paraneoplastic or autoimmune (anti-Hu-associated)
    Sjogren syndrome
    Vitamin B_6 toxicity
    Vitamin E deficiency

Inherited generalized symmetric sensory and motor polyneuropathies
Charcot-Marie-Tooth disease type 1, 2, 3, and X Familial amyloidosis Hereditary predisposition to pressure palsies (focal and symmetric)
Asymmetric generalized sensory and motor polyneuropathies
Diabetes mellitus Lyme disease Sarcoidosis Vasculitis
Mononeuropathies
Compression and entrapment neuropathies Diabetes mellitus Vasculitis

Reprinted from Cleveland Clinic Center for Continuing Education. Peripheral neuropathy. Available at: https://www.clevelandclinicmeded.com/medicalpubs/diseasemanagement/neurology/peripheral-neuropathy/

Educational Objective
Differentiate among the many etiologies of peripheral neuropathy in patients with diabetes mellitus.

Reference(s)
Poncelet AN. An algorithm for the evaluation of peripheral neuropathy. *Am Fam Physician.* 1998;15;57(4):755-764. PMID: 9490998

Azhary H, Farooq MU, Bhanushali M, Majid A, Kassab MY. Peripheral neuropathy: differential diagnosis and management. *Am Fam Physician.* 2010;81(7):887-892. PMID: 20352146

Ryan M, Ryan SJ. Chronic inflammatory demyelinating polyneuropathy: considerations for diagnosis, management, and population health. *Am J Manag Care.* 2018;24(Suppl 17):S371-S379. PMID: 30312032

Rakocevic G, Floeter MK. Autoimmune stiff person syndrome and related myelopathies: understanding of electrophysiological and immunological processes. *Muscle Nerve.* 2012;45(5):623-634. PMID: 22499087

13 ANSWER: C) Discuss the potential value of genetic counseling/testing for the parents and fetus

Congenital adrenal hyperplasia (CAH) due to 21-hydroxylase deficiency is one of the most common autosomal recessive disorders. CAH is caused by pathogenic variants in the *CYP21A2* gene. More severe 21-hydroxylase enzyme deficiency results in classic CAH with salt-wasting adrenal crisis or adrenal insufficiency at birth or soon after birth and ambiguous genitalia in females. Less severe 21-hydroxylase enzyme deficiency results in nonclassic CAH without adrenal insufficiency. Nonclassic CAH presents with precocious puberty or symptoms of androgen excess and irregular menses similar to that observed in polycystic ovary syndrome. In classic CAH, glucocorticoids and mineralocorticoids are required to replace deficiency, whereas in nonclassic CAH, the goal of glucocorticoid treatment in childhood/adolescence is to stop further pubertal development, to optimize growth potential, and to lower androgen excess while also avoiding iatrogenic glucocorticoid excess.

Although reduced fertility rates are reported in women with CAH, this is in part due to fewer women trying to conceive. Pregnancy rates can be as high as 60% to 80% in this patient population. Only 10% to 25% of women with CAH try to conceive. Multiple factors contribute to decreased desire to conceive, including suboptimal surgical construction resulting in vaginal stenosis or anxiety regarding body image and sexual function. It is generally recommended that women with CAH have a gynecologic examination, especially if they have a history of genital surgery. This patient is asymptomatic, but given her history, it would be reasonable to recommend examination before trying to conceive.

Androgen excess can also interfere with ovulation. When trying to conceive, glucocorticoid replacement in classic CAH ideally prevents the morning ACTH rise to more effectively decrease 17-hydroxyprogesterone, androgen, and progesterone concentrations that interfere with ovulation and implantation. Dexamethasone (Answer A) is typically associated with more adverse effects of cortisol excess such as weight gain and worsening insulin resistance and would need to be stopped as soon as pregnancy is diagnosed because it can cross the placenta into the fetal circulation.

Longer-acting glucocorticoids (eg, prednisone or prednisolone) might be prescribed at night, especially when trying to conceive, to help lower progesterone levels (ideally to <0.6 ng/mL [<2 nmol/L]), which has been shown to increase the likelihood of pregnancy. However, 17-hydroxyprogesterone does not need to be normalized when treating CAH in adults regardless of whether they are trying to conceive, as this tends to lead to overtreatment. Thus, its measurement (Answer D) would not change management. Ideally, after discontinuing oral contraceptives but before trying to conceive, treatment optimization can be monitored with measurement of progesterone in the follicular phase (Answer E), but it would not be helpful while this patient is still on oral contraceptives.

Preconception counseling should include discussion about the potential value of genetic counseling and testing for the parents and fetus (Answer C). Genetic counseling is important to inform the parents about the risk of having a child with CAH if the father is a carrier and to discuss how this information can be used to consider prenatal testing and treatment of a female fetus. If the patient has not yet had genetic testing herself, then determining her genotype would be helpful in assessing possible pregnancy outcomes/severity of pathogenic variants. The couple should also be counseled about the implications for a female fetus if the father is a carrier. Prenatal dexamethasone treatment can prevent virilization of a female fetus and reduce the chance that genital surgery will be needed. The parents should also be informed of the potential for prenatal testing through chorionic villus sampling at 12 to 13 weeks' gestation to determine both the baby's sex and the *CYP21A2* genotype. Maternal plasma can also be used less invasively and earlier at 4.5 weeks' gestation to identify the *SRY* gene in circulating cell-free fetal DNA. Early identification of a male fetus would allow prompt discontinuation of dexamethasone. There is controversy regarding overtreatment of unaffected fetuses until testing has determined the sex and genotype of the fetus, as the long-term effects of high-dosage dexamethasone on an unaffected fetus are unknown. Women with CAH and their partners might opt out of genetic testing if they know they would not proceed with prenatal dexamethasone treatment. Prenatal dexamethasone treatment of a female fetus of a woman with CAH or a woman who has a child with CAH is still experimental and should only be considered after informed consent for an IRB-approved clinical trial.

In summary, before trying to conceive, this patient should ideally have a gynecologic examination, possible genetic counseling/testing, and optimization of her follicular-phase progesterone once off oral contraceptives (via adjustments of her glucocorticoid replacement regimen). She should not discontinue the oral contraceptive and start trying to conceive yet (Answer B).

Educational Objective
Provide prepregnancy counseling and outline treatment considerations for a woman with classic congenital adrenal hyperplasia.

Reference(s)
Ng SM, Stepien KM, Krishan A. Glucocorticoid replacement regimens for treating congenital adrenal hyperplasia. *Cochrane Database Syst Rev*. 2020;3:CD012517. PMID: 32190901

Speiser PW, Arlt W, Auchus RJ, et al. Congenital adrenal hyperplasia due to steroid 21-hydroxylase deficiency: an Endocrine Society clinical practice guideline. *J Clin Endocrinol Metab*. 2018;103(11):4043-4088. PMID: 30272171

Casteràs A, De Silva P, Rumsby G, Conway GS. Reassessing fecundity in women with classical congenital adrenal hyperplasia (CAH): normal pregnancy rate but reduced fertility rate. *Clin Endocrinol (Oxf)*. 2009;70(6):833-837. PMID: 19250265

Chandran SR, Loh LM. The importance and implications of preconception genetic testing for accurate fetal risk estimation in 21-hydroxylase congenital adrenal hyperplasia (CAH). *Gynecol Endocrinol*. 2019;35(1):28-31. PMID: 30044156

14 ANSWER: D) Right adrenalectomy

This patient's clinical presentation is strongly suggestive of primary aldosteronism with (1) resistant hypertension (uncontrolled blood pressure despite treatment with at least 3 agents at reasonable dosages [one of which would usually be a diuretic, but previously discontinued here because of marked hypokalemia]), and (2) persistent hypokalemia despite treatment with ramipril and potassium supplementation.

When plasma renin is suppressed and the aldosterone concentration is greater than 20 ng/dL (>555 pmol/L) in a patient with a history of hypokalemia, confirmatory testing (Answer E) such as saline infusion, oral salt loading, fludrocortisone suppression, or captopril challenge is not required.

CT has documented a 2.5-cm adrenal lesion. Although the baseline Hounsfield units are above the threshold normally expected for an adenoma (<10 Hounsfield units), postcontrast findings are very reassuring (absolute washout 83.3% [≥60% is consistent with an adenoma], relative washout 50% [≥40% is consistent with an adenoma]). There is therefore no indication for further imaging with adrenal MRI (Answer C).

Once surgery is being contemplated for primary aldosteronism, adrenal venous sampling (Answer A) performed by an experienced radiologist is usually recommended to distinguish between unilateral and bilateral adrenal disease. However, it has been proposed that in limited circumstances, it is reasonable to proceed directly to surgery (Answer D), and this patient is an example of such a case by virtue of the following characteristics:

- Age <35 years
- Spontaneous hypokalemia
- Marked aldosterone excess
- Unilateral adrenal lesion(s) with radiologic features of a cortical adenoma on adrenal CT

Accordingly, following institution of mineralocorticoid receptor antagonist therapy to optimize blood pressure control and normalize serum potassium, this patient was referred for successful curative surgery. It is important to note, however, that some endocrinologists contend that a lateralizing procedure should be considered in all cases. Unfortunately, high-quality adrenal venous sampling is not widely available, and other approaches (eg, molecular PET imaging with 11C-metomidate) are being explored to try and remove this bottleneck to potential curative surgery.

Familial hyperaldosteronism type 1 (glucocorticoid-remediable aldosteronism) is inherited in an autosomal dominant manner and is a rare cause of primary aldosteronism (≤1%). Affected individuals harbor a chimeric gene in which the promoter region of *CYP11B1* (encoding 11β-hydroxylase) is fused to the coding region of *CYP11B2* (aldosterone synthase), resulting in ACTH-driven hyperaldosteronism. Presentation can be variable, but early-onset resistant hypertension and premature cardiovascular events are often seen in affected families. The possibility of glucocorticoid-remediable aldosteronism and other forms of familial hyperaldosteronism should be considered in all younger patients presenting with primary aldosteronism. However, in this vignette, there is no personal or family history to point to an inherited basis, hypokalemia is marked (in glucocorticoid-remediable aldosteronism, hypokalemia is less common in the absence of diuretic therapy), and the findings on adrenal CT are not typical of glucocorticoid-remediable aldosteronism (normal or hyperplastic glands). Genetic testing for glucocorticoid-remediable aldosteronism (Answer B) is generally reserved for patients with primary aldosteronism onset at a young age (<20 years) and/or a family history of primary aldosteronism or stroke at a young age (<40 years).

Educational Objective
Determine whether additional confirmatory testing is required to establish the diagnosis and/or determine lateralization in primary aldosteronism.

Reference(s)
Funder JW, Carey RM, Mantero F, et al. The management of primary aldosteronism: case detection, diagnosis, and treatment: an Endocrine Society clinical practice guideline. *J Clin Endocrinol Metab.* 2016;101(5):1889-1916. PMID: 26934393

Vaduva P, Bonnet F, Bertherat J. Molecular basis of primary aldosteronism and adrenal Cushing syndrome. *J Endocr Soc.* 2020;4(9):bvaa075. PMID: 32783015

15 ANSWER: A) Continue alendronate

Although the indications to initiate osteoporosis therapy are well delineated by clinical guidelines, the decision to interrupt or switch to an alternative class of antifracture treatment is much less well established. Oral bisphosphonates, including alendronate, risedronate, and ibandronate, are generally considered frontline therapy for most patients based on overall benefit-risk assessment (efficacy, tolerability, and cost) compared with selective estrogen receptor modulators (raloxifene and bazedoxifene), parenteral antiresorptive agents (zoledronic acid, ibandronate, and denosumab), and anabolic agents (teriparatide, abaloparatide, and romosozumab). In addition, there is evidence to support the interruption of therapy after a period of treatment (5 years for oral bisphosphonates and 3 years for intravenous bisphosphonates), with the expectation of bone mineral density stability and continued fracture risk reduction for a period of time after discontinuation. Nonetheless, there remains uncertainty as to whether there is a threshold of bone mineral density at which treatment may no longer be indicated to meaningfully reduce the risk of fracture. This approach, dubbed "treat to target," postulates that additional therapy with an FDA-approved medication may not be necessary once an individual attains a bone density T-score greater than –2.5 (ie, osteopenia), with some expert opinion suggesting that a T-score greater than –2.0 is more desirable. This approach, however, has not been validated in a robust, prospective manner.

The absence of definitive evidence notwithstanding, clinicians can derive guidance from existing evidence that individuals who would be deemed at high risk of fracture, based on bone mineral density or a high estimated 10-year risk of major osteoporotic fracture, may well benefit from either continuation of therapy or a switch to an alternative antifracture agent. Specifically, a major osteoporotic fracture risk greater than 23% over 10 years at the conclusion of a 5-year course of alendronate appears to identify postmenopausal women who would benefit from continuation of therapy (Answer A), as would be the case for this woman. There is also evidence to support continuation of therapy in patients who remain osteoporotic at the femoral neck, which is also reflected by this patient's bone mineral density results. There may also be a rationale for reducing the dosage of alendronate (ie, 70 mg every 2 weeks), which is supported by the original Fracture Intervention trial (FIT-2) that confirmed vertebral fracture efficacy with an alendronate dosage of 5 mg administered daily for the first 2 years. Given this evidence, initiation of a drug holiday (Answer D) does not appear to be appropriate for this patient.

Although switching to an alternative antifracture therapy could also be considered in patients deemed to be at a continued high risk of fracture, there is overwhelming evidence that the effect of the parathyroid analogue teriparatide (Answer C) on bone mineral density is significantly blunted in patients who have received immediately antecedent long-term bisphosphonate therapy. While raloxifene (Answer E) is an FDA-approved antifracture therapy that could be considered for this patient, it has not been shown to reduce the risk of hip or nonvertebral fractures in randomized clinical trials.

Finally, measurement of skeletal biomarkers such as the bone resorption product C-telopeptide (Answer B) and the bone formation marker bone-specific alkaline phosphatase has been advocated as potentially helpful in osteoporosis management, based on their ability to predict bone mineral density change and fracture risk reduction in large groups of patients in randomized controlled trials of FDA-approved antifracture therapies. Nonetheless, there is not sufficient evidence to date that the use of bone biomarkers can predict such skeletal outcomes in individual patients, most likely in large part because of significant inherent biologic variability.

Educational Objective
Determine candidacy of a postmenopausal woman for a bisphosphonate holiday based on bone mineral density and FRAX-based criteria (major fracture risk).

Reference(s)
Bauer DC, Schwartz A, Palermo L, et al. Fracture prediction after discontinuation of 4 to 5 years of alendronate therapy: the FLEX study. *JAMA Intern Med.* 2014;174(7):1126-1134. PMID: 24798675

Eastell R, Rosen CJ, Black DM, Cheung AM, Murad MH, Shoback D. Pharmacological management of osteoporosis in postmenopausal women: an Endocrine Society* clinical practice guideline. *J Clin Endocrinol Metab.* 2019;104(5):1595-1622. PMID: 30907953

Black DM, Schwatz A, Bauer D, et al. Predicting fracture risk during a bisphosphonate holiday in the FIT Long-term Extension (FLEX) Study: comparison of a custom risk tool vs FRAX. Abstract 1089. Presented at: Annual Meeting of the American Society for Bone and Mineral Research; September 20-23, 2019; Orlando, FL.

16 ANSWER: E) Cyclosporine

Posttransplant hyperlipidemia is a common problem seen after solid and nonsolid organ transplant, and its prevalence ranges from 30% to 87% depending on the type of transplant. Hypercholesterolemia increases this population's cardiovascular risk, which contributes to increased cardiac death, increased nonfatal myocardial infarction, and possibly to allograft injury as a nonimmune risk factor. Nonmodifiable risk factors that increase an individual's likelihood of developing posttransplant hyperlipidemia include advancing age, pretransplant hyperlipidemia, family history of hyperlipidemia, male sex, and kidney dysfunction. Identifying patients who develop this condition is important, as pharmacologic interventions have been shown to lower cardiovascular risk and improve a patient's outcome after transplant.

The 4 main categories of immunosuppressants used are calcineurin inhibitors, antimetabolites, mTOR inhibitors, and corticosteroids. The most commonly prescribed calcineurin inhibitors are cyclosporine (Answer E) and tacrolimus. They raise LDL cholesterol by binding to the LDL receptor, increasing the activity of hepatic lipase, and decreasing bile acid synthesis. Their effect is dosage dependent. Tacrolimus produces fewer lipid disturbances than does cyclosporine. Sirolimus is an mTOR inhibitor that mainly increases triglycerides by impairing the action of lipoprotein lipase and increasing the secretion of VLDL. Its effect is also dosage dependent. Corticosteroids are known for increasing both LDL cholesterol and triglycerides. Corticosteroids raise LDL cholesterol by decreasing the synthesis of the LDL receptor and increasing the activity of HMG-CoA reductase; they raise triglycerides by decreasing the activity of lipoprotein lipase and increasing the activity of fatty acid synthase. The antimetabolites azathioprine and mycophenolate sodium do not cause any change in lipid profiles. This patient's lipid profile shows that the only lipid value that has changed is LDL cholesterol. Therefore, cyclosporine is the most likely cause. If prednisone (Answer D) were the culprit, an increase in both LDL cholesterol and triglycerides would be expected.

Hypothyroidism (Answer A) causes hypercholesterolemia due to increased synthesis and decreased degradation of LDL cholesterol. However, TSH elevations less than 14.9 mIU/L with a normal free T_4 level are not associated with cholesterol abnormalities. This patient's LDL-cholesterol changes cannot be attributed to her abnormal TSH.

Dyslipidemia associated with weight gain (Answer B) presents as increased LDL cholesterol and triglycerides and decreased HDL cholesterol. The only abnormality in this patient's lipid profile is her elevated LDL cholesterol, so weight gain is not the best explanation.

Topiramate (Answer C) is not known to cause dyslipidemia.

Educational Objective
Explain the effect cyclosporine has on cholesterol metabolism.

Reference(s)
Agarwal A, Prasad GVR. Post-transplant dyslipidemia: mechanisms, diagnosis and management. *World J Transplant.* 2016;6(1):125-134. PMID: 27011910

Bamgbola O. Metabolic consequences of modern immunosuppressive agents in solid organ transplantation. *Ther Adv Endocrinol Metab.* 2016;7(3):110-127. PMID: 27293540

Hueston WJ, Pearson WS. Subclinical hypothyroidism and the risk of hypercholesterolemia. *Ann Fam Med.* 2004;2(4):351-355. PMID: 15335135

17 ANSWER: E) Review the daily insulin delivery data for further information

In 2017, a panel of experts convened to discuss standardized reporting of continuous glucose monitoring metrics. In 2019, the panel defined goals for use in clinical practice. They determined that "time in ranges" as a metric of glycemic control provided more information than hemoglobin A_{1c}, and they established target percentages of time in various glycemic ranges individualized for different populations such as pregnant women or older patients at higher risk.

For the typical population, the target glucose goal is 70 to 180 mg/dL (3.9-10.0 mmol/L) for at least 70% of the time. Users of continuous glucose monitoring should not have glucose concentrations less than 70 mg/dL (<3.9 mmol/L) more than 4% of the day (1 hour) or less than 54 mg/dL (<3.0 mmol/L) more than 1% of the day (15 minutes). Glucose concentrations should not be greater than 180 mg/dL (>10.0 mmol/L) more than 25% of the time and not be greater than 250 mg/dL (>13.9 mmol/L) more than 5% of the time. The coefficient of variation can be used to discuss glycemic variability. A target of less than 36% (some experts recommend <33%) is an indicator of lower risk for hypoglycemia.

This vignette contains an example of an ambulatory glucose profile, a template for data presentation and visualization of time in range, low and high blood glucose values, and coefficient of variation. If one were only to review the ambulatory glucose profile summary, the most likely conclusion would be that no therapy change is needed to the pump settings, as the patient is meeting all the standardized clinical goals and has a low coefficient of variation. However, this vignette highlights a significant discrepancy between total daily dose by hourly basal setting vs what is actually being delivered and thus stresses the need to review all data presented rather than just the summary reports. Currently, this patient is in automode more than 90% of the time, so his risk for hypoglycemia is low. However, if he had to convert to manual mode, his risk for recurrent hypoglycemia would be high. If one were to review the daily hourly dose delivered in automode (not shown in the vignette), one would see the actual basal hourly dose delivered is significantly less than the set hourly rate. This is implied by the difference in his calculated total daily basal dose of 28.53 units and the reported average daily basal dose of 23.65 units. Thus, maintaining the current settings (Answer A) is incorrect.

The delivered basal daily dose is already at 57% of the total daily insulin dose, and typically the bolus dose should be 50% or more of the total daily dose. Therefore, modifying the insulin-to-carbohydrate ratio from 1:12 to 1:13 (Answer B) is incorrect, as the basal rate must be reduced, not the carbohydrate ratio.

Setting a temporary basal rate or placing the pump in "exercise mode" at a time of day when the patient is more active (Answer C), although a good technique, would not address the main issue in this case, which is his excessive basal rates when in manual mode. Likewise, reducing the basal rate during only part of the day (Answer D) is also incorrect, in part because the indicated change is insufficient and also because the actual basal delivery throughout the day must be reviewed to determine the timing and magnitude of needed changes in programmed basal rates as highlighted by the severely low value 3 weeks ago. In both of those scenarios, one should review the actual 24-hour basal delivery.

The correct answer is to gather more information by reviewing hourly daily delivery (Answer E), which would show significantly less basal insulin delivered throughout the day and overnight and lead to the conclusion to reduce the basal rate across the board by 20% to limit risk for hypoglycemia when not in automode.

Educational Objective
Interpret insulin pump and continuous glucose monitoring data to make recommendations for care in patients with diabetes mellitus.

Reference(s)
Battelino T, Danne T, Bergenstal RM, et al. Clinical targets for continuous glucose monitoring data interpretation: recommendations from the International Consensus on Time in Range. *Diabetes Care.* 2019;42(8):1593-1603. PMID: 31177185

Bergenstal RM, Ahmann AJ, Bailey T, et al. Recommendations for standardizing glucose reporting and analysis to optimize clinical decision making in diabetes: the ambulatory glucose profile (AGP). *Diabetes Technol Ther.* 2013;15(3):198-211. PMID: 23448694

18 ANSWER: C) Switch to denosumab

This postmenopausal woman has severe osteoporosis (very low T-scores and recent vertebral compression fragility fractures) in the setting of chronic intermittent glucocorticoid use and longstanding oral bisphosphonate therapy for her osteoporosis (8 years of alendronate treatment). She is at high risk of future fracture, and as with any other patient with osteoporosis, she should be counseled on fall prevention. In addition, an individualized therapeutic plan should be developed based on a discussion of the risks and benefits of the currently available osteoporosis treatment options, with the most appropriate drug chosen given her comorbidities and clinical findings. Her declining bone mineral density and the occurrence of new vertebral compression fractures despite adherence to alendronate therapy are consistent with therapy failure. Therefore, continuing alendronate (Answer A) should not be recommended.

While switching to osteoanabolic therapy such as teriparatide (PTH 1-34) (Answer D) may be an attractive choice, her history of recurrent kidney stones and mild hypercalcemia should raise concern for primary hyperparathyroidism, thus eliminating this as the best option. In addition, several studies have confirmed that there is some blunting in bone mineral density increases when teriparatide is given to patients who were previously treated with bisphosphonates.

Romosozumab is a monoclonal antibody to sclerostin, an endogenous inhibitor of bone formation. In 2019, the US FDA approved romosozumab for the treatment of postmenopausal osteoporosis, and it has a black box warning of the potential risk of myocardial infarction, stroke, and cardiovascular death. Romosozumab should not be initiated in patients who have had a myocardial infarction or stroke within the preceding year. Since this patient had a stroke 6 months ago, switching to romosozumab (Answer E) would not be appropriate at this time.

Switching to zoledronic acid (Answer B), an intravenous bisphosphonate, would not be the best choice in this case given the patient's long-term bisphosphonate use and borderline renal function. Zoledronic acid is contraindicated in the setting of chronic kidney disease when the estimated glomerular filtration rate is less than 35 mL/min per 1.73 m^2.

Denosumab is a fully human monoclonal antibody to the receptor activator of nuclear factor kappaB ligand (RANKL). By blocking the binding of RANKL to RANK, it reduces osteoclast formation, function, and survival, which results in decreased bone resorption and increased bone density. Switching to denosumab (Answer C), which is a potent antiresorptive agent that is not excreted by the kidneys, would be the most appropriate recommendation for this patient. Studies assessing transitioning from oral bisphosphonates to denosumab have demonstrated improved efficacy in increasing bone mineral density compared with continuing bisphosphonate therapy. Denosumab is administered by subcutaneous injection once every 6 months. Because of emerging concerns about an increased risk of vertebral fracture after discontinuation of denosumab, a "drug holiday" would not be appropriate, and the need for indefinite administration of denosumab or switching to an alternative therapy, if possible, should be discussed with patients before its initiation. Denosumab may induce significant hypocalcemia in patients with renal impairment. Ensuring an adequate amount of calcium and vitamin D supplementation is critical to avoid this complication, especially in patients who have conditions that predispose to hypocalcemia such as chronic kidney disease or malabsorption syndromes. Denosumab should not be given to patients with preexisting hypocalcemia until it is corrected.

Educational Objective
Recommend the most appropriate osteoporosis treatment for a patient in whom bisphosphonate therapy has failed.

Reference(s)
Carey JJ. What is a 'failure' of bisphosphonate therapy for osteoporosis? *Cleve Clin J Med*. 2005;72(11):1033-1039. PMID: 16315442

Leder BZ. Optimizing sequential and combined anabolic and antiresorptive osteoporosis therapy. *JBMR Plus*. 2018;2(2):62-68. PMID: 30283892

19 ANSWER: E) Serum estradiol measurement

Gynecomastia is defined as the unilateral or bilateral enlargement of the glandular tissue of the male breast exceeding 0.2 to 0.8 in (0.5-2.0 cm). The diagnosis requires palpation to distinguish true gynecomastia (felt as a firm or rubbery disk of tissue) from pseudogynecomastia or lipomastia associated with obesity. Gynecomastia must also be distinguished from rare male breast cancer, presenting typically as a unilateral hard, nontender mass that may be accompanied by dimpling of the skin, nipple discharge, and axillary lymphadenopathy. Common physiologic causes of gynecomastia include puberty and aging. Relatively common pathologic causes include hypogonadism and drugs (eg, spironolactone or 5α-reductase inhibitors).

Marked gynecomastia as in this case is unusual and is not compatible with aging alone. Several clues in this case vignette point to excess estrogen exposure as the most likely cause. Thus, serum estradiol measurement (Answer E) is correct. The clues include (1) biochemically marked secondary hypogonadism due to estradiol-mediated central suppression of the hypothalamic-pituitary-testicular axis; (2) elevated SHBG (estradiol increases SHBG); and (3) relatively good bone mineral density despite the biochemical hypogonadism. The effects of testosterone on skeletal health in men are largely indirect via aromatization to estradiol. In this man, estradiol was markedly elevated at 270 pg/mL (10-40 pg/mL [SI: 991.2 pmol/L (36.7-146.8 pmol/L)]). Causes for elevated estradiol include exposure to exogenous sources or increased endogenous estradiol. Increased endogenous estradiol is caused by increased aromatization of androgens produced in excess from either testicular sources (eg, Leydig/Sertoli-cell tumor) or adrenal sources (eg, feminizing adrenocortical tumors). Sometimes increased sex steroid production can be caused by pathologic secretion of hCG, usually produced by a testicular or extratesticular germ-cell tumor. In this case, the patient admitted to ingesting oral estradiol, between 2 to 4 mg daily, which he obtained from the Internet. He did not wish to go into reasons for doing so, but he did not endorse clinical features of gender dysphoria.

Of note, the patient was clinically and biochemically euthyroid. Gynecomastia, usually mild, is not uncommon in men with hyperthyroidism. This is because hyperthyroidism is associated with increased aromatization of androgens to estrogens, as well as increased SHBG. Given that SHBG binds testosterone more avidly than estradiol, increased SHBG concentrations lead to an increased free estradiol-to-free testosterone ratio, further aggravating the gynecomastia.

Prolactin excess can be associated with modest gynecomastia due to the associated secondary hypogonadism. In hypogonadism, both serum testosterone and serum estradiol are reduced, and gynecomastia can arise due to reduced testosterone-mediated estradiol antagonism in the breast glandular tissue. However, prolactin excess would not explain the marked gynecomastia, the increased SHBG, and the relative preservation of bone mineral density. Therefore, measuring prolactin (Answer A) is incorrect.

Feminizing adrenal tumors are very rare, usually aggressive, and may cosecrete adrenal androgens (such as DHEA-S) and glucocorticoids. In a review of 52 cases, 98% of patients had gynecomastia, 58% had a palpable abdominal tumor, and 52% had testicular atrophy. However, the overall clinical presentation in this case (generally well, absence of cushingoid features) is not typical for this rare condition, Thus, measuring DHEA-S (Answer B) is not the most important initial test. There is no reason to suspect a testicular tumor, so testicular ultrasonography (Answer C) is not indicated. While many men with Klinefelter syndrome are either diagnosed late in life or never at all, Klinefelter syndrome presents with primary hypogonadism. Moreover, the degree of the gynecomastia, reported history of fertility, and relatively good bone density make this diagnosis unlikely. Thus, karyotype analysis (Answer D) is incorrect.

Of note, while individuals with aromatase excess syndrome can present with gynecomastia, it is a very rare inherited disorder characterized by prepubertal gynecomastia, accelerated bone age, and early growth arrest. It is not a differential diagnostic consideration in this case.

Some patients are bothered by gynecomastia, either because of pain, tenderness, or embarrassment. Gynecomastia proceeds through 3 stages. The initial proliferative phase is typically associated with pain. Gynecomastia that has been present for a year or longer usually progresses to a fibrotic stage that is less likely to resolve or respond to medical therapy. There are very few controlled clinical trials in this area, which is a shortcoming given that gynecomastia, especially in earlier stages, is characterized by a relatively high spontaneous resolution rate. In hypogonadal men, painful gynecomastia may respond to testosterone treatment. In eugonadal men, selective estrogen receptor modulators have been used, with some evidence for tamoxifen, used off label, in an analysis of 6 studies that included 109 patients. A reduction in gynecomastia size was reported in 80% of patients. If there is persistent pain or embarrassment in patients with longstanding gynecomastia, surgical removal of breast tissue may need to be considered, but it is very important that the surgery is performed by an experienced breast surgeon to optimize success and minimize procedural complications.

Educational Objective
Evaluate and manage gynecomastia.

Reference(s)
Braunstein GD. Gynecomastia. *N Engl J Med.* 1993;18;328(7):490-495. PMID: 8421478

Gruntmanis U, Braunstein GD. Treatment of gynecomastia. *Curr Opin Investig Drugs.* 2001;2(5):643-649. PMID: 11569940

Ali SN, Jayasena CN, Sam AH. Which patients with gynaecomastia require more detailed investigation? *Clin Endocrinol (Oxf).* 2018;88(3):360-363. PMID: 29193251

20 ANSWER: B) Perform a 72-hour fast

The first consideration when evaluating hypoglycemia is to establish the Whipple triad, which includes (1) symptoms consistent with hypoglycemia, (2) documentation of low plasma glucose when symptoms are present, and (3) resolution of symptoms when the glucose level is increased. The Whipple triad cannot be assessed definitively in this vignette since only a fingerstick glucose value (not plasma glucose value) was documented while the patient was symptomatic. The next consideration, especially given her history of gastric bypass surgery, is to assess whether the hypoglycemia occurs postprandially or when fasting.

Postbariatric hypoglycemia typically occurs more than 1 year following surgery. Symptoms are usually postprandial, occurring 1 to 3 hours after a high carbohydrate-containing meal. If the symptoms are postprandial, a mixed-meal challenge (Answer A) can be done as a provocative test. However, a mixed-meal challenge would not be the right choice in this case since the patient is experiencing fasting hypoglycemia, not postprandial hypoglycemia. Oral glucose tolerance testing (Answer C) should be avoided in patients who have had upper gastrointestinal surgery, including Roux-en-Y gastric bypass. The large glucose load is not well tolerated and may cause symptoms of dumping syndrome. Dietary change to a carbohydrate-restricted diet (Answer E) is recommended for the management of postbariatric hypoglycemia. In this case, since hypoglycemia is not triggered by a meal, dietary change is not the best next step.

An alternative cause for hypoglycemia should be sought if symptoms develop within 6 to 12 months following surgery. An alternative cause should also be sought if hypoglycemia is experienced overnight, in the fasting state, or following physical activity. In this vignette, the hypoglycemia occurs in the fasting state and overnight, so a thorough investigation for an alternative cause for hypoglycemia should be undertaken.

Establishing fasting hypoglycemia (with plasma blood glucose) while the patient is symptomatic is the first step in the evaluation and will help establish the Whipple triad. In addition, when the patient has blood glucose concentration less than 45 mg/dL (<2.5 mmol/L), other laboratory measurements should be obtained, including proinsulin, C-peptide, β-hydroxybutyrate, insulin, and insulin antibodies, as well as a sulfonylurea/meglitinide screen. Eliciting hypoglycemia can be attempted after an overnight fast; however, extending the fast up to 72 hours may be necessary (Answer B).

Insulin antibodies (Answer D) can cause hypoglycemia, often in the postprandial state. Although this is a reasonable test to order as part of the broader assessment, it is not a comprehensive evaluation and is not the best next step in this patient's management.

Educational Objective
Assess hypoglycemia following bariatric surgery.

Reference(s)
Selehi M, Vella A, McLaughlin T, Patti M-E. Hypoglycemia after gastric bypass surgery: current concepts and controversies. *J Clin Endocrinol Metab.* 2018;103(8):2815-2826. PMID: 30101281

21

ANSWER: E) Recommend no additional action now

The diagnosis of adrenal insufficiency is based on documenting a frankly low morning serum cortisol concentration (<3.0 μg/dL [<82.8 nmol/L]) in a patient with normal wake/sleep pattern. Patients with symptoms and a morning serum cortisol value between 3.0 and 15.0 μg/dL (82.8-413.8 nmol/L) require some form of dynamic testing, such as a cosyntropin-stimulation test or an insulin tolerance test. In patients with adrenal insufficiency, the plasma ACTH level distinguishes between primary adrenal insufficiency (elevated ACTH) and secondary adrenal insufficiency (low or inappropriately normal ACTH).

This patient has evidence of secondary adrenal insufficiency based on low levels of both cortisol and ACTH. While secondary adrenal insufficiency can be part of hypopituitarism, it is extremely rare to have isolated ACTH deficiency in the setting of pituitary pathology (with the exception of hypophysitis caused by immune checkpoint inhibitor therapy, which this patient has not received). This patient has isolated ACTH deficiency, as demonstrated by her normal thyroid axis, appropriately elevated FSH given her age, and normal prolactin. The most frequent cause of isolated ACTH deficiency is prolonged exogenous glucocorticoid therapy.

While patients are likely to volunteer a history of oral glucocorticoid therapy, other means of administration may be missed if a patient is not specifically asked. The most frequent cause is the repeated administration of intraarticular glucocorticoids, but other routes of administration, such as inhaled or even rectal glucocorticoids, can also be responsible. This patient is being treated with budesonide for her collagenous colitis. Budesonide is a powerful glucocorticoid. Its affinity for glucocorticoid receptors is 195 times greater than that of hydrocortisone and 15 times greater than that of prednisolone. However, despite oral administration, budesonide is considered a "topical" glucocorticoid due to a 90% first-pass hepatic metabolism, resulting in low systemic bioavailability (except in patients with portosystemic shunt, such as those with portal hypertension). While budesonide does not often suppress the hypothalamic-pituitary-adrenal axis, several cases have been reported.

This patient's budesonide dosage is currently being reduced, and she has symptoms of adrenal insufficiency. The most likely cause of her ACTH deficiency is budesonide therapy. As she is symptomatic and there is no easy way to measure the budesonide serum level (a synthetic glucocorticoid screening test is not widely available), oral glucocorticoid replacement therapy should be initiated, and her hypothalamic-pituitary-adrenal axis must be reevaluated after budesonide therapy is stopped. Therefore, at this point, no additional action is needed (Answer E). In general, to assess recovery of the hypothalamic-pituitary-adrenal axis, early-morning serum cortisol and plasma ACTH are measured every 2 months. A rise in ACTH is the first sign of axis recovery.

Should this patient's adrenal insufficiency persist for a long time after budesonide discontinuation, or if she shows any signs or symptoms of a pituitary mass, pituitary MRI (Answer C) may be indicated in the future. Isolated ACTH deficiency is very rare in pituitary disease, so pituitary MRI, which may identify an unrelated pituitary incidentaloma, is not needed.

As she has secondary adrenal insufficiency, measuring adrenal antibodies (Answer A) would not be appropriate.

Although oral ketoconazole is a possible cause of adrenal insufficiency, ketoconazole cream has not been associated with adrenal adverse effects. Thus, stopping use of the ketoconazole cream (Answer B) is incorrect. Additionally, ketoconazole directly inhibits the function of several adrenal enzymes and would therefore be a cause of primary adrenal insufficiency (with elevated plasma ACTH).

Methenamine is an antibiotic used to prevent and treat infections of the urinary tract. It is not associated with adrenal disease. Thus, stopping methenamine (Answer D) is not necessary.

Educational Objective
List the multiple causes of steroid-induced adrenal insufficiency.

Reference(s)

Paragliola RM, Papi G, Pontecorvi A, Corsello SM. Treatment with synthetic glucocorticoids and the hypothalamus-pituitary-adrenal axis. *Int J Mol Sci.* 2017;18(10):2201. PMID: 29053578 10.3390/ijms18102201

Arntzenius A, van Galen L. Budesonide-related adrenal insufficiency. *BMJ Case Rep.* 2015:bcr2015212216. PMID: 26430235

22 ANSWER: E) Pheochromocytoma

This patient presents with an incidentally discovered adrenal mass that has radiographic characteristics suggestive of a lipid-poor and contrast-avid tumor. The differential diagnosis includes a lipid-poor adenoma, an adrenocortical carcinoma, an asymptomatic pheochromocytoma, and less likely, an extraadrenal metastasis.

The radiographic characteristics of an adrenal mass are critical in determining its etiology and evaluating whether it is benign or potentially malignant. Each imaging modality can provide similar and complementary information. Reassuring features that are suggestive of a benign adrenal mass include round and uniform shape, homogenous appearance, high lipid content (eg, low attenuation on unenhanced CT [<10 Hounsfield units] or loss of signal on out-of-phase sequencing on MRI), and high contrast washout on delayed contrast CT imaging (absolute washout on delayed imaging >60%). Small size (generally <4 cm) is usually reassuring, but it is not a reliable feature. Lack of fluorodeoxyglucose-avidity on PET scan is also generally reassuring.

Features that raise concern for a malignant process include larger size (>4 or 6 cm), irregular shape or contour, heterogeneous content, calcifications, low lipid content on CT or lack of signal dropout on in-phase and out-of-phase MRI imaging, poor washout on delayed contrast CT imaging, and fluorodeoxyglucose-avidity on PET scan. A benign pheochromocytoma usually has poor lipid content and poor washout on delayed contrast CT imaging and may also have very high contrast uptake on CT. However, pheochromocytomas generally present as slow-growing masses with a round contour and shape and with substantial elevations in metanephrines, even in the absence of overt episodic and hyperadrenergic symptoms. Further, pheochromocytomas often have very high early attenuation following contrast administration, as was the case here. Therefore, based on the radiographic characteristics, this adrenal mass may represent a lipid-poor adenoma, pheochromocytoma, or a primary or extraadrenal malignancy. Importantly, a substantial proportion of pheochromocytomas are now diagnosed after being incidentally discovered on imaging, rather than presenting with classic hyperadrenergic symptoms.

Metanephrines are the stable and inactive metabolites of catecholamines that provide the highest sensitivity and specificity for diagnosing pheochromocytoma and paraganglioma. Thus, the 2- to 3-fold elevations in this patient's metanephrines strongly suggest that she could have a pheochromocytoma, even in the absence of symptoms. Mild elevations in normetanephrine levels, and less frequently metanephrine levels, typically less than 2 times above the upper limit of the reference range, are often seen and attributed to false-positive results due to catecholamine-reuptake inhibitors such as venlafaxine. Thus, it is possible that these biochemical abnormalities could be attributable to venlafaxine use. However, in the absence of other steroid production to suggest an adrenocortical carcinoma (Answer A), the elevated metanephrines and the radiographic characteristics suggest that the most likely etiology is pheochromocytoma (Answer E). This patient underwent an adrenalectomy, which revealed a 2.0-cm pheochromocytoma.

The high unenhanced attenuation and poor washout of this mass exclude a lipid-rich adenoma (Answer C) and a cyst (Answer B). A lipid-poor adenoma (Answer D) is a consideration; however, the elevated metanephrines are diagnostic of pheochromocytoma.

Educational Objective
Identify the radiographic characteristics of an incidentally discovered pheochromocytoma.

Reference(s)

Lenders LW, Duh QY, Eisenhofer G, et al; Endocrine Society. Pheochromocytoma and paraganglioma: an Endocrine Society clinical practice guideline. *J Clin Endocrinol Metab.* 2014;99(6):1915-1942. PMID: 24893135

Fassnacht M, Arlt W, Bacos I, et al. Management of adrenal incidentalomas: European Society of Endocrinology clinical practice guideline in collaboration with the European Network for the Study of Adrenal Tumors. *Eur J Endocrinol.* 2016;175(2):G1-G34. PMID: 27390021

Vaidya A, Hamrahian A, Bancos I, Fleseriu M, Ghayee HK. The evaluation of incidentally discovered adrenal masses. *Endocr Pract.* 2019;25(2):178-192. PMID: 30817193

23 ANSWER: D) Start gemfibrozil, 600 mg twice daily

Management of hypertriglyceridemia consists of addressing the etiology (when known), pursuing a nonpharmacologic approach, and, in selected patients, adding a pharmacologic agent. Nonpharmacologic approaches centered on dietary changes are recommended for all patients with high triglycerides. Patients should be educated on which foods and/or drinks elevate triglycerides, and they should be counseled to avoid simple carbohydrates such as white bread, white rice, white pasta, and sugary drinks (eg, juices, regular soda, and sweet tea). Alcohol intake should also be avoided. Ideally, patients with hypertriglyceridemia should meet with a registered dietitian to receive dietary counseling. Hypertriglyceridemia is linked to increased cardiovascular disease and acute pancreatitis.

Pharmacologic options to lower triglycerides vary if treating moderate (500-999 mg/dL [5.65-11.29 mmol/L]) to severe (≥1000 mg/dL [≥11.30 mmol/L]) hypertriglyceridemia vs mild hypertriglyceridemia (150-499 mg/dL [1.70-5.64 mmol/L]). Fibrates and high-dosage omega-3 fatty acids should be considered if the triglyceride concentration is greater than 500 mg/dL (>5.65 mmol/L) with the goal of avoiding acute pancreatitis. The risk of acute pancreatitis is greater when the triglyceride concentration is higher than 1000 mg/dL (>11.30 mmol/L). For selected patients who have mild hypertriglyceridemia, high-dosage omega-3 fatty acids can be recommended. However, the initial focus for these patients should be to lower LDL cholesterol to goal. If, after that, their triglyceride concentration is still mildly elevated, adding high-dosage omega-3 is indicated.

Fibrates, including fenofibrate and gemfibrozil, activate the α-subunit of peroxisome proliferator–activated receptors. This activation leads to decreased production of apolipoprotein CIII (a lipoprotein lipase inhibitor), reduced secretion of VLDL cholesterol, and reduced hepatic triglyceride production. Regarding triglyceride-lowering effects, fenofibrate lowers triglycerides by an average of 40%, whereas gemfibrozil lowers triglycerides by an average of 48%. Fenofibrate dosages range from 30 mg to 200 mg daily, while gemfibrozil dosages range from 600 mg daily to 600 mg twice daily. When prescribing both medications, clinicians must bear in mind that dosages should be adjusted based on the patient's renal function, as these medications are excreted via the urine. Only fenofibrate may reversibly increase serum creatinine, and this laboratory change does not require additional workup. Renal dosage adjustment for fenofibrate starts when an individual's estimated glomerular filtration rate is less than 60 mL/min per 1.73 m^2. The patient in this vignette has stage 3 chronic kidney disease; therefore, she is not a candidate for full-dosage fenofibrate (Answer C). However, she could take a smaller dosage of fenofibrate, which could be a preferred option as fenofibrate is dosed daily compared with gemfibrozil, which is dosed twice daily and thus increases the patient's burden. In comparison, renal dosage adjustment for gemfibrozil starts when a patient has stage 4 chronic kidney disease. Thus, prescribing gemfibrozil, 600 mg twice daily (Answer D), is the best next step of the listed options.

This case also shows that coadministration of a fibrate and a statin is an option when clinically indicated. Clinicians should monitor for muscle-related adverse effects when adding a fibrate to the regimen of a patient who is already taking a statin. Gemfibrozil's interaction with atorvastatin, rosuvastatin, and pitavastatin is minor. High-dosage omega-3 fatty acids could be another reasonable treatment option for this patient. The exact mechanism by which omega-3 fatty acids lower triglycerides is not well understood. However, it is postulated that it must be similar to the way fibrates work. High-dosage omega-3 fatty acids lower triglycerides by 20% to 50% depending on the preparation that is used.

Ezetimibe (Answer B) is a cholesterol absorption inhibitor that works by blocking the cholesterol transport protein, Niemann-Pick C1-like 1. Ezetimibe lowers LDL cholesterol by 18%. It has no direct effect on triglycerides, so it would not be a good choice for this patient.

Low- to moderate-intensity statins lower triglycerides by 10%, while high-intensity statins can lower triglycerides by 28%. Atorvastatin, 20 mg daily, and pravastatin, 40 mg daily (Answer A), are both moderate-intensity statins. Therefore, switching from atorvastatin to pravastatin would not provide any additional triglyceride lowering.

Colestipol (Answer E), as well as all other bile acid sequestrants, should be avoided in patients with triglyceride concentrations greater than 300 to 500 mg/dL (3.39-5.65 mmol/L), as it can further raise triglycerides.

Educational Objective
Prescribe adequate triglyceride-lowering therapy, bearing in mind a patient's kidney function.

Reference(s)

Kelly MS, Beavers C, Bucheit JD, Sisson EM, Dixon DL. Pharmacologic approaches for the management of patients with moderately elevated triglycerides (150-499 mg/dL). *J Clin Lipidol.* 2017;11(4):872-879. PMID: 28669686

Berglund L, Brunzell JD, Goldberg AC, et al; Endocrine Society. Evaluation and treatment of hypertriglyceridemia: an Endocrine Society clinical practice guideline. *J Clin Endocrinol Metab.* 2012;97(9):2969-2989. PMID: 22962670

Wiggins BS, Saseen JJ, Morris PB. Gemfibrozil in combination with statins-is it really contraindicated? *Curr Atheroscler Rep.* 2016;18(4):18. PMID: 26932225

24 ANSWER: B) Hyperthyroidism

The most likely cause of this patient's gynecomastia is hyperthyroidism (Answer B). His clinical presentation, specifically his increased anxiety, weight loss, mild thyroid gland enlargement, and resting tremor, is suggestive of hyperthyroidism. Gynecomastia occurs in 10% to 40% of men with hyperthyroidism and resolves in most cases with restoration of euthyroidism. Gynecomastia is defined as an enlargement of the mammary glands in men and results from a relative or absolute excess of estrogens or a relative or absolute deficiency of androgens. In hyperthyroidism, increased serum SHBG and progesterone levels and increased aromatization of androgens to estrogens are potential factors contributing to the development of gynecomastia.

Hypogonadism (Answer A) is a relatively common cause of gynecomastia, but it is not the most likely etiology in this patient with normal testicular size and no signs or symptoms of hypogonadism. Gynecomastia is seen more frequently with primary hypogonadism than with secondary hypogonadism, and it occurs as a result of testosterone deficiency (due to a loss of androgen-mediated inhibition of breast growth) and from LH excess (leading to increased aromatization to estrogens). In secondary hypogonadism, the production of both estradiol and testosterone decreases as a result of deficient LH. However, gynecomastia may occur because of an imbalance in the estradiol-to-testosterone ratio resulting from the preserved adrenocortical production of estrogen precursors.

A testicular germ-cell tumor (Answer C) is not the most likely cause of gynecomastia in this patient. Although a palpable mass may not be present on testicular examination in men with germ-cell tumors, rapid-onset gynecomastia with breast pain and tenderness are characteristic clinical findings that are not described in this vignette. Testicular germ-cell tumors that cause gynecomastia do so through the production of intact hCG, which stimulates Leydig-cell aromatase activity and increases the conversion of androgen precursors to estrogens. Non–germ-cell tumors of the testes, including Leydig- and Sertoli-cell tumors, can induce gynecomastia through the same mechanism, while Leydig-cell tumors also secrete estradiol in excess.

Although the patient does report an increase in gym participation, his clinical presentation is not particularly suspicious for anabolic androgenic steroid use (Answer E). In addition to gynecomastia, clinical hallmarks of anabolic androgen abuse include acne and decreased testicular size in the setting of normal virilization. Gynecomastia occurs mainly as a result of increased aromatization of exogenous androgen (testosterone or androstenedione) to estrogens.

Most cases of gynecomastia are benign and do not increase the risk for malignancy; however, breast cancer (Answer D) is important to distinguish from gynecomastia. Usually this distinction can be made based on physical examination findings alone. Breast cancer is typically unilateral and located eccentric to the nipple-areolar complex, while gynecomastia is usually subareolar. Breast cancers are also often nonmobile and can be associated with skin changes or regional lymphadenopathy.

Educational Objective
Diagnose hyperthyroidism as a cause of gynecomastia.

Reference(s)

Narula HS, Carlson HE. Gynaecomastia--pathophysiology, diagnosis and treatment. *Nat Rev Endocrinol.* 2014;10(11):684-698. PMID: 25112235

Sansone A, Romanelli F, Sansone M, Lenzi A, Di Luigi L. Gynecomastia and hormones. *Endocrine.* 2017;55(1):37-44. PMID: 27145756

25 ANSWER: E) Romosozumab

While there is well-established guidance on the indication for pharmacotherapy in a postmenopausal woman with osteoporosis, there has been, to date, somewhat less certainty regarding the choice of antifracture agent. Recently, however, comprehensive systematic reviews and analyses by professional organizations, including the Endocrine Society and the American Association of Clinical Endocrinologists, have provided more specific guidance to practicing clinicians. These guidelines are generally predicated on the degree of bone mineral density deficit, presence of prior low-trauma fractures and, appropriately by extension, the patient's overall level of fracture risk. In addition, a greater degree of bone mineral density improvement in the total hip does appear to robustly predict higher fracture risk reduction, based on a comprehensive analysis of subject level data as reported by the Foundation for the National Institutes of Health Bone Quality Project. In light of this evidence, consideration should be given primarily to the use of an anabolic or potent parenteral antiresorptive therapy in a patient with a very high fracture risk, such as the patient in this vignette.

On the basis of the degree of fracture risk and bone mineral density deficit in this patient, initiation of an anabolic therapy would be indicated. Indeed, this patient's risk of major osteoporotic fracture is even higher than reported, as discordantly lower bone density in the spine vs the hip confers additional risk. This is based on evidence demonstrating a roughly 10% increase in major fracture risk for every rounded standard deviation difference between the lumbar spine and hip (femoral neck or total) T-score. For this patient, the 1.5 SD difference rounds to 2, which, multiplied by 0.1, equals 0.2. Her major fracture risk is then multiplied by 0.2 ($26 \times 0.2 = 5.2$), which is added to the baseline major fracture risk to give an adjusted estimate ($26 + 5.2 = 31.2\%$). In guiding this patient on the most appropriate therapeutic choice, there are no definitive head-to-head comparative data between anabolic therapies that confirm a superior agent. Nonetheless, the sclerostin antibody romosozumab (Answer E) improves bone mineral density more than other available anabolic therapies (based on clinical trial data), through both anabolic and antiresorptive effects. Thus, it is the appropriate choice for this patient. Teriparatide (Answer C), which confers an anabolic but proresorptive effect as well, based on its mechanism of action through stimulation of the PTHR1 receptor, is a potential anabolic option for this patient. The increase in urinary calcium excretion caused by the drug would, however, render it a secondary choice to romosozumab in this patient with preexisting nephrolithiasis. The PTHrP analogue abaloparatide leads to less urinary calcium excretion and could be an option in this patient, particularly since romosozumab is not universally available in all countries.

While oral bisphosphonates are generally considered frontline therapy in patients with a low or even moderate risk of osteoporotic fractures based on current recommendations, romosozumab is a superior choice over alendronate (Answer A) in this patient based on the ARCH trial (Treatment of Postmenopausal Women With Osteoporosis), which confirmed significant reductions in clinical, hip, and nonvertebral fractures in patients who received romosozumab for 1 year followed by alendronate vs those who received alendronate for 2 years. Denosumab (Answer D) is considered a frontline therapy in patients at high risk of fracture based on robust and long-term clinical trial experience. Nonetheless, the lack of head-to-head data with romosozumab notwithstanding, a more established approach to this patient would be sequential therapy with romosozumab followed by denosumab as demonstrated in the FRAME study (Fracture Study in Postmenopausal Women With Osteoporosis), which showed consolidation of bone mineral density improvement and fracture risk reduction in postmenopausal women with osteoporosis. Furthermore, although sequential denosumab-to-romosozumab therapy has not been studied, patients treated with PTH analogues given after denosumab experience paradoxical bone mineral density loss, possibly due to initial augmentation of osteoclast activation that occurs with denosumab cessation. The lack of such data at this time therefore renders the option of initiating denosumab with plans to switch to romosozumab an inferior choice for this patient.

Finally, raloxifene (Answer B) reduces the risk of vertebral fractures in postmenopausal women with osteoporosis, but it does not reduce the risk of hip or nonvertebral fractures based on primary outcome evidence from available randomized controlled trials.

Educational Objective
Recommend the best treatment for a postmenopausal woman with severe osteoporosis (romosozumab).

Reference(s)

Bouxsein ML, Eastell R, Lui LY, et al; FNIH Bone Quality Project. Change in bone density and reduction in fracture risk: a meta-regression of published trials. *J Bone Miner Res.* 2019;34(4):632-642. PMID: 30674078

Eastell R, Rosen CJ, Black DM, Cheung AM, Murad MH, Shoback D. Pharmacological management of osteoporosis in postmenopausal women: an Endocrine Society* clinical practice guideline. *J Clin Endocrinol Metab.* 2019;104(5):1595-1622. PMID: 30907953

Leslie WD, Lix LM, Johansson H, Oden A, McCloskey E, Kanis JA. Spine-hip discordance and fracture risk assessment: a physician-friendly FRAX enhancement. *Osteoporos Int.* 2011;22(3):839-847. PMID: 20959961

Saag KG, Petersen J, Brandi ML, et al. Romosozumab or alendronate for fracture prevention in women with osteoporosis. *N Engl J Med.* 2017;377(15):1417-1427. PMID: 28892457

Cosman F, Crittenden DB, Adachi JD, et al. Romosozumab treatment in postmenopausal women with osteoporosis. *N Engl J Med.* 2016;375(16):1532-1543. PMID: 27641143

26 ANSWER: B) Glutamic acid decarboxylase 65 antibody assessment

Unfortunately, this patient was not recognized as having diabetes before pregnancy, which resulted in hyperglycemia during the first trimester of pregnancy. This almost certainly contributed to congenital cardiac defects in her baby. At the time of diagnosis, she had obesity, and type 2 diabetes mellitus seemed to be a reasonable diagnosis. Interestingly, she was very sensitive to insulin and developed hypoglycemia. Her regimen was therefore switched to metformin during the pregnancy. Now, despite weight loss and excellent glucose control, she reports postprandial hyperglycemia if she does not take metformin. This situation should prompt consideration of an alternative diagnosis.

One possibility could be maturity-onset diabetes of the young (MODY). However, these monogenic causes of diabetes are often inherited in an autosomal dominant manner, which is not evident in this patient's family history. Thus, genetic testing for pathogenic variants in the *HNF1A* gene (Answer C) or *GCK* gene (Answer E) would be an incorrect next step. Furthermore, patients with *HNF1A*-related MODY respond to sulfonylureas, but not as well to other agents such as insulin and metformin. Patients with *GCK*-related MODY often have mild fasting hyperglycemia as their only manifestation and may not require treatment.

Another diagnostic possibility is that this patient may have an autoimmune basis for diabetes that is slowly progressive, usually referred to as latent autoimmune diabetes in adults (LADA). While the precise definition of LADA is debated, the Immunology of Diabetes Society has established 3 main criteria: (1) adult age of onset (>30 years); (2) presence of any islet-cell autoantibody; and (3) absence of insulin requirement for at least 6 months after diagnosis. However, there is heterogeneity in the rate of β-cell destruction and disease progression. Thus, the fact that this patient does not use insulin does not necessarily exclude the possibility that she may have an autoimmune basis for her diabetes. Her family history is strongly positive for other autoimmune conditions. C-peptide measurement (Answer A) is not likely to be helpful for diagnostic purposes, given the absence of insulin requirement. Testing autoantibody titers would be the most direct way to establish the diagnosis of LADA, but insulin autoantibody testing (Answer D) may be falsely positive, although it is acknowledged that recombinant human insulins are less immunogenic than previously used animal insulins. Thus, among the answer choices, testing for glutamic acid decarboxylase (GAD) 65 autoantibodies (Answer B) would be the best way forward. Indeed, this patient had positive GAD 65 autoantibodies with a titer of 102 IU/mL (normal <5 IU/mL).

Interestingly, multicenter studies have shown that 2% to 14% of patients considered to have type 2 diabetes have autoantibodies that are consistent with a diagnosis of LADA, with rates higher in studies of northern European populations and lower in African American, Hispanic, and Arab populations. Additionally, the rate of autoantibody positivity is even higher in patients younger than 35 years (up to 25%), and there are now reports of LADA-like syndromes in children (ie, autoimmune diabetes that progresses to insulin requirement very slowly). Regarding disease progression, studies suggest that persons with diagnosed type 2 diabetes who have positive islet-cell antibodies have impaired β-cell function at diagnosis compared with patients with type 2 diabetes who do not have islet-cell antibodies, but that β-cell function is not as reduced as it is in persons with type 1 diabetes (as measured by response of C-peptide to a glucose infusion). However, over time, β-cell responsiveness decreases in individuals who have LADA. The decline is variable, and studies suggest that β-cell failure, described as undetectable C-peptide, may occur as late as 12 years after diagnosis.

Returning to the question of C-peptide measurement, once LADA is diagnosed, a recent expert consensus statement suggests that random C-peptide measurement may be used to guide treatment such that low levels of C-peptide (<0.9 ng/mL [<0.3 nmol/L]) prompt institution of insulin therapy (multiple daily injection regimen), while patients with higher levels (>2.11 ng/mL [>0.7 nmol/L]) may be treated per type 2 diabetes guidelines. C-peptide concentrations between those values are considered to be in a grey area.

Educational Objective
Diagnose latent autoimmune diabetes in adults or autoimmune diabetes in which β-cell failure is slowly progressive.

References
Stenstrom G, Gottsater A, Bakhtadze E, Berger B, Sundkvist G. Latent autoimmune diabetes in adults: definition, prevalence, beta-cell function, and treatment. *Diabetes*. 2005;54(Suppl 2):S68-S72. PMID: 16306343

Buzzetti R, Tuomi T, Mauricio D, et al. Management of latent autoimmune diabetes in adults: a consensus statement from an International Expert Panel. *Diabetes*. 2020;69(10):2037-2047. PMID: 32847960

27 ANSWER: C) Achieve euthyroidism with antithyroid drugs and then recommend total thyroidectomy

Graves disease is the most common cause of hyperthyroidism in women during the third and fourth decades of life. Biochemical findings include suppressed TSH, elevated free T_4 and/or elevated free T_3 (T_3>>T_4), and elevated thyroid-stimulating immunoglobulin antibodies. Thyroid-stimulating immunoglobulin antibodies distinguish this condition from other causes of hyperthyroidism. Thyroid scan shows homogeneously increased radiotracer uptake in both thyroid lobes and 24-hour thyroid uptake is elevated. Graves disease can affect organs and parts of the body besides the thyroid, including eyes, skin, and/or extremities. Orbitopathy (ophthalmopathy) in patients with hyperthyroidism is characteristic of Graves disease. Graves orbitopathy can be present in 20% of patients with Graves hyperthyroidism, but only 5% have moderate to severe disease. The incidence of Graves orbitopathy peaks in the fifth and sixth decades of life. The degree of hyperthyroidism, existence of Graves orbitopathy, size of the thyroid gland, and comorbidities (older age, cardiovascular disease) influence decision-making in the management of Graves disease. In addition to β-adrenergic blockers, treatment options include antithyroid drugs vs radioiodine treatment vs total thyroidectomy.

Antithyroid drugs or thyroidectomy do not appear to have a negative impact on the course of orbitopathy. After each of these choices, the serum thyroid-stimulating immunoglobulin concentration decreases. In contrast, radioiodine therapy appears to affect the development or worsening of orbitopathy related to a sustained increase in thyroid-stimulating immunoglobulin levels compared with antithyroid drugs or surgery. Therefore, radioiodine treatment should not be recommended in patients with Graves disease who have active moderate to severe orbitopathy. Antithyroid drugs or surgery are the preferred options. Recent data suggest that long-term antithyroid medication is safe in the management of Graves disease and can influence the remission rate. In the case of a patient refusing surgery (or having medical contraindication) and not being able to tolerate antithyroid drugs, glucocorticoid administration should be provided concurrent with radioiodine treatment to decrease the orbitopathy exacerbation. The recommendation is to initiate prednisone, 30 to 40 mg orally daily, and taper off within 6 to 8 weeks. The European Thyroid Association recommends intravenous steroids for moderate to severe active orbitopathy. Patients with Graves disease receiving radioiodine treatment should be advised about cigarette smoking cessation and avoiding pregnancy for the first 6 months after radioiodine treatment, as well as the importance of maintaining the TSH concentration within the euthyroid range before conception. Cigarette smoking increases the incidence of symptomatic Graves orbitopathy, increases the risk of worsening orbitopathy after radioiodine treatment, and reduces the efficacy of steroid therapy. The severity of Graves orbitopathy is defined in the table.

Table. Defining the Severity of Graves Orbitopathy

Severity of orbitopathy	Features
Mild	- Lid retraction <2 mm - Mild involvement of soft tissues - Proptosis <3 mm above upper normal limit for race - No or intermittent diplopia - No corneal exposure - Normal optic nerve
Moderate	- Lid retraction ≥2 mm - Moderate involvement of soft tissues - Proptosis ≥3 mm above upper normal limit for race - Inconstant diplopia - Mild corneal irritation - Normal optic nerve
Severe	- Lid retraction ≥2 mm - Severe involvement of soft tissues - Proptosis ≥3 mm above upper normal limit for race - Constant diplopia - Mild corneal exposure - Normal optic nerve
Sight-threatening	- Severe corneal exposure and compression of the optic nerve

While evaluating for proptosis, upper normal limits for race are defined as follows:
- Asian: female/male, 16 mm/17 mm (Thai) or 18.6 mm (Chinese)
- White: female/male, 19 mm/21 mm
- Black: female/male, 23 mm/24 mm

Active orbitopathy is defined by the clinical activity score. At the initial visit, a 7-point clinical activity score is reviewed and 1 point is given for each item present:
- Pain behind the globe in the last 4 weeks
- Pain with eye movement in the last 4 weeks
- Redness of the eyelids
- Redness of the conjunctiva
- Eyelid swelling
- Chemosis
- Inflammation of the caruncle

At a follow-up visit, 3 more items are reviewed and 1 point is given for each item present:
- Increase in proptosis ≥2 mm
- Decreased eye movements ≥5 degrees in any one direction
- Decreased visual acuity ≥1 line on Snellen chart

Graves orbitopathy is considered active in patients with a clinical activity score of 3 or higher at the initial assessment and 4 or higher at the follow-up assessment.

The patient in this vignette has Graves disease with active moderate Graves orbitopathy and an enlarged thyroid gland without compressive symptoms. Therefore, performing neck CT (Answer A) is not recommended. The best treatment strategy is to achieve euthyroidism with antithyroid drugs and then perform total thyroidectomy (Answer C). Due to her active moderate Graves orbitopathy and her large goiter, radioiodine treatment (Answer B) should not be recommended. SSKI (Answer D) is usually not given as a sole treatment, but SSKI, 5 drops 3 times daily, is usually prescribed for 5 days before thyroidectomy to decrease the vascularity to the thyroid gland and decrease the bleeding risk during thyroidectomy. Thyroid scan (Answer E) is not necessary to confirm the diagnosis, as an elevated thyroid-stimulating immunoglobulin concentration is consistent with Graves disease.

Educational Objective
Manage hyperthyroidism in a patient with moderate to severe Graves orbitopathy (ophthalmopathy).

Reference(s)
Ross DS, Burch HB, Cooper DS, et al. 2016 American Thyroid Association guidelines for diagnosis and management of hyperthyroidism and other causes of thyrotoxicosis. *Thyroid*. 2016;26(10):1343-1421. PMID: 27521067

Bartalena L, Baldeschi L, Boboridis K, et al. The 2016 European Thyroid Association/European group on graves orbitopathy guidelines for the management of graves orbitopathy. *Eur Thyroid J*. 2016;5(1):9-26. PMID: 27099835

Laurberg P, Berman DC, Bulow Pedersen I, et al. Incidence and clinical presentation of moderate to severe graves' orbitopathy in a Danish population before and after iodine fortification of salt. *J Clin Endocrinol Metab*. 2012;97(7):2325-2332. PMID: 22518849

Azizi F, Abdi H, Amouzegar A. Control of Graves hyperthyroidism with very long-term methimazole treatment: a clinical trial. *BMC Endocr Disord*. 2021;21(1):16. PMID: 33446181

28
ANSWER: C) Insulin glargine, 20 units once daily, and regular insulin, 8 units every 6 hours

Evidence of poor outcomes in hospitalized patients with hyperglycemia has led to the development of a revised approach to the inpatient management of diabetes. Insulin therapy is the current standard of care in the inpatient setting. When patients are consuming regular meals and experiencing hyperglycemia, insulin therapy administered via the traditional basal-bolus approach is indicated. While the approach is similar in patients receiving continuous enteral nutrition, a few issues must be considered.

Patients should receive a dose of basal insulin that is appropriate for their body weight and/or their current total daily insulin dose. Very lean, insulin-sensitive patients, elderly patients, or patients with new hyperglycemia (no history of diabetes) may receive conservative dosing (~0.3 units/kg per day). Patients with normal body weight or who are overweight and have a history of diabetes are typically given 0.4 to 0.5 units/kg per day. Patients with obesity who have a history of diabetes, are receiving glucocorticoids, or are known to be very insulin resistant typically receive 0.6 to 0.8 units/kg per day (or more). Renal function should also be considered when determining insulin doses. Impaired renal clearance of insulin prolongs the half-life of circulating insulin and often results in decreased insulin requirements. A decrease in the metabolic clearance rate of insulin is observed in patients with an estimated glomerular filtration rate less than 40 mL/min per 1.73 m^2, and a significant prolongation of the insulin half-life is observed when the rate falls below 20 mL/min per 1.73 m^2.

Once the total daily insulin dose is determined (either calculated using weight-based dosing, the current total daily dose of intravenous insulin, or taking an average of the 2), a 50/50 distribution of the patient's total daily insulin requirement is generally administered via a basal-bolus regimen. However, many clinicians suggest that the regimen be more heavily weighted to bolus coverage in patients receiving continuous enteral nutrition, and that less basal insulin be provided (30%-40% basal and 60%-70% bolus) because of the frequent interruption of enteral nutrition that can occur in the inpatient setting. Insulin is usually administered via a once-daily dose of basal insulin and scheduled doses of regular or short-acting insulin every 6 hours to be given while enteral nutrition is being administered. A correction dose of short-acting insulin is also usually added to the scheduled doses of bolus insulin.

An inadequate dose of basal insulin results in hyperglycemia when the regularly scheduled doses of bolus insulin are stopped (ie, when continuous enteral nutrition is interrupted). If the dose of basal insulin is too high (Answer A), it will likely result in the development of hypoglycemia should the enteral nutrition be stopped or interrupted. The patient's total daily insulin dose was 50 units while receiving intravenous insulin. A reasonable basal dose of subcutaneous insulin would be 30% to 40% of the total daily dose (15-20 units), and the bolus dose would be 60% to 70% (30-35 units), divided into 4 regularly scheduled doses administered every 6 hours (~7-9 units every 6 hours) when using regular insulin, or divided into 6 regularly scheduled doses administered every 4 hours when using faster-acting insulin analogues (insulin aspart, insulin lispro, etc). The only answer choice listed that contains both a basal and bolus schedule of insulin doses, with a reasonable distribution of insulin doses (~30%-40% basal and 60%-70% bolus), is Answer C (insulin glargine, 20 units once daily, and regular insulin, 8 units every 6 hours).

Administering insulin glargine, 50 units once daily, and insulin aspart, correction dosing every 6 hours (Answer B) is incorrect because it does not include regularly scheduled doses of bolus insulin (only correction doses, and the dose of basal insulin is too high. Administering insulin glargine, 25 units subcutaneously twice daily (Answer D) is incorrect because there are no scheduled doses of bolus insulin, and the patient would be at high risk of hypoglycemia should the continuous enteral nutrition be interrupted while he is receiving a dose of basal insulin that is 100% of his current total daily insulin dose. Administering insulin glargine, 50 units once daily, and insulin aspart, 6 units every 6 hours (Answer E) is incorrect because the basal and bolus insulin doses are well above the patient's current total daily insulin dose. Given his current level of glycemic control (130-190 mg/dL [7.2-10.5 mmol/L]), such doses would be inappropriate.

Mixed insulin (70/30 insulin NPH/insulin regular) administered 2 to 3 times daily is an additional approach to managing hyperglycemia in patients receiving continuous enteral nutrition. This program allows lowering or eliminating 1 of the doses for the increasingly common tube-feeding programs in rehabilitation centers or patients' homes that entail discontinuation of tube feeding for 6 to 8 hours. The main issue with this approach is the lack of basal insulin coverage in patients for whom continuous enteral nutrition (and thus insulin doses) must be withheld for prolonged periods. Accordingly, an alternative approach is to administer NPH insulin twice daily to provide basal coverage, and regular insulin every 6 to 8 hours to cover the carbohydrate content of the continuous enteral nutrition. Regimens comprised of 70/30 mixed insulin or NPH and regular insulin may also be more advantageous in some situations where the cost of insulin therapy is an additional issue that must be considered.

Educational Objective
Manage glycemic control with multiple daily insulin injections in patients with diabetes mellitus who are receiving continuous enteral nutrition.

Reference(s)

American Diabetes Association. 15. Diabetes care in the hospital: standards of medical care in diabetes—2020. *Diabetes Care.* 2020;43(Suppl 1):S193-S202. PMID: 31862758

Mabrey ME, Barton AB, Corsino L, et al. Managing hyperglycemia and diabetes in patients receiving enteral feedings: A health system approach. *Hosp Pract* (1995). 2015;43(2):74-78. PMID: 25744356

Gosmanov AR, Umpierrez GE. Management of hyperglycemia during enteral and parenteral nutrition therapy. *Curr Diab Rep.* 2013;13(1):155-162. PMID: 23065369

Cortinovis F, Cassibba S, Colombo O. Blood glucose control in enteral nutrition: strategy for the treatment of hyperglycemia in patients receiving enteral nutrition. *Diet Nutri Crit Care.* 2014:1-12.

Hsia E, Seggelke SA, Gibbs J, Rasouli N, Draznin B. Comparison of 70/30 biphasic insulin with glargine/lispro regimen in non-critically ill diabetic patients on continuous enteral nutrition therapy. *Nutr Clin Pract.* 2011;26(6):714-717. PMID: 22205560

Leahy JL. Insulin management of diabetic patients on general medical and surgical floors. *Endocr Pract.* 2006;12(Suppl 3):86-90. PMID: 16905523

Eberhard Ritz, Marcin Adamczak, Andrzej Wiecek. Carbohydrate metabolism in kidney disease and kidney failure. In: Kopple JD, Massry SG, Kalantar-Zadeh K, eds. *Nutritional Management of Renal Disease.* Academic Press; 2013:17-30.

29 ANSWER: D) Perform a progesterone withdrawal test

A pituitary macroadenoma was diagnosed when this patient developed secondary amenorrhea, which resolved after surgical tumor resection. Now, she has developed secondary amenorrhea after a recent pregnancy. Secondary amenorrhea is defined as no menses for more than 3 months in women with a history of regular menses or for more than 6 months in women with irregular menses. Primary amenorrhea is diagnosed in adolescence or young adulthood if there is a history of delayed menarche after age 15 years. Although the most common causes of secondary amenorrhea include polycystic ovary syndrome or hypothalamic amenorrhea, her history of stereotactic radiosurgery places her at greater risk for developing secondary hypogonadism. Studies vary in the reported rates and timing of hypopituitarism after stereotactic radiosurgery—from 24% to 40%. Risk increases over time, generally starting 3 to 5 years after therapy. Selecting stereotactic radiosurgery for residual adenoma growth allowed for an interval when she could try to conceive before the effects of radiation affected pituitary function. The development of hypopituitarism after repeat surgery might have occurred earlier and affected her ability to successfully conceive again.

The key question in this case is whether the patient has enough estrogen present or requires estrogen replacement. Therefore, using a combined oral contraceptive (Answer E) containing estrogen will induce a period if there are no structural abnormalities, but this would not determine estrogen status.

The progesterone withdrawal test mimics the luteal phase of an ovulatory cycle to assess whether there is enough endogenous estrogen present to develop an endometrial lining and result in a menstrual period within 10 days of completing the progesterone 10-day treatment. Therefore, the best next step would be to perform a progesterone withdrawal test (Answer D). At the same time, withdrawal bleeding makes it less likely that an anatomic abnormality is preventing menstrual bleeding. In addition, given that she has had no period for 6 months, it would prevent endometrial hyperplasia if she is having anovulatory cycles with estrogen present rather than secondary hypogonadism. It can also be a treatment for women with anovulatory amenorrhea with estrogen present, and it is recommended to have a withdrawal bleed every 3 months if there are no spontaneous menses.

Although pelvic ultrasonography (Answer C) could also be reassuring if the endometrial lining is thicker than 4 mm (confirming enough estrogen is present), it has also been 6 months of amenorrhea since she finished lactation, so preventing the development of endometrial hyperplasia is important. Similarly, measurement of FSH and estradiol (Answer A) might demonstrate very low estradiol concentrations, but this would not offer a potential treatment of the endometrial lining. If estradiol is present but on the low side or just slightly lower than normal, additional diagnostic testing would be required.

Because her residual adenoma has demonstrated stability after stereotactic radiosurgery, pituitary MRI (Answer B) is less likely to guide diagnosis and treatment at this time. Of note, her pituitary macroadenoma was diagnosed at a young age, so the diagnosis of familial isolated pituitary adenoma might have been considered, especially if there were a family history of pituitary adenomas. Although pathogenic variants in the AIP gene are inherited in an autosomal dominant manner, only 20% to 30% of individuals with a pathogenic variant develop a pituitary adenoma. Even if this patient had familial isolated pituitary adenoma, tumors are not more likely to recur after treatment.

Educational Objective
Evaluate secondary amenorrhea after treatment of a nonsecreting pituitary macroadenoma.

Reference(s)
Cordeiro D, Xu Z, Mehta G, et al. Hypopituitarism after gamma knife radiosurgery for pituitary adenomas: a multicenter, international study. *J Neurosurg.* 2019;131(4):1188-1196. PMID: 31369225

Gordan CM, Ackerman KE, Berga SL, et al. Functional hypothalamic amenorrhea: an Endocrine Society clinical practice guideline. *J Clin Endocrinol Metab.* 2017;102(5):1413-1439. PMID: 28368518

30 ANSWER: D) Thyrotropinoma

This patient has numerous symptoms and signs consistent with thyrotoxicosis. She also has a small, symmetric goiter, but no pathognomonic eye signs to indicate an autoimmune basis despite the family history of primary hypothyroidism in her mother.

The serum free T_4 and free T_3 levels are both clearly elevated, which is consistent with the clinical picture. However, serum TSH is not suppressed (<0.1 and typically <0.01 mIU/L) as should be the case in primary hyperthyroidism. At this point, it is necessary to consider the possible causes of hyperthyroxinemia with nonsuppressed TSH, which include:

1. Increased thyroid hormone–binding capacity (leading to increased total T_4 and total T_3, but typically normal free hormone levels (eg, due to oral estrogen therapy, pregnancy)
2. Laboratory assay interference
    a) Falsely elevated free thyroid hormones
        i. Heterophilic antibodies
        ii. Antiiodothyronine antibodies
        iii. Familial dysalbuminemic hyperthyroxinemia
    b) Falsely nonsuppressed TSH:
        i. Heterophilic or human antianimal antibodies
        ii. Macro-TSH
3. Thyroxine replacement therapy (including poor adherence)
4. Medications (eg, amiodarone, heparin, biotin)
5. Nonthyroidal illness (including acute psychiatric disorders)
6. Thyrotropinoma (TSH-secreting pituitary adenoma)
7. Resistance to thyroid hormone due to a loss-of-function pathogenic variant in the *THRB* gene
8. Disorders of thyroid hormone transport or metabolism

In the absence of confounding medications or intercurrent illness, the next step is to exclude assay interference. Here the laboratory has already undertaken appropriate analyses and confirmed true hyperthyroxinemia with nonsuppressed TSH.

This excludes familial dysalbuminemic hyperthyroxinemia (Answer B) as the underlying diagnosis. In this condition, thyroid hormone–binding capacity ($T_4 \pm T_3$) is increased due to a pathogenic variant in the gene encoding albumin (albumin is 1 of the 3 major binding proteins for T_4 and T_3). Total thyroid hormone levels are therefore raised, even though the patient is euthyroid. In addition, measured free hormone levels may also be artifactually high due to interference by the mutant albumin variant in commonly used 1-step laboratory assays. However, some 2-step assays or less commonly available gold standard methods (eg, equilibrium dialysis, mass spectrometry) confirm biochemical euthyroidism.

Only when assay interference has been excluded should rarer causes be considered, such as a TSH-secreting pituitary adenoma (thyrotropinoma) (Answer D) or resistance to thyroid hormone (due to a loss-of-function pathogenic variant in the human thyroid hormone receptor β gene [*THRB*]) (Answer C). Distinguishing between thyrotropinoma and *THRB*-related resistance to thyroid hormone typically requires a combination of investigations (*see table*).

Table. Distinguishing Between Thyrotropinoma and *THRB*-Related Resistance to Thyroid Hormone

Investigation	Thyrotropinoma	Resistance to thyroid hormone (THRB-resistance to thyroid hormone)
Serum SHBG	Increased (but may be normal if cosecretion of GH)	Normal
Serum α-subunit	Increased/normal	Normal
Thyrotropin-releasing hormone stimulation test (not available in all countries)	Absent/attenuated TSH response	Preserved/exaggerated TSH response
Pituitary MRI	Adenoma (although some microadenomas may not be visualized on standard MRI sequences)	Normal (but incidentalomas in 10%-15% as per the general population)

In this patient, serum SHBG is elevated and the TSH response to thyrotropin-releasing hormone is absent, both of which strongly point towards a TSH-secreting pituitary adenoma. Although the serum α-subunit level is normal, this does not exclude a thyrotropinoma. Microthyrotropinomas may not be readily visualized on standard clinical MR sequences (analogous to corticotropinomas in Cushing disease), and additional imaging may be required to localize the causative lesion. This patient's presentation is therefore still most likely due to a thyrotropinoma despite the unremarkable MRI findings.

Although there is a family history of thyroid dysfunction, we are told this is primary hypothyroidism. In addition, in hyperthyroxinemia with nonsuppressed TSH due to *THRB*-related resistance to thyroid hormone, SHBG is typically normal, reflecting hepatic resistance, and the TSH response to thyrotropin-releasing hormone is preserved or exaggerated.

The presentation is not consistent with primary hyperthyroidism due to a toxic multinodular goiter (Answer E) or surreptitious exogenous thyroxine ingestion (Answer A), both of which would be expected to cause TSH suppression.

Educational Objective
Describe the key steps in the laboratory and radiologic investigation of a patient with apparent hyperthyroxinemia and nonsuppressed TSH.

Reference(s)

Khoo S, Lyons G, McGowan A, et al. Familial dysalbuminaemic hyperthyroxinaemia interferes with current free thyroid hormone immunoassay methods. *Eur J Endocrinol.* 2020;182(6):533-538. PMID: 32213658

Gurnell M, Visser T, Beck-Peccoz PB, Chatterjee VKK. Resistance to thyroid hormone. In: JL Jameson JL, De Groot LJ, eds. *Endocrinology.* 7th ed. Saunders Elsevier; 2015:1649-1665.

Koulouri O, Gurnell M. TSH-secreting pituitary adenomas. In: Huhtaniemi I, Martini L, eds. *Encyclopedia of Endocrine Diseases.* 2nd ed. Academic Press; 2018:261-266.

31 ANSWER: C) Refer for intravenous iron infusion

Iron deficiency is a common complication of Roux-en Y gastric bypass surgery for several reasons. The excluded proximal duodenum is a major site of iron absorption; combined with a low-acid environment and commonly experienced food aversion to meat, this contributes to the development of iron deficiency. In addition, about 50% of women who undergo bariatric surgery are of reproductive age and lose blood through monthly menstrual periods. The prevalence of iron deficiency following Roux-en Y gastric bypass is estimated to be between 20% and 50% and is more common in premenopausal women. The reported prevalence of iron deficiency in men after gastric bypass is approximately 17%. Patients with preexisting iron deficiency and concurrent B12 deficiency are at high risk of developing significant iron deficiency after surgery. Iron deficiency may or may not be associated with anemia. The decision to treat should therefore be based on symptoms attributable to iron deficiency, including fatigue and reduced exercise tolerance.

The general recommendation for iron intake following gastric bypass surgery is 45 to 60 mg of elemental iron daily. Iron supplementation is often required to meet this need, especially in light of dietary restrictions and physiologic changes that limit efficient absorption of dietary iron. Oral iron is better absorbed when taken with vitamin C, while calcium supplements and high-calcium foods can decrease absorption and should be taken separately from iron supplements.

Patients who develop iron deficiency after Roux-en Y gastric bypass should first be started on oral iron supplements. After bariatric surgery, it can be difficult for patients to tolerate oral iron supplementation because of commonly experienced gastrointestinal adverse effects. Although increasing her oral iron supplementation (Answer A) at this time is reasonable, she has already developed symptomatic iron deficiency anemia despite taking what should be an adequate amount of oral iron. When response to oral iron supplementation is poor, or if a patient develops symptomatic iron deficiency anemia, intravenous iron administration (Answer C) is the best next step. The ferritin level should be measured in 3 months to ensure an adequate biochemical response. Repeating the iron infusion is appropriate if the patient's ferritin level remains low. Of note, new-onset hypophosphatemia has been reported in patients receiving ferric carboxymaltose after gastric bypass surgery through a mechanism involving renal phosphate wasting via FGF-23.

Patients should also be screened for other sources of blood loss, including losses from the gastrointestinal tract and the genitourinary system. If the patient has persistent iron deficiency anemia despite adequate iron supplementation, upper and lower endoscopies for occult gastrointestinal bleeding (Answer B) can be considered. However, this would not be the first step in a young patient with a clear risk factor for iron deficiency (Roux-en-Y gastric bypass). Women with heavy menstrual blood flow may benefit from a referral to gynecology to discuss management strategies. Although patients who undergo gastric bypass surgery may be deficient in thiamine and folate, deficiencies of these vitamins do not manifest as microcytic anemia. Thus, prescribing thiamine (Answer D) or folate supplementation (Answer E) is not the best next step.

Educational Objective

Explain how gastric bypass anatomy predisposes to iron deficiency and formulate a management plan.

Reference(s)

Decker GA, Swain JM, Crowell MD, Scolapio JS. Gastrointestinal and nutritional complications after bariatric surgery. *Am J Gastroenterol.* 2007;102(11):2571-2580; quiz 2581. PMID: 17640325

Parrott J, Frank L, Rabena R, Craggs-Dino L, Isom KA, Greiman L. American Society for Metabolic and Bariatric Surgery Integrated Health Nutritional Guidelines for the Surgical Weight Loss Patient 2016 Update: Micronutrients. *Surg Obes Relat Dis.* 2017;13(5):727-741. PMID: 28392254

Schoeb M, Räss A, Frei N, Aczél S, Brändle M, Bilz S. High risk of hypophosphatemia in patients with previous bariatric surgery receiving ferric carboxymaltose: a prospective cohort study. *Obes Surg.* 2020;30(7):2659-2666. PMID: 32221822

32 ANSWER: C) Subacute thyroiditis

This patient's most likely diagnosis is subacute thyroiditis (Answer C). Subacute (granulomatous) thyroiditis, also called de Quervain or painful thyroiditis, is an uncommon cause of thyrotoxicosis that often begins with a prodrome of low-grade fever, pharyngitis, and other symptoms of an upper respiratory infection. This is followed by the development of bilateral or unilateral thyroid pain that radiates to the jaw or ear and can be associated with dysphagia. When initially unilateral, the pain typically migrates to the contralateral lobe over subsequent days to weeks. On physical examination, the thyroid gland may be enlarged up to 3 to 4 times normal size and is characteristically tender to palpation. Elevated erythrocyte sedimentation rate and C-reactive protein are characteristic laboratory findings.

Suppurative thyroiditis (Answer D), also called acute infectious thyroiditis, is an important diagnostic consideration in patients presenting with signs and symptoms suggestive of subacute thyroiditis. Pain and tenderness in suppurative thyroiditis are unilateral and a palpable fluctuant mass may be present. When the diagnosis is unclear, such as in cases of unilateral thyroid pain or when leukocytosis is present, prompt evaluation with ultrasonography is needed and FNA should be considered to obtain material for stains and cultures. Although the patient is an intravenous drug user, neck ultrasonography had no findings suggestive of an abscess but did demonstrate diffuse heterogeneity, which is characteristic of subacute thyroiditis. In contrast, the ultrasonographic appearance of thyroid abscess-like structures in the setting of infectious thyroiditis is shown (*see images*). The patient described in the associated case report was immunocompromised; the infectious organism was identified as coccidioidomycosis.

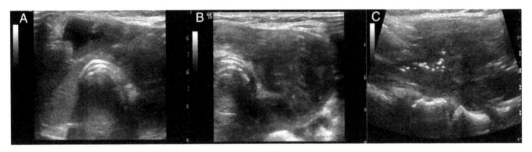

Reprinted from: McAninch EA, Xu C, Lagari VS, Kim BW. Coccidiomycosis thyroiditis in an immunocompromised host post-transplant: case report and literature review. *J Clin Endocrinol Metab*. 2014;99(5):1537-1542.

The pathogenesis of subacute thyroiditis is not completely understood, but it is thought to be related to a viral infection or a postviral inflammatory reaction occurring in genetically predisposed individuals, particularly with the HLA-B35 haplotype. Subacute thyroiditis is thought to occur seasonally with a higher incidence in summer and has been associated with coxsackievirus, adenovirus, measles, mumps, and more recently with SARS-CoV-2 infection. Thyroid dysfunction with subacute thyroiditis usually follows a typical pattern of thyrotoxicosis, transient euthyroidism, hypothyroidism, and return to euthyroidism. Thyroid autoimmunity does not have a central role in this disorder and thus recurrence is rare following recovery. There is no role for the use of thionamide drugs (methimazole) in the management of subacute thyroiditis because it is not a disorder of increased thyroid hormone production. Nonsteroidal antiinflammatory drugs and glucocorticoids are used to mitigate inflammatory symptoms related to subacute thyroiditis. Glucocorticoids may be associated with a shorter time to symptom resolution. Neither Graves disease (Answer A) nor autoimmune thyroiditis (Hashimoto) (Answer B) is the most likely diagnosis in this patient. Graves disease causes hyperthyroidism resulting from TSH receptor antibody–mediated activation of the TSH receptor. Autoimmune thyroiditis most often causes hypothyroidism, but it can be associated with episodes of painless or postpartum thyroiditis. Both typically cause the same pattern of thyroid dysfunction seen in subacute thyroiditis; however, pain is notably absent and recovery to euthyroidism may not occur. Neither Graves disease nor autoimmune thyroiditis would be associated with a history of recent viral illness or result in recurrent fevers over a period of weeks.

This patient's clinical presentation is also inconsistent with that of thyroid lymphoma (Answer E), which usually presents with a rapidly enlarging mass in a patient with preexisting autoimmune thyroiditis. The characteristic ultrasonographic appearance of thyroid lymphoma is a large hypoechoic mass with marked posterior acoustic enhancement.

Educational Objective
Diagnose subacute thyroiditis.

Reference(s)

Brancatella A, Ricci D, Viola N, Sgrò D, Santini F, Latrofa F. Subacute thyroiditis after Sars-COV-2 infection. *J Clin Endocrinol Metab*. 2020;105(7):dgaa276. PMID: 32436948

Fatourechi V, Aniszewski JP, Fatourechi GZ, Atkinson EJ, Jacobsen SJ. Clinical features and outcome of subacute thyroiditis in an incidence cohort: Olmsted County, Minnesota, study. *J Clin Endocrinol Metab*. 2003;88(5):2100-2105. PMID: 12727961

Sato J, Uchida T, Komiya K, et al. Comparison of the therapeutic effects of prednisolone and nonsteroidal anti-inflammatory drugs in patients with subacute thyroiditis. *Endocrine*. 2017;55(1):209-214. PMID: 27688010

McAninch EA, Xu C, Lagari VS, Kim BW. Coccidiomycosis thyroiditis in an immunocompromised host post-transplant: case report and literature review. *J Clin Endocrinol Metab*. 2014 May;99(5):1537-1542. PMID: 24606101

33 ANSWER: A) Basic metabolic panel and serum β-hydroxybutyrate measurement

Until recently, this patient was doing very well from a diabetes management perspective. However, the severe restriction of carbohydrate intake that occurred when he initiated the ketogenic diet, in addition to his current SGLT-2 inhibitor therapy, resulted in development of diabetic ketoacidosis. Patients taking SGLT-2 inhibitor therapy must be counseled on the risk of diabetic ketoacidosis, particularly when initiating low-carbohydrate diets, as well as in situations where oral intake is significantly decreased because of acute illness, medical testing, etc. Patients sometimes initiate very aggressive dietary programs without consulting their team of medical professionals, so counseling and education at the time of SGLT-2 inhibitor initiation is critical. Ketogenic diets are high-fat, moderate-protein, low-carbohydrate dietary patterns in which the body's principal energy source is fat. The traditional ketogenic diet for the treatment of epilepsy consists of 90% of calories from fat, although less restrictive versions have also been used. Generally, ketogenic eating plans not intended for the treatment of epilepsy can be described by the following breakdown of calories from macronutrients: ~60%-85% fat, ~15%-30% protein, ~5%-10% carbohydrate.

The best next step is to obtain a basic metabolic panel and measure serum β-hydroxybutyrate (Answer A) (as well as stop the SGLT-2 inhibitor therapy). Arterial blood gas assessment would also help in the diagnosis and management. The basic metabolic panel would help to identify a reduced bicarbonate level and electrolyte and kidney function abnormalities that are commonly observed in patients with diabetic ketoacidosis. Serum β-hydroxybutyrate should be measured, as it will be helpful in making the correct diagnosis in this patient. The level of β-hydroxybutyrate in the setting of nutritional or starvation ketosis is generally far lower than what is usually observed in a state of diabetic ketoacidosis.

While a urine analysis (Answer D) would be helpful to investigate for a urinary tract infection, the patient did not report dysuria or hematuria. The urinalysis would reveal qualitative levels of ketonuria and glucosuria because of his current diet and SGLT-2 inhibitor therapy, but it would not reveal his underlying state of diabetic ketoacidosis. Ketonuria occurs in patients who are following ketogenic dietary programs (starvation ketosis) and/or receiving SGLT-2 inhibitor therapy, and glucosuria would be observed in any patient taking an SGLT-2 inhibitor.

The more problematic question for patients with diabetes following a ketogenic diet is how to distinguish between desired nutritional ketosis and diabetic ketoacidosis. Many patients taking SGLT-2 inhibitors or following a very low-carbohydrate diet have some degree of ketosis noted in their urine or blood, but the level seen in the setting of diabetic ketoacidosis would be expected to be much higher. According to Volek and Phinney, blood ketone levels anywhere from 0.5 to 3.0 mmol/L are expected in nutritional ketosis, with the higher end of the range (1.5-3.0 mmol/L) being optimal. Although these levels are not high enough to indicate diabetic ketoacidosis, they can still be seen as a potential warning sign. As such, the larger clinical picture should be considered. Typical blood ketone levels observed in diabetic ketoacidosis are usually 10 to 20+ mmol/L. Patients must be educated regarding additional signs of diabetic ketoacidosis, including nausea, vomiting, and difficulty breathing. In addition, cases of ketoacidosis in patients without diabetes who are adhering to very low-carbohydrate diets have been reported.

Although C-peptide (Answer B) may be helpful in identifying a state of insulin deficiency, it would not establish the diagnosis of diabetic ketoacidosis in this patient. Insulin, and thus C-peptide levels, are reduced in patients following a very strict low-carbohydrate diet.

CT of the abdomen and pelvis (Answer C) would be premature at this point in the evaluation. Diagnostic laboratory testing should generally preclude the ordering of imaging studies. Pancreatic cancer can certainly present with weight loss and gastrointestinal symptoms, but the course of these symptoms is generally more prolonged. This patient reports onset of symptoms just 5 days ago, and his weight loss was intentional.

Obtaining a point-of-care blood glucose value (Answer E) would not be that helpful, as it may be within the normal range in patients with diabetic ketoacidosis in the setting of SGLT-2 inhibitor therapy, commonly referred to as "euglycemic diabetic ketoacidosis."

The potential mechanisms whereby adjunctive therapy with SGLT-2 inhibitors may promote ketosis and increase the risk of ketoacidosis are depicted (*see figure*).

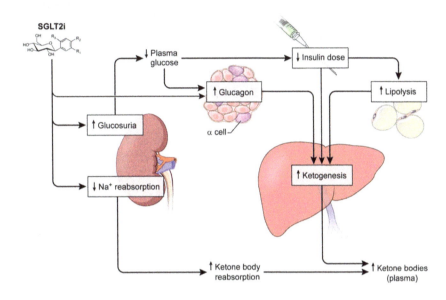

Reprinted from Taylor SI, Blau JE, Rother KI. SGLT2 inhibitors may predispose to ketoacidosis. *J Clin Endocrinol Metab.* 2015;100(8):2849-2852.

Educational Objective
Evaluate and manage patients with suspected diabetic ketoacidosis in the setting of SGLT-2 inhibitor therapy.

Reference(s)
Kossoff EH, Zupec-Kania BA, Amark PE, et al. Practice Committee of the Child Neurology Society; International Ketogenic Diet Study Group. Optimal clinical management of children receiving the ketogenic diet: recommendations of the International Ketogenic Diet Study Group. *Epilepsia.* 2009;50(2):304-317. PMID: 18823325

Carmen M, Safer DL, Saslow LR, et al. Treating binge eating and food addiction symptoms with low-carbohydrate ketogenic diets: a case series. *J Eat Disord.* 2020;8:2. PMID: 32010444

Hayami T, Kato Y, Kamiya H, et al. Case of ketoacidosis by a sodium-glucose cotransporter 2 inhibitor in a diabetic patient with a low-carbohydrate diet. *J Diabetes Investig.* 2015;6(5):587-590. PMID: 26417418

Pankaj S, Isley W. Ketoacidosis during a low-carbohydrate diet. *N Engl J Med.* 2006;354(1):97-98. PMID: 16394313

Chalasani S, Fischer J. South Beach Diet associated ketoacidosis: a case report. *J Med Case Rep.* 2008;2:45. PMID: 18267031

Chen T-Y, Smith W, Rosenstock JL, Lessnau K-D. A life-threatening complication of Atkins diet. *Lancet.* 2006;367(9514):958. PMID: 16546552

Peters AL, Buschur EO, Buse JB, Cohan P, Diner JC, Hirsch IB. Euglycemic diabetic ketoacidosis: a potential complication of treatment with sodium-glucose cotransporter 2 inhibition. *Diabetes Care.* 2015;38(9):1687-1693. PMID: 26078479

Taylor SI, Blau JE, Rother KI. SGLT2 inhibitors may predispose to ketoacidosis. *J Clin Endocrinol Metab.* 2015;100(8):2849-2852. PMID: 26086329

Volek JS, Phinney SD. *The Art and Science of Low Carbohydrate Performance.* Beyond Obesity LLC; 2012.

34

ANSWER: D) Primary aldosteronism

The most common cause of hypertension and hypokalemia is primary aldosteronism (Answer D), although this condition is grossly underdiagnosed and underrecognized. In the context of hypertension and hypokalemia, primary aldosteronism should be the leading diagnosis until proven otherwise.

Primary aldosteronism is a syndrome of renin-independent aldosterone production wherein aldosterone is produced even though renin and angiotensin II are suppressed despite intravascular volume expansion, and often despite hypokalemia. Although conventionally primary aldosteronism has been considered to be a rare cause of endocrine hypertension that presents with resistant hypertension and hypokalemia, it is important to note that the prevalence of primary aldosteronism is much higher than previously considered, and that it can be present even in the absence of resistant hypertension or hypokalemia. Although the possibility of having primary aldosteronism has often been defined by having aldosterone concentrations or aldosterone-to-renin ratio values that are higher than certain prespecified thresholds, emerging studies have consistently shown that primary aldosteronism is a syndrome that manifests across a severity spectrum. Furthermore, aldosterone production is variable throughout the day and aldosterone concentrations can fluctuate across ranges that may not always be perceived to be "high." Therefore, primary aldosteronism is best recognized as a syndrome of inappropriate aldosterone production; that is, aldosterone production when renin is suppressed, when volume is expanded or blood pressure is high, and/or when serum potassium is low.

The prevalence of primary aldosteronism is at least 6% to 22% in patients with hypertension, 28% in patients with hypertension and hypokalemia, and nearly 90% in patients with hypertension and a serum potassium concentration less than 2.5 mEq/L (<2.5 mmol/L). In contrast, less than 3% of patients with hypertension and hypokalemia are ever screened for primary aldosteronism in clinical practice, highlighting the large gap in awareness and clinical implementation. The public health consequences of these missed diagnoses are important since primary aldosteronism is a major contributor to cardiovascular diseases that can be effectively treated with surgical and medical therapies to mitigate this risk.

This patient's history of hypertension and hypokalemia should immediately trigger consideration of primary aldosteronism. The presence of suppressed plasma renin activity further strengthens the possibility of this diagnosis. The fact that the initial aldosterone concentration was 5.2 ng/dL (144.2 pmol/L) should not exclude primary aldosteronism since aldosterone values can fluctuate hour-to-hour, be lower in the setting of hypokalemia, and be influenced by concomitant medications. One option is to repeat testing after withdrawing antihypertensive medications, normalizing serum potassium with oral repletion, and first thing in the morning; this process is laborious and can entail several weeks of effort. Another more practical option is to repeat the screening evaluation with a recalibrated consideration for inappropriate aldosterone production or to conduct a dynamic confirmatory test. On a repeated measurement another day, this patient's aldosterone concentration was 9.5 ng/dL (263.5 pmol/L) with a plasma renin activity less than 0.6 ng/mL per h, underscoring the inappropriate aldosterone production in the setting of hypertension and renin suppression. To maximize the sensitivity of the diagnosis, aldosterone levels as low as 5.0 to 6.0 ng/dL (138.7-166.4 pmol/L) can be considered to be a positive screen in the setting of hypertension, hypokalemia, and renin suppression. This patient underwent recommended dynamic confirmatory testing—in this case, an oral sodium-suppression test—which showed that despite sodium-loading and volume expansion, his aldosterone production remained high and did not suppress (urine sodium excretion of 223 mEq/24 h and aldosterone excretion of 22 μg/24 h [normal <12 μg/24 h]). This result confirmed the diagnosis of primary aldosteronism.

Idiopathic resistant hypertension (Answer B) is a diagnosis of exclusion and should not be considered in a patient with hypokalemia until primary aldosteronism, or other endocrine causes of hypertension, are thoroughly evaluated. Studies in presumptive idiopathic resistant hypertension have shown that mineralocorticoid receptor antagonists are strikingly effective at lowering blood pressure. In fact, many patients with resistant hypertension who respond to mineralocorticoid receptor antagonists have low renin and inappropriate aldosterone production, thereby suggesting that they may instead have a mild form of primary aldosteronism.

Consumption of real licorice (Answer A) can cause a syndrome of apparent mineralocorticoid excess (Answer E). Glycyrrhetinic acid is an inhibitor of 11β-hydroxysteroid dehydrogenase type 2. 11β-Hydroxysteroid dehydrogenase type 2 is normally coexpressed with the renal mineralocorticoid receptor and converts cortisol to the inactive cortisone. In this manner, 11β-hydroxysteroid dehydrogenase type 2 prevents cortisol-induced mineralocorticoid receptor activation. When 11β-hydroxysteroid dehydrogenase type 2 is inhibited, cortisol becomes the dominant ligand of the mineralocorticoid receptor. Because it circulates in approximately 1000-fold higher concentrations than aldosterone, it can induce a potent syndrome of hypertension and hypokalemia with suppression of both renin and aldosterone. The diagnosis of this syndrome further requires some confirmation of glycyrrhetinic acid consumption. Although licorice consumption is common in many parts of the world, consumption of sufficient amounts of glycyrrhetinic acid to induce a chronic form of apparent mineralocorticoid excess is rare.

Liddle syndrome (Answer C) is a consequence of activating pathogenic variants in the gene encoding the epithelial sodium channel resulting in excess sodium reabsorption, volume expansion, and hypokalemia. This condition is rare, is typically diagnosed at a young age, and presents with undetectable circulating aldosterone.

Educational Objective
Diagnose primary aldosteronism.

Reference(s)
Vaidya A, Carey RM. Evolution of the primary aldosteronism syndrome: updating the approach. *J Clin Endocrinol Metab.* 2020;105(12):dgaa606. PMID: 32865201

Funder JW, Carey RM, Mantero F, et al. The management of primary aldosteronism: case detection, diagnosis, and treatment: an Endocrine Society clinical practice guideline. *J Clin Endocrinol Metab.* 2016;101(5):1889-1916. PMID: 26934393

Edelman ER, Butala NM, Avery LL, Lundquist AL, Dighe AS. Case 30-2020: a 54-year-old man with sudden cardiac arrest. *N Engl J Med.* 2020;383(13):1263-1275. PMID: 32966726

35 ANSWER: B) Refer to endocrine surgery for bilateral neck exploration

Hypercalcemia is one of the most common conditions that prompts endocrinology consultation. Most patients presenting as outpatients with hypercalcemia have a benign condition, with the most frequent etiology being primary hyperparathyroidism. Indeed, this patient presents with evidence of hypercalcemia with concomitant intact PTH elevation. In addition, she has anatomic evidence of a possible single parathyroid adenoma, which is noted in approximately 85% to 90% of patients presenting with primary hyperparathyroidism. The caveat, however, in this patient's history is a diagnosis of bipolar disorder with concurrent and long-term use of lithium carbonate.

Lithium is a divalent cation that binds to the calcium-sensing receptor, thereby shifting the calcium set point curve for PTH release to the right. This results in a higher ambient calcium level necessary for suppression of PTH release. In addition, lithium modifies the renal tubular response to PTH, generally resulting in normal or low urinary calcium excretion. These effects can cause hypercalcemia on a consistent or intermittent basis in a large number of treated patients. Indeed, the prevalence of lithium-associated hypercalcemia in patients with bipolar disorder approximated 26% in one large retrospective series. Consistent with a global effect on parathyroid chief-cell stimulation, the incidence of multigland involvement in patients with hyperparathyroidism who are on lithium is substantial, with more than half of patients having evidence of multigland involvement. Indeed, the recurrence rate following resection of a single parathyroid adenoma in patients on chronic lithium therapy is substantially higher than that of patients undergoing single-gland resection for a diagnosis of traditional primary hyperparathyroidism (~16% vs 2%). Given these observations, current evidence supports bilateral neck exploration (Answer B) in patients presenting with hyperparathyroidism who are on long-term lithium therapy to effect the greatest likelihood of long-term cure. More advanced imaging techniques, such as 4D computerized imaging, provide paired anatomic and functional information about candidate parathyroid lesions that can help guide surgical management. Based on a higher risk for reoperation due to lack of cure or subsequent relapse, referral for directed minimally invasive neck exploration (Answer A) is not appropriate for this patient.

Pathogenic variants in the *CASR* gene (Answer C) that cause familial hypocalciuric hypercalcemia also result in a shift of the calcium response curve of PTH release to the right, resulting—similarly to what has been observed with lithium—in a higher serum calcium level required for suppression of PTH release. However, the absence of low calcium excretion, normal serum magnesium (often elevated in patients with familial hypocalciuric hypercalcemia due to enhanced renal magnesium absorption), and history of long-term lithium use in this patient preclude the need for genetic testing for familial hypocalciuric hypercalcemia.

This patient's calcium elevation is above the threshold for indication for surgical referral, based on existing guidelines for the management of asymptomatic hyperparathyroidism. More importantly, she is symptomatic and there is evidence for significant improvement in quality of life in patients who undergo surgical resection and cure with lithium-associated hyperparathyroidism. Thus, conservative management with follow-up biochemical monitoring (Answer E) is not appropriate for this patient. Likewise, treatment with an oral bisphosphonate (Answer D), while protecting against bone mineral density loss in patients with classic primary hyperparathyroidism, is not indicated based on this patient's normal bone density and no expectation of meaningful fracture risk reduction.

Although not included as a potential approach, the use of a calcium-sensing receptor agonist such as cinacalcet may be helpful for patients who are not surgical candidates and who cannot discontinue lithium. In addition, discontinuation of lithium is generally not an option for these patients because of concerns of exacerbating their bipolar disorder and because the effects of lithium often persist upon discontinuation in patients on long-term therapy.

Educational Objective
Diagnose multigland involvement in a patient with primary hyperparathyroidism secondary to long-term lithium use.

Reference(s)
Meehan AD, Udumyan R, Kardell M, Landén M, Järhult J, Wallin G. Lithium-associated hypercalcemia: pathophysiology, prevalence, management. *World J Surg.* 2018;42(2):415-424. PMID: 29260296

Norlén O, Sidhu S, Sywak M, Delbridge L. Long-term outcome after parathyroidectomy for lithium-induced hyperparathyroidism. *Br J Surg.* 2014;101(10):1252-1256. PMID: 25043401

36 ANSWER: B) Endogenous excess insulin production

The patient in this vignette presents for evaluation of hypoglycemia. The Whipple triad has been fulfilled. The triad includes (1) symptoms consistent with hypoglycemia, (2) documentation of low plasma glucose when symptoms are present, and (3) resolution of symptoms when the glucose level is increased. Establishing the Whipple triad is important because isolated low blood glucose measurements may or may not be indicative of underlying pathology. In ill-appearing patients, the cause of hypoglycemia is often more obvious, but in well-appearing patients such as this young woman, further evaluation to determine etiology is necessary.

Laboratory evaluation should be performed when the patient is symptomatic, as was done in this case. Since she was symptomatic overnight and in the fasting state, appropriate testing was done after an overnight fast. Sometimes the fast must be extended up to 72 hours. If the patient describes predominantly postprandial hypoglycemia, then the first test can be a mixed-meal challenge.

Review of the laboratory values in this vignette gives insight into the possible etiology. She had inappropriately normal insulin and C-peptide levels when her glucose concentration was 32 mg/dL (1.8 mmol/L). Hypoglycemia induced by a non–islet-tumor (Answer A) is a rare presentation in patients with malignancy. Characteristically, insulin levels are low in this condition. Hypoglycemia in this setting is mostly seen with mesenchymal tumors (eg, fibrosarcoma) or epithelial tumors (eg, hepatocellular carcinoma). The primary mechanism appears to be production of excess incompletely processed IGF-2 ("big IGF-2"). Big IGF-2 stimulates insulin receptors and increases glucose use. The resulting hypoglycemia leads to lower plasma insulin levels. Big IGF-2 also lowers glucagon and GH levels (and hence IGF-1). Therefore, IGF-2/IGF-1 levels are elevated. In this patient, insulin is inappropriately normal for the degree of hypoglycemia, and the IGF-1 level is normal. A non–islet-cell tumor as a cause of hypoglycemia in this patient is therefore unlikely.

Although patients with adrenal insufficiency (Answer C) can present with hypoglycemia, it is unlikely in this patient because her plasma cortisol concentration is greater than 15 μg/dL (>413.8 nmol/L).

Insulin autoimmune syndrome (also known as Hirata disease) (Answer D) is characterized by hyperinsulinemic hypoglycemia and elevated insulin autoantibodies in patients with no previous exposure to exogenous insulin or other pancreas pathology. It was first described in a Japanese population and occurs more frequently in patients of East Asian ancestry and is rarely diagnosed in White patients in western countries. Hypoglycemia in insulin autoimmune syndrome is often postprandial, but it can be seen in the fasting state. Another form of autoimmune hypoglycemia can be mediated by insulin receptor antibodies. In this White patient with primarily fasting hypoglycemia, insulin autoimmune syndrome is an unlikely etiology for hypoglycemia, and it can be ruled out by checking insulin antibody levels.

The presence of elevated insulin raises the possibility of surreptitious insulin use (Answer E). However, the inappropriately normal C-peptide level for the degree of hypoglycemia makes this etiology less likely. Use of a sulfonylurea or meglitinide would present with high insulin and C-peptide levels, but this patient's medication screen was negative. Endogenous insulin production (Answer B) is therefore the most likely etiology for her hypoglycemia. Laboratory findings suggestive of endogenous insulin production (when the medication screen is negative, plasma blood glucose is <55 mg/dL [<3.1 mmol/L], and the patient is symptomatic) include the following:

- Insulin >3 µIU/mL (>20.8 pmol/L)
- C-peptide >0.6 ng/mL (>0.2 nmol/L)
- β-hydroxybutyrate <2700 µmol/L at the end of the fast

Glycemic response to intravenous glucagon: at least 25 mg/dL (1.4 mmol/L) to 1 mg of glucagon
In this vignette, the insulin, C-peptide, and β-hydroxybutyrate levels meet the criteria for endogenous insulin excess and additional evaluation for insulinoma should be pursued.

Educational Objective
Guide the evaluation for suspected insulinoma.

Reference(s)
Cryer PE, Axelrod L, Grossman AB, et al. Evaluation and management of adult hypoglycemic disorders: an Endocrine Society clinical practice guideline.
 J Clin Endocrinol Metab. 2009;94(3):709-728. PMID: 19088155

Placzkowski KA, Vella A, Thompson GB, et al. Secular trends in the presentation and management of functioning insulinoma at the Mayo Clinic, 1987-2007.
 J Clin Endocrinol Metab. 2009;94(4):1069-1073. PMID: 19141587

37 ANSWER: C) Increased testosterone concentrations in the milk

Transgender men and gender-diverse individuals with a uterus can become pregnant and lactate. If an individual initiates gender-affirming therapy prior to trying to conceive, testosterone should be discontinued before conception and throughout the pregnancy. Transgender and gender-diverse individuals who carry a pregnancy often want to provide their baby with human milk for the well-established benefits to the baby and lactating parent. The desire to lactate is balanced by consideration of difficulties in latching or milk production related to masculinizing chest surgery, the desire to restart gender-affirming testosterone therapy, and the potential for triggering gender dysphoria (ie, distress caused by incongruence between primary and secondary sex characteristics and gender identity). Awareness of lactating tissue, usage of the gendered term *breastfeeding* instead of the preferred term *chestfeeding*, or the process of chestfeeding itself might contribute to dysphoria.

In a study of cisgender lactating women treated with testosterone vaginal cream (dosage not reported), sublingual drops (dosage not reported), or 100-mg subcutaneous pellet implantation, milk testosterone concentrations did not exceed 10 ng/L, the infants' circulating testosterone concentrations were not increased, and no adverse effects to the infants were documented during 7 months of observation. The low oral bioavailability of testosterone most likely explains why increased testosterone concentrations in human milk did not affect the infants. No available data support a correlation between testosterone concentrations in milk and circulating testosterone concentrations in nursing infants (thus, Answer D is incorrect). Circulating testosterone concentrations were not measured in the cisgender lactating women in that study, but they would be predicted to be lower than male-range concentrations typically achieved with gender-affirming testosterone therapy. If testosterone were detectable in the milk of cisgender women on lower-dosage testosterone therapy, it could be assumed there would most likely be increased testosterone concentrations in the milk of transgender men taking gender-affirming testosterone dosages (thus, Answer C is correct).

In the limited reports available, masculinization of babies of transgender men taking testosterone therapy while chestfeeding (Answer B) has not been observed. While masculinization of the infant seems less likely due to low oral bioavailability, this potential risk should be discussed. There are no data regarding the role of testosterone administration route or whether transdermal testosterone vs injectable therapy (Answer E) is preferred in transgender/gender-diverse individuals who are lactating. However, in the aforementioned study, there did not seem to be a difference in testosterone concentrations or effects in the infants of cisgender women receiving testosterone by oral, subcutaneous, or vaginal routes.

Because testosterone can decrease serum prolactin and inhibit lactation, especially if taken before the milk supply is well established, discussion with transgender and gender-diverse individuals who are considering gender-affirming testosterone therapy while lactating should include the possibility of reduced milk production (Answer A). However, the single case report of a lactating transgender man who continued lactation after starting testosterone therapy 21 months postpartum did not report any decrease in milk production for 15 months or any increase in the child's testosterone concentrations. It is thought that establishing lactation for many months before initiating testosterone might decrease the risk for reduced or limited milk supply.

Educational Objective
Counsel a transgender man regarding chestfeeding and postpartum reinitiation of gender-affirming testosterone therapy.

Reference(s)
Center of Excellence for Transgender Health, Department of Family and Community Medicine, University of California San Francisco. Guidelines for the Primary and Gender-Affirming Care of Transgender and Gender Nonbinary People. 2nd ed. Deutsch MB, ed. June 2016. Available at: www.transhealth.ucsf.edu/guidelines. Accessed for verification November 2020.

Hembree WC, Cohen-Kettenis PT, Gooren L, et al. Endocrine treatment of gender-dysphoric/gender-incongruent persons: an Endocrine Society clinical practice guideline. *J Clin Endocrinol Metab.* 2017;102(11):3869-3903. PMID: 28945902

Glaser RL, Newman M, Parsons M, Zava D, Glaser-Garbrick D. Safety of maternal testosterone therapy during breast feeding. *Int J Pharm Compd.* 2009;13(4):314-317. PMID: 23966521

Section on Breastfeeding. Breastfeeding and the use of human milk. *Pediatrics.* 2012;129(3):e827-e841. PMID: 22371471

MacDonald T, Noel-Weiss J, West D, et al. Transmasculine individuals' experiences with lactation, chestfeeding, and gender identity: a qualitative study. *BMC Pregnancy and Childbirth.* 2016;16:106. PMID: 27183978

McDonald TK. Lactation care for transgender and non-binary patients: empowering clients and avoiding aversives. *J Hum Lact.* 2019;35(2):223-226. PMID: 30920857

Light AD, Obedin-Maliver J, Sevelius JM, Kerns JL. Transgender men who experienced regnancy after female-to-male gender transitioning. *Obstet Gynecol.* 2014;124(6):1120-1127. PMID: 25415163

38 ANSWER: A) Measure serum TSH

Lithium is one of the most widely prescribed medications for treating bipolar disorder, and it reduces the risk of suicide in this patient population. The starting dosage is usually 300 mg 2 to 3 times daily. The total daily dose can be increased by 300 mg to 600 mg based on response and tolerability. The serum lithium level should be monitored, so it is maintained in the therapeutic range and toxicity is avoided. Lithium is contraindicated in patients with sodium depletion, dehydration, significant renal impairment, psoriasis, or cardiovascular disease. Lithium can cause many adverse effects unrelated to toxicity and may affect the thyroid gland, kidneys, and parathyroid glands. In addition, lithium can cause tremor, nausea, loose stools/diarrhea, cardiac dysrhythmias, and weight gain. Thyroid-related adverse effects include hypothyroidism, goiter, chronic autoimmune thyroiditis, and hyperthyroidism. Lithium inhibits thyroid hormone release from the thyroid gland, reduces iodine trapping within the gland, and inhibits thyroid hormone synthesis. Before initiating lithium in a patient with bipolar disorder, serum TSH should be measured. TSH should then be measured 3 months after medication initiation and every 6 to 12 months thereafter.

In this vignette, the patient's lithium dosage was further increased due to her symptoms. Her serum TSH concentration was normal before adjustment of the lithium dosage; after the dosage increase, she started experiencing symptoms consistent with hypothyroidism (fatigue, feeling unmotivated, and weight gain). She also has a mild goiter and bradycardia. As lithium is known to cause hypothyroidism, her serum TSH should be measured now (Answer A).

TPO antibodies (Answer C) should be checked before the initiation of lithium therapy, as the presence of TPO antibodies can further predict the development of hypothyroidism. This patient has a goiter and if her thyroid gland increases in size, thyroid ultrasonography (Answer E) would be warranted.

Lithium has other adverse endocrine effects, including hypercalcemia with elevated serum PTH leading to hyperparathyroidism. This medication increases calcium reabsorption from the kidneys and alters the set point of receptors that sense calcium in parathyroid cells, which shifts the set point of the calcium-PTH curve to the right. The extracellular calcium-sensing receptor has a role in PTH synthesis, PTH secretion, and cellular proliferation. It is possible that a patient may also have a parathyroid adenoma or multiple parathyroid diseases causing hypercalcemia and hyperparathyroidism in addition to lithium treatment. However, patients receiving lithium usually have hypocalciuria through the inhibition of renal cyclic adenosine monophosphate (cAMP). In the case of mild hypercalcemia, such patients are followed and if there is severe hypercalcemia, lithium can be switched to another mood stabilizer, calcimimetic therapy (cinacalcet) can be initiated, or parathyroidectomy can be offered.

Lithium can decrease the glomerular filtration rate and cause nephrogenic diabetes insipidus (a urinary concentrating defect) in approximately 20% of patients, resulting in polyuria (urine output >3 L/day), dehydration, thirst, and compensatory polydipsia. Aquaporins are water channels that are expressed in the renal tubules and collecting ducts. The activation of aquaporins stimulates water resorption in the renal collecting ducts leading to lower urine volume. Binding of antidiuretic hormone to the vasopressin receptor (V2 receptor) stimulates expression of aquaporins in the kidney. Lithium inhibits expression of these aquaporins in the renal collecting duct, and thereby polyuria ensues. The most severe adverse effect of lithium is the development of end-stage renal disease, but this is rare. Kidney function should be monitored every 3 to 6 months in patients treated with lithium.

This patient's basic panel was normal recently and her lithium therapy has not affected her kidney function or her electrolytes. In addition, she has no nocturia and has not reported polyuria and polydipsia. Therefore, there is no need to assess urine osmolality (Answer B) or PTH and calcium levels (Answer D).

Other adverse effects, including tremor and weight gain, are worth reviewing. Lithium-induced tremor happens in early treatment and is also seen with lithium toxicity. Reducing the lithium dosage sometimes helps improve tremor. The mechanism of lithium-induced weight gain is not well established, but affected patients should be advised to watch their diet while taking lithium.

Educational Objective
Explain the adverse endocrine effects of lithium treatment.

Reference(s)
Lazarus JH. Lithium and thyroid. *Best Pract Res Clin Endocrinol Metab.* 2009;23(6):723-733. PMID: 19942149

Gupta S, Khastgir U. Drug information update. Lithium and chronic kidney disease: debates and dilemmas. *BJPsych Bull.* 2017(41);216-220. PMID: 28811917

Meehan AD, Udumyan R, Kardell M, Landen M, Jarhult J, Wallin G. Lithium-associated hypercalcemia: pathophysiology, prevalence, management. *World J Surg.* 2018;42(2):415-424. PMID: 29260296

39 ANSWER: B) Initiate oral cinacalcet therapy

Primary hyperparathyroidism is typically characterized by hypercalcemia in the setting of inappropriately normal or elevated PTH levels. When hypercalcemia develops because of autonomous parathyroid function and excessive PTH secretion after longstanding secondary hyperparathyroidism (such as in patients with end-stage kidney disease and after kidney transplant), this is referred to as tertiary hyperparathyroidism.

The elderly patient in this vignette presents with moderate symptomatic chronic hypercalcemia, elevated PTH, and hypercalciuria, all of which are consistent with a diagnosis of primary hyperparathyroidism. This patient should be treated since she is symptomatic, but her age and cardiopulmonary comorbidities make her a poor surgical candidate. Thus, referring for parathyroid surgery (Answer E) would not be the best option.

In patients with symptomatic hypercalcemia who are unable to undergo parathyroidectomy, oral cinacalcet (Answer B) is the treatment of choice. Cinacalcet is a calcimimetic agent that activates the calcium-sensing receptor in the parathyroid gland, thereby inhibiting PTH secretion. Cinacalcet is effective in lowering, and often normalizing, serum calcium and increasing serum phosphate in patients with primary hyperparathyroidism. Cinacalcet is indicated for the treatment of hypercalcemia in adult patients with primary hyperparathyroidism for whom parathyroidectomy would be indicated on the basis of serum calcium levels, but who are unable to undergo parathyroidectomy. Common adverse effects include nausea, diarrhea, myalgias, dizziness, and paresthesias, unfortunately requiring discontinuation of the medication on occasion.

Immediate treatment with subcutaneous calcitonin therapy (Answer A) or an intravenous bisphosphonate infusion such as intravenous pamidronate (Answer D) would be indicated in a patient with acute severe hypercalcemia (albumin-corrected calcium >14 mg/dL [>3.5 mmol/L]), but not in a mildly symptomatic individual with chronic moderate hypercalcemia (total albumin-corrected calcium between 12 and 14 mg/dL [3.0-3.5 mmol/L]). An acute rise of these moderate concentrations may cause profound symptoms, which would require more aggressive therapy.

Finally, while subcutaneous denosumab therapy (Answer C) is an approved treatment for osteoporosis, it has no role in the treatment of chronic hypercalcemia secondary to primary hyperparathyroidism.

Educational Objective
Recommend cinacalcet for the treatment of chronic moderate hypercalcemia in a symptomatic patient with primary hyperparathyroidism who is not a surgical candidate.

Reference(s)
Marcocci C, Bollerslev J, Khan AA, Shoback DM. Medical management of primary hyperparathyroidism: proceedings of the fourth International Workshop on the Management of Asymptomatic Primary Hyperparathyroidism. *J Clin Endocrinol Metab.* 2014;99(10):3607-3618. PMID: 25162668

Sensipar. Prescribing information. Amgen; 2004. Accessed May 2021. https://www.pi.amgen.com/~/media/amgen/repositorysites/pi-amgen-com/sensipar/sensipar_pi_hcp_english.pdf

40 ANSWER: C) Cabergoline therapy

Dopaminergic agents are the mainstay of treatment of prolactin-secreting adenomas. Prolactin normalization occurs in about 90% of patients, and a significant percentage of patients also have tumor shrinkage. Therefore, medical therapy is usually the first-line treatment of these tumors, particularly if they are large and therefore unlikely to be fully cured by surgery. The 2 medications approved in this setting are bromocriptine and cabergoline. Bromocriptine is a D1 and D2 dopamine receptor agonist. It has a short half-life and must be administered daily. Cabergoline is a more specific D2 dopamine receptor agonist. It has a longer half-life, allowing for weekly or biweekly administration. Cabergoline is superior to bromocriptine in terms of efficacy and fewer adverse effects. This patient presented with a very high prolactin level and hypopituitarism. His response to cabergoline was very good, but hypogonadism persisted and testosterone therapy was added. He now presents with new behavioral changes.

Impulse control disorders are being increasingly recognized as an adverse effect of dopaminergic therapy in addition to the more common adverse effects such as gastrointestinal symptoms (eg, nausea and vomiting), hypotension, and dizziness. Impulse control disorders may be due to overstimulation of the mesolimbic dopamine 3 receptors in the central dopaminergic reward system. While initially reported in as many as one-fifth of patients with Parkinson disease and restless legs syndrome (possibly due to the high dosage of dopaminergic agents used to treat these diseases), impulse control disorders are now recognized to occur in patients taking dosages typically used to treat prolactinoma. These behaviors include hypersexuality, compulsive shopping and gambling, stealing, risky behaviors, binge eating, and punding (repetitive performance of tasks, such as collecting, sorting, and disassembling and assembling objects). Apart from the dopaminergic drug dosage, male sex has been identified as a risk factor for developing an impulse control disorder in most studies, while younger age and being unmarried has been identified only in some studies. The dopamine agonist dosage in reported prolactinoma cases is variable, and these symptoms have been described with cabergoline and bromocriptine (and quinagolide, which is not available in the United States). Currently, it is unknown whether the risk is higher with one drug vs the others or whether a dosage threshold exists. Therefore, it is advisable to inform patients and their families about possible impulse control disorders before initiating dopaminergic therapy and to ask patients about this potential adverse effect during follow-up visits.

In this patient, the behavior changes coincided with the start of cabergoline therapy (Answer C), and this is the most likely cause. His management will be challenging, as he has had a great response to cabergoline. Surgery is unlikely to be curative because of the adenoma's large size. One possible approach, given the already present hypopituitarism, could be radiation therapy, which is quite effective in preventing tumor growth.

Although his free T$_4$ level is higher than normal, this abnormality is marginal. Despite occasional past reports of thyrotoxicosis being associated with criminal behavior, this association is not well proven. Thus, excessive thyroid hormone replacement dosage (Answer A) is incorrect.

While glucocorticoids (Answer B) have been associated with psychosis ("steroid psychosis"), this adverse effect usually occurs with much higher dosages than those used for replacement (and with dosages higher than that of the incorrectly prescribed prednisone). Additionally, this patient does not have psychotic symptoms.

His serum testosterone concentration is normal, so an excessive testosterone dosage (Answer D) is incorrect.

Finally, it would be very coincidental to have developed new bipolar disorder (Answer E), as the age of onset generally ranges from childhood to 50 years, with a mean age of approximately 21 years. A new bipolar disorder diagnosis at this patient's age would be very unlikely.

Educational Objective
Identify the potential behavioral adverse effects of dopaminergic agents.

Reference(s):
Athanasoulia-Kaspar AP, Popp KH, Stalla GK. Neuropsychiatric and metabolic aspects of dopaminergic therapy: perspectives from an endocrinologist and a psychiatrist. *Endocr Connect.* 2018;7(2):R88-R94. PMID: 29378769.

Barake M, Klibanski A, Tritos NA. Management of endocrine disease: impulse control disorders in patients with hyperpolactinemia treated with dopamine agonists: how much should we worry? *Eur J Endocrinol.* 2018;179(6):R287-R296. PMID: 30324793

41 ANSWER: C) Measure C-peptide and glucose

Type 1 diabetes mellitus is an autoimmune disease that causes destruction of pancreatic β cells. Not everyone who presents in diabetic ketoacidosis has type 1 diabetes. Patients with type 2 diabetes, including those with type 2 ketosis-prone diabetes, can present in diabetic ketoacidosis. Making the correct diabetes diagnosis is important to guide long-term management. Several systems have been developed to assist the provider with making the correct diagnosis, including the "Aβ system" (antibodies/β cells). Determining the presence or absence of antibodies and the presence or absence of β-cell function are useful diagnostic tools.

Autoantibodies for type 1 diabetes include islet-cell antibodies (against cytoplasmic proteins in the β cell) (ICA), glutamic acid decarboxylase antibodies (GAD), insulin autoantibodies (IAA), insulinoma 2–associated antibodies (IA-2A), and zinc transporter 8 antibodies (ZnT8). Not all individuals develop insulinopenic diabetes in the setting of autoantibodies. Less than 5% of individuals who carry only 1 autoantibody progress to type 1 diabetes. Residual β-cell function can be assessed by production of C-peptide. C-peptide is a short 31–amino acid polypeptide that connects insulin's A-chain to its B-chain in the proinsulin molecule and is released in amounts equal to that of endogenous insulin.

The patient in this vignette presented in diabetic ketoacidosis and has a family history of autoimmune diseases; thus, type 1 diabetes is a possible diagnosis. However, she has obesity and a family history of type 2 diabetes, so ketosis-prone type 2 diabetes is also in the differential. Proceeding immediately to therapy (Answers D and E) is incorrect. Neither this patient's antibody status nor her current ability to make insulin (β-cell function) has been determined. C-peptide was measured during her hospitalization, but as it was ordered when she was experiencing significant glucose toxicity, it may have been low in that acute state. Although glucose was measured at the same time (205 mg/dL [11.4 mmol/L]), the sample was drawn in a post-acute setting (diabetic ketoacidosis just resolved). Thus, the effect of glucose toxicity to suppress β-cell function must be considered. Measuring C-peptide now (Answer C) is appropriate to evaluate her current endogenous production, and it may also be the most critical assessment to determine appropriate therapy. As she is currently taking exogenous insulin, measuring insulin levels (Answer A) would not be helpful. While assessing for diabetes autoantibodies may help predict the future need for insulin and is indicated, measuring IAA (Answer B) is incorrect. IAA is often the first antibody to appear in children, but it is important to recognize that once patients have been receiving insulin injections for a few weeks, nearly all develop insulin antibodies. Thus, IAA measurement after initiating insulin injections cannot be used as a marker of immune-mediated diabetes. Measuring GAD and/or other antibodies would be a correct choice in addition to C-peptide measurement, but it was not offered as an answer option.

Some patients with type 1 diabetes retain or regain the ability to produce insulin and may require no insulin or less insulin and respond to insulin-sparing diabetes medications for varying durations. This period is often referred to as the "honeymoon period" or remission of type 1 diabetes. The duration of this remission and the ability to continue to produce insulin is heterogeneous, with some individuals rapidly losing all insulin-producing capability and some retaining some production of insulin for decades after diagnosis. Lower hemoglobin A_{1c}, older age of onset, higher frequency of the HLA-DR3 genotype, and responsiveness to a mixed-meal tolerance test are some of the noted factors that are associated with the ability to retain some β-cell function.

Educational Objective
Describe the broad clinical spectrum of diabetes mellitus and explain how to use C-peptide as a tool for management.

Reference(s)
Atkinson MA, Eisenbarth GS, Michels AW. Type 1 diabetes. *Lancet*. 2014;383(9911):69-82. PMID: 23890997

Keenan HA, Sun JK, Levine J, et al. Residual insulin production and pancreatic ß-cell turnover after 50 years of diabetes: Joslin Medalist Study. *Diabetes*. 2010;59(11):2846-2853. PMID: 20699420

Greenbaum CJ, Beam CA, Boulware D, et al. Fall in C-peptide during first 2 years from diagnosis: evidence of at least two distinct phases from composite Type 1 Diabetes TrialNet data. *Diabetes*. 2012;61(8):2066-2073. PMID: 22688329

Maldonado M, Hampe CS, Gaur LK, et al. Ketosis-prone diabetes: dissection of a heterogeneous syndrome using an immunogenetic and beta cell functional classification, prospective analysis, and clinical outcomes. *J Clin Endocrinol Metab*. 2003;88(11):5090-5098. PMID: 14602731

Buzzetti R, Tuomi T, Mauricio D, et al. Management of latent autoimmune diabetes in adults: a consensus statement from an International Expert Panel. *Diabetes*. 2020;69(10):2037-2047. PMID: 32847960

42 ANSWER: D) Whole-body bone scintigraphy

Prostate cancer is among the most common cancers in men worldwide. Androgen-deprivation therapy (ADT) is a cornerstone treatment that improves survival in the setting of metastatic disease. ADT reduces circulating testosterone and estradiol levels into the castrate range, which causes severe hypogonadism. The profound sex steroid deficiency accelerates age-related bone loss by 5- to 10-fold and increases fracture risk by 30%. Bisphosphonates increase bone mineral density during ADT, but evidence of antifracture benefit is currently limited to denosumab. While ADT is initially effective in controlling the disease, castrate-resistant prostate cancer emerges after a median of 2 to 3 years, necessitating intensification of treatment. For example, abiraterone, an inhibitor of androgen synthesis, improves survival in metastatic castrate-resistant prostate cancer, presumably due to suppression of extratesticular androgen production occurring in the adrenal glands and/or in prostate cancer tissue. Prostate cancer most commonly metastasizes to bone, particularly the long bones, axial skeleton, and pelvis. Given the bone trophism of prostate cancer, bone scintigraphy (Answer D) is part of routine staging.

Of note, this patient initiated denosumab only several years after ADT was initially commenced, and his baseline DXA scan revealed significant osteoporosis. Metabolic bone screen at that time was normal, suggesting that his osteoporosis was largely caused by ADT, which could have been mitigated by starting osteoporotic drug therapy earlier. Indeed, international guidelines recommend that bone health (including DXA) be assessed at the time ADT is commenced and periodically thereafter. Unfortunately, observational studies indicate that a minority of men undergo DXA within 12 months of ADT commencement, suggesting that, as in this case, timely diagnosis and treatment of ADT-associated osteoporosis does not occur in most patients.

This patient had stable bone mineral density for the first 3 years after starting denosumab treatment. However, after 2 more years of denosumab therapy, his bone mineral density increased massively, by 140% at the lumbar spine. The T-score increased from −3.2 to +5.6 over this 2-year period (*see image in the vignette stem*). This was the result of a much greater increase in bone mineral content than bone area in both the lumbar spine and femoral neck. The very large and parallel change in bone mineral density and bone mineral content, coupled with the small increases in bone area on DXA scans, especially in the context of rising bone remodeling markers and elevated alkaline phosphatase, were unlikely due to the effect of antiresorptive therapy alone and are instead consistent with a true increase in mineralized bone due to osteoblastic metastases. Therefore, performing whole-body bone scintigraphy is the best option.

In this case, whole-body bone scintigraphy revealed avid tracer retention throughout the skeleton consistent with diffuse skeletal disease, leading to a so-called superscan (*see image*). A "superscan" is a phenomenon where the metastatic process is so diffuse that virtually all of the radiotracer is concentrated in the skeleton, with little or no activity in the soft tissues or urinary tract. This can be misinterpreted as normal uptake if the radiotracer is symmetrically distributed throughout the skeleton and the absence of soft tissue or urinary tract uptake is not appreciated. The bone scintigraphy findings in this patient could be mistaken for demonstrating only a few sites of metastases with the asymmetrically increased uptake in the shoulders, the right fifth rib, and the sacrum. However, the lack of renal activity (*see image arrows*) and soft-tissue activity in the bone scan in the context of accelerated bone remodeling despite denosumab dosed to treat osteoporosis is consistent with a diffuse metastatic process. Remarkably, the patient reported no bone pain. PSA was markedly elevated (238 ng/mL [238 μg/L]). He was referred back to his urologist who increased the denosumab dosage to 120 mg subcutaneously monthly to treat his skeletal metastases. Abiraterone with prednisolone was initiated and leuprorelin was continued.

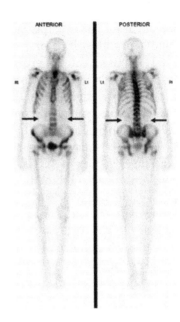

There is no indication to determine the trabecular bone score (Answer E), a commercially available software add-on for late-generation DXA systems that has been cleared by the US FDA for use as a complement to DXA analysis and clinical examination for assessment of fracture risk and monitoring the effects of therapy. Trabecular bone score has not been shown to be clinically useful to monitor the skeletal effects of denosumab.

Likewise, abnormalities in serum calcium (Answer A), serum 25-hydroxyvitamin D (Answer B), or serum 1,25-dihydroxyvitamin D (Answer C) would not explain the clinical picture and are not the most important diagnostic tests. However, serum calcium and 25-hydroxyvitamin D should be measured, especially because some patients with active osteoblastic metastases may have "consumption hypocalcemia," especially in the context of serum 25-hydroxyvitamin D deficiency and antiresorptive treatment. Calcium and 25-hydroxyvitamin D intake should be carefully optimized.

Finally, of note, this patient has mild anemia, a common adverse effect of ADT, due to the lack of erythropoietic actions of testosterone.

Educational Objective
Manage bone health in men receiving androgen-deprivation therapy and recognize pitfalls of DXA measurements in patients with prostate cancer.

Reference(s)
Cheung Y-M, Ramchand SK, Grossmann M. Pitfalls in bone density monitoring in prostate cancer during anti-resorptive treatment. *Osteoporos Int.* 2018;29(7):1665-1670. PMID: 29666893

Russell N, Grossmann M. Management of bone and metabolic effects of androgen deprivation therapy. *Urol Oncol.* 2018;S1078-S1439(18)30389-2. PMID: 30446463

43 ANSWER: B) Adrenal hyperandrogenism

This male patient has classic congenital adrenal hyperplasia secondary to 21-hydroxylase deficiency, which induces a syndrome of primary adrenal insufficiency, as well as a syndrome of adrenal androgen excess. The primary adrenal insufficiency results in a deficiency in cortisol and aldosterone with a concomitant elevation in ACTH. Elevated ACTH stimulates adrenal steroidogenesis, which leads to elevated 17-hydroxyprogesterone and adrenal androgen production. Treatment of primary adrenal insufficiency can be achieved by providing supplemental glucocorticoid and mineralocorticoid (in this case, hydrocortisone and fludrocortisone). This treatment can prevent the morbid consequences of adrenal insufficiency. However, balancing the dosage of glucocorticoids to adequately treat adrenal insufficiency and simultaneously lowering ACTH can be challenging. Inadequate dosing of glucocorticoids can cause adrenal insufficiency, excess ACTH action, and adrenal hyperandrogenism. In contrast, excess dosing of glucocorticoids can suppress ACTH action and adrenal hyperandrogenism but at the expense of inducing Cushing syndrome. Balancing these 2 scenarios is one of the major challenges in treating patients with congenital adrenal hyperplasia and can require different strategies depending on the patient's life stage (childhood vs adulthood) and goals of care.

The consequences of excess ACTH include not only adrenal hyperandrogenism but also an increased risk of adrenal rest tumors. Adrenal hyperandrogenism in a male may induce premature puberty but can also induce secondary hypogonadism. In this case, the patient's very high androstenedione concentrations were aromatized to estrone and resulted in suppression of gonadotropins, which consequently decreased testosterone production and spermatogenesis. Thus, the most likely cause of this patient's infertility is adrenal hyperandrogenism (Answer B). This process may be reversible with increased glucocorticoid dosing, particularly nocturnal dosing to suppress morning elevations in ACTH. In this case, the patient was treated with methylprednisolone, 2 to 3 mg every night at bedtime, in addition to his current regimen, and after 6 months, this normalized his testosterone, increased the sperm count, and improved sperm morphology. The patient and his partner were counseled on the value of genetic testing to prognosticate the probability that their child may have congenital adrenal hyperplasia. He and his wife were able to achieve a spontaneous pregnancy after 10 months of this treatment.

Although a pituitary tumor (Answers A and D) could be the cause of secondary hypogonadism, this possibility should not be pursued until the more likely culprit of adrenal hyperandrogenism is addressed. Testicular adrenal rest tumors (Answer E) are certainly a possibility and could represent an additional source of infertility. For this reason, routine testicular ultrasonography is recommended. However, the main culprit to address is adrenal hyperandrogenism. Klinefelter syndrome (Answer C) causes primary, rather than secondary, hypogonadism.

Educational Objective
Identify the cause of hypogonadism in a man with classic congenital adrenal hyperplasia.

Reference(s)
Merke DP, Auchus RJ. Congenital adrenal hyperplasia due to 21-hydroxylase deficiency. *N Engl J Med*. 2020;383(13):1248-1261. PMID: 32966723

Speiser PW, Arlt W, Auchus RJ, et al. Congenital adrenal hyperplasia due to steroid 21-hydroxylase deficiency: an Endocrine Society clinical practice guideline. *J Clin Endocrinol Metab*. 2018;103(11):4043-4088. PMID: 30272171

44 ANSWER: C) Autoimmune atrophic gastritis with pernicious anemia

Autoimmune atrophic gastritis with pernicious anemia (Answer C) is the most likely diagnosis in this patient with autoimmune thyroid disease, an increasing levothyroxine dosage requirement, vitiligo, glossitis, peripheral neuropathy, and macrocytic anemia. Among patients with autoimmune thyroid disease, up to 20% have parietal-cell antibody positivity. Parietal-cell antibodies are not specific for pernicious anemia and can also be found in patients without any autoimmune disease. However, a prospective study of patients with both autoimmune thyroid disease and parietal-cell antibodies demonstrates that up to 25% of patients go on to develop histologic evidence of autoimmune gastritis within 5 years. The pathogenesis of autoimmune atrophic gastritis involves the autoimmune destruction of the gastric parietal cells, leading to hypochlorhydria and eventual achlorhydria, gastric atrophy, and an increased risk for gastric cancer. Reduced gastric acid secretion can lead to iron deficiency and microcytic anemia. Increase in gastric pH is also the likely mechanism for the increased levothyroxine dosage requirements observed in many patients with autoimmune atrophic gastritis. Pernicious anemia can occur in conjunction with autoimmune atrophic gastritis due to loss of intrinsic factor leading to reduced vitamin B_{12} absorption. Clinical findings include macrocytic anemia, glossitis, peripheral neuropathy, hypersegmented neutrophils, thrombocytopenia, and elevated methylmalonic acid.

Reduced absorption of vitamin B_{12} is a known consequence of long-term metformin therapy (Answer D); however, this medication would be unlikely to cause clinically apparent vitamin B_{12} deficiency so soon after its initiation. In addition, metformin is not known to affect the absorption of levothyroxine, although several studies have demonstrated a TSH suppressive action of metformin in patients with subclinical or overt hypothyroidism.

Medications that decrease gastric acid, such as proton-pump inhibitors and H_2 blockers may also contribute to reduced vitamin B_{12} absorption because gastric acid has a role in the dissociation of vitamin B_{12} from food proteins. Proton-pump inhibitors have also been associated with reduced absorption of levothyroxine, most likely related to their effects on gastric acidity. However, absorption of levothyroxine has not been shown to be significantly affected by shorter-acting H_2 blockers, such as ranitidine (Answer E).

There is no reason to suspect nonadherence to levothyroxine therapy (Answer A). The patient's refill history supports good adherence, and her hemoglobin A_{1c} level indicates adequate control of her diabetes with metformin and lifestyle changes, providing evidence that she is engaged in her health care.

Consumptive hypothyroidism (Answer B) is a rare cause of hypothyroidism that is most often observed in infants but has also been reported in adults, including athyreotic patients. Hypothyroidism results as a consequence of increased deiodination of T_4 to metabolically inactive reverse T_3 in the context of large vascular hepatic tumors (hemangiomas) that express high levels of type 3 iodothyronine deiodinase (D3). Consumptive hypothyroidism is not the most likely cause of the higher levothyroxine dosage requirements seen in this patient given the rarity of this diagnosis in adults and the fact that it would not provide an explanation for the patient's signs and symptoms of B_{12} deficiency.

Educational Objective
Recognize autoimmune atrophic gastritis with pernicious anemia in a patient with vitiligo and hypothyroidism due to Hashimoto thyroiditis.

Reference(s)
Checchi S, Montanaro A, Pasqui L, et al. L-thyroxine requirement in patients with autoimmune hypothyroidism and parietal cell antibodies. *J Clin Endocrinol Metab.* 2008;93(2):465-469. PMID: 18042648

Fallahi P, Ferrari SM, Ruffilli I, Antonelli A. Reversible normalisation of serum TSH levels in patients with autoimmune atrophic gastritis who received L-T4 in tablet form after switching to an oral liquid formulation: a case series. *BMC Gastroenterol.* 2016;16:22. PMID: 26965518

Huang SA, Fish SA, Dorfman DM, et al. A 21-year-old woman with consumptive hypothyroidism due to a vascular tumor expressing type 3 iodothyronine deiodinase. *J Clin Endocrinol Metab.* 2002;87(10):4457-4461. PMID: 12364418

Robertson HMA, Narayanaswamy AKP, Pereira O, et al. Factors contributing to high levothyroxine doses in primary hypothyroidism: an interventional audit of a large community database. *Thyroid.* 2014;24(12):1765-1771. PMID: 25203248

45 ANSWER: B) Lipoprotein lipase deficiency

This patient has familial chylomicronemia syndrome. Familial chylomicronemia syndrome is an autosomal recessive condition caused by pathogenic variants in genes encoding 1 or more of the following 5 proteins: lipoprotein lipase (Answer B), apolipoprotein CII, apolipoprotein AV, lipase maturation factor 1, and glycosylphosphatidylinositol anchored HDL binding protein 1. Homozygous or compound heterozygous pathogenic variants lead to accumulation of chylomicrons secondary to impaired clearance. The prevalence of familial chylomicronemia syndrome is estimated to be 1 in 1 million individuals. However, in some populations, such as French Canadians, the prevalence is higher. Clinical features of familial chylomicronemia syndrome include epigastric abdominal pain that radiates to the back, nausea, vomiting, hepatosplenomegaly, eruptive xanthomas, and lipemia retinalis. The most serious complication of familial chylomicronemia syndrome is recurrent pancreatitis. Patients with familial chylomicronemia syndrome have fasting triglyceride concentrations greater than 1000 mg/dL (>11.30 mmol/L), and their plasma has a milky appearance. The diagnosis is made clinically in most cases, as genetic testing and measurement of post-heparin LPL activity are not readily available. Management of familial chylomicronemia syndrome centers on restriction of dietary fat intake to less than 10 to 30 g daily. Affected patients do not respond to traditional pharmacologic options for hypertriglyceridemia such as fibrates, omega-3 fatty acids, or statins.

Familial hypercholesterolemia is a genetic disease inherited in an autosomal dominant manner that results in high levels of LDL cholesterol. The high LDL-cholesterol levels predispose to premature atherosclerotic cardiovascular disease if the condition is untreated. Pathogenic variants in the genes encoding the following proteins are responsible for most cases of familial hypercholesterolemia: LDL receptor (Answer A), apolipoprotein B_{100} (Answer D), and PCSK9.

Dysbetalipoproteinemia is a genetic disorder due to pathogenic variants in the gene encoding apolipoprotein E (Answer C) with a prevalence of 1 in 1000 to 1 in 5000. Apolipoprotein E is found in chylomicrons, chylomicron remnants, VLDL, intermediate-density lipoprotein, and HDL. There are 3 apolipoprotein E alleles: *E2*, *E3*, and *E4*. Each individual inherits 2 alleles. Most people have 2 *E3* alleles. E3 is the ligand for the LDL receptor, and it promotes uptake of remnants to the liver. Most individuals with familial dysbetalipoproteinemia have 2 *E2* alleles. The *E4* allele is associated with Alzheimer disease. Patients with dysbetalipoproteinemia have high levels of VLDL and intermediate-density lipoproteins, which lead to elevations of total cholesterol and triglycerides with an approximate 2:1 molar ratio. Physical examination findings include palmar xanthomas, orange discoloration of skin creases, and tuberoeruptive xanthomas on elbows and knees. Affected individuals are at increased risk of premature atherosclerotic cardiovascular disease.

Apolipoprotein CIII is a small protein that inhibits lipoprotein lipase and hepatic lipase. Inhibition of lipoprotein lipase leads to higher triglycerides. Defective apolipoprotein CIII (Answer E) leads to lower triglycerides, which would not be consistent with the values in this vignette.

Educational Objective
Identify lipoprotein lipase deficiency as an etiology of familial chylomicronemia syndrome.

Reference(s)
Chait A, Eckel RH. The chylomicronemia syndrome is most often multifactorial: a narrative review of causes and treatment. *Ann Intern Med.* 2019;170(9):626-634. PMID: 31035285

Paquette M, Bernard S, Hegele RA, Baass A. Chylomicronemia: differences between familial chylomicronemia syndrome and multifactorial chylomicronemia. *Atherosclerosis.* 2019;283:137-142. PMID: 30655019

Brown WV, Goldberg I, Duell B, Gaudet D. Round table discussion: familial chylomicronemia syndrome: diagnosis and management. *J Clin Lipidol.* 2018;12(2):254-263. PMID: 29534878

Koopal C, Marais AD, Visseren FLJ. Familial dysbetalipoproteinemia: an underdiagnosed lipid disorder. *Curr Opin Endocrinol Diabetes Obes.* 2017;24(2):133-139. PMID: 28098593

Norata GD, Tsimikas S, Pirillo A, Catapano AL. Apolipoprotein C-III: from pathophysiology to pharmacology. *Trends Pharmacol Sci.* 2015;36(10):675-687. PMID: 26435212

46 ANSWER: E) Monitor calcium, albumin, and PTH levels every 6 months

Isolated intact PTH elevation with concomitantly normal albumin-adjusted serum calcium is commonly encountered in clinical practice, although its clinical significance is often uncertain. In patients without a history of known autonomous parathyroid disease, the clinical evaluation must address several clinical parameters that can result in secondary PTH elevation, including chronic renal insufficiency, vitamin D deficiency, and magnesium deficiency. Additionally, PTH elevation in patients with a history of surgically remediated primary hyperparathyroidism, as is the case with this particular patient, raises the concern over disease persistence or recurrence.

There is emerging evidence that persistent PTH elevation following successful parathyroidectomy for primary hyperparathyroidism is not uncommon, occurring in upwards of 25% to 50% of patients. Identified factors that appear to predict a higher likelihood of normocalcemic PTH elevation postoperatively include lower 25-hydroxyvitamin D levels, preexisting renal insufficiency, and a higher concentration of intact PTH preoperatively. There are conflicting data to support larger parathyroid adenoma size as a predictor of persistent PTH elevation. Based on available evidence, there does not appear to be a higher rate of recurrent disease in patients with persistent PTH elevation, although long-term prospective studies addressing this are lacking. Given these observations, the most appropriate course for this patient is expectant management with follow-up biochemical monitoring (Answer E). By extension, referral back to endocrine surgery for another neck exploration (Answer A) would be inappropriate. Furthermore, reoperation if clinically indicated for this patient in the future, would be best directed by comprehensive anatomic imaging such as 4-dimensional CT of the neck, given the challenges of successful reexploration because of postoperative scarring. Performance of dedicated imaging (Answer B), however, is not indicated now.

Cinacalcet (Answer D) is a calcium-sensing receptor agonist that is FDA approved for the management of severe secondary hyperparathyroidism in patients with chronic renal insufficiency, as well as in patients with parathyroid carcinoma. It is also approved for use in patients with primary hyperparathyroidism who are not deemed surgical candidates due to significant comorbidities. This patient, however, is normocalcemic with isolated PTH elevation, and she would not benefit from normalization of her PTH level based on available evidence.

Activated vitamin D analogues such as calcitriol (Answer C) and paricalcitol are approved for use in patients with PTH elevation in the context of advanced renal insufficiency. Additionally, the use of these agents is central to the management of inherited or acquired hypoparathyroidism with hypocalcemia. This approach, however, is not pertinent to this particular patient's care.

Educational Objective
Manage persistent PTH elevation in a patient following successful parathyroidectomy for primary hyperparathyroidism.

Reference(s)
Carsello CB, Yen TWF, Wang TS. Persistent elevation in serum parathyroid hormone levels in normocalcemic patients after parathyroidectomy: does it matter? *Surgery.* 2012;152(4):575-581. PMID: 23021134

Caldwell M, Laux J, Clark M, Kim L, Rubin J. Persistently elevated PTH after parathyroidectomy at one year: experience in a tertiary referral center. *J Clin Endocrinol Metab.* 2019;104(10):4473-4480. PMID: 31188435

47 ANSWER: B) Perform a glucagon-stimulation test

Patients who undergo skull base radiation (regardless of which kind) are at high risk for developing hypopituitarism. Hypopituitarism may happen many years after radiation, so lifetime surveillance is required. Generally, but not always, GH secretion is the first pituitary function that is lost when the pituitary is damaged. While IGF-1 measurement may help in the diagnosis of GH deficiency, it can be normal in patients who have obvious GH deficiency according to stimulation tests. This is particularly true for males, who can have a normal serum IGF-1 level in up to 50% of cases of acquired GH deficiency. Therefore, to diagnose GH deficiency, one must rely on GH-stimulation tests. Tests are not uniformly available in different countries. Their interpretation is complicated by the fact that, in general, peak GH is inversely proportional to BMI. Hence, the diagnosis of GH deficiency is more difficult to establish in patients who are overweight.

The gold standard GH-stimulation test is the insulin tolerance test. However, it requires close medical supervision and has some contraindications (age >65 years, history of coronary artery disease or seizures). While the combination of GHRH + arginine is widely used in Europe and countries around the world, GHRH is not available in the United States. The glucagon-stimulation test is widely used in the United States, but it has the downsides of sometimes being unpleasant (due to nausea and occasional vomiting) and being very long (4 hours, as about 6% of the GH peaks occur in the fourth hour). Macimorelin was recently approved by the US FDA for GH-stimulation testing. Macimorelin is used at the oral dose of 0.5 mg/kg, and blood is drawn 30, 45, 60, and 90 minutes after administration. The US FDA has set a cutoff of normal GH response (peak GH) at 2.8 ng/mL (2.8 µg/L), a rather low value that is meant to reduce the risk of false-positive results. Therefore, based on the FDA recommendation, this patient does not have GH deficiency (particularly in view of his low BMI, although this test seems to be less BMI-dependent than others). However, macimorelin (a ghrelin agonist) is thought to stimulate GH secretion acting directly on the somatotroph cells. Because postradiation hypopituitarism is a hypothalamic disease, it may take many years (>5) to be reflected in the atrophy of the somatotroph cells. Therefore, early in the disease, a test that assesses the function of the somatotroph cells may be falsely normal. This has been clearly proven for the GHRH + arginine test, and it is most likely true for the ghrelin test. Therefore, given the patient's persistent symptoms, a stimulation test that assesses the function of the entire GHRH-GH axis would be advised. The only test listed in the answers that fits this characteristic is the glucagon-stimulation test (Answer B), but an insulin tolerance test would also be appropriate and, in fact, would be the best test where available if no contraindication is present. Given this patient's low BMI, the interpretation of a positive glucagon-stimulation test would be a peak GH value less than 3.0 ng/mL (<3.0 µg/L). If his BMI were between 25 and 30 kg/m^2, the cutoff would be debatable (1.0 or 3.0 ng/mL [1.0 or 3.0 µg/L]). For a patient with a BMI above 30 kg/m^2, the cutoff should be 1.0 ng/mL (1.0 µg/L). Reassuring the patient that he has normal pituitary function (Answer A) would not yet be appropriate.

Early studies have established the macimorelin dose of 0.5 mg/kg as the most appropriate, and no additional information would be gained by repeating the test with a higher dose (Answer C).

Measurement of IGFBP-3 (a protein part of the circulating heterotrimer with IGF-1 and acid-labile subunit) (Answer D) is not helpful in the diagnosis of GH deficiency.

Finally, an arginine-stimulation test (Answer E) is not a good test to diagnose adult GH deficiency, as arginine is a weak stimulus of GH secretion.

Educational Objective
Explain the mechanism of action and limitations of the macimorelin GH-stimulation test.

Reference(s)

Garcia JM, Biller BMK, Korbonits M, et al. Macimorelin as a diagnostic test for adult GH deficiency. *J Clin Endocrinol Metab.* 2018;103(8):3083-3093. PMID: 29860473

Garcia JM, Biller BMK, Korbonits M, et al. Sensitivity and specificity of the macimorelin test for diagnosis of AGHD. *Endocr Connect.* 2021;10(1):76-83. PMID: 33320108

Yuen KCJ, Biller BMK, Radovick S, et al. American Association of Clinical Endocrinologists and American College of Endocrinology guidelines for management of growth hormone deficiency in adults and patients transitioning from pediatric to adult care. *Endocr Pract.* 2019;25(11):1191-1232. PMID: 31760824

Darzy KH, Aimaretti G, Wieringa G, HR Gattamaneni H, Ghigo E, Shalet SM. The usefulness of the combined growth hormone (GH)-releasing hormone and arginine stimulation test in the diagnosis of radiation-induced GH deficiency is dependent on the post-irradiation time interval. *J Clin Endocrinol Metab.* 2003;88(1):95-102. PMID: 12519836

48 ANSWER: B) Continuous glucose monitoring

Achieving excellent glycemic control before pregnancy and maintaining good glucose control throughout pregnancy are important for preventing adverse neonatal outcomes. With the advent of technologies such as continuous glucose monitoring (CGM) and insulin pumps, patients have more options to help them achieve the glycemic targets in pregnancy set by major medical societies. In patients with cystic fibrosis–related diabetes, few data are available to directly address this clinical question. As these patients are often managed similarly to those with type 1 diabetes, it is reasonable to extend conclusions from studies in pregnant patients with type 1 diabetes.

In the CONCEPTT trial, participants with type 1 diabetes who were planning pregnancy (110 patients) or who were early in pregnancy (215 patients) were randomly assigned to use CGM or to continue usual capillary blood glucose testing with a recommendation to test glucose levels at least 7 times daily. This is the largest such study published, as previous studies were smaller or involved older CGM technology. Compared with outcomes in patients doing 7-point glucose testing by fingerstick, pregnant patients in the CGM group had small but significant improvements in glycemic control at 34 weeks' gestation as measured by hemoglobin A_{1c} (–0.19%), glycemic variability, and time in target range. Most importantly, patients in the CGM group had a significantly lower proportion of newborns large for gestational age (odds ratio, 0.51), and their babies were less likely to have neonatal hypoglycemia (odds ratio, 0.45) or be admitted to the neonatal intensive care unit for more than 24 hours (odds ratio, 0.48). Thus, while the glycemic improvement was quite modest with CGM use in pregnant women, the risk of neonatal complications was much reduced. Patients who were planning to become pregnant did not show any apparent benefit. Thus, increasing self-monitoring of blood glucose (Answer E), while certainly advisable, is not the best next step. This patient should begin CGM (Answer B).

In a separate, prespecified analysis of 248 pregnant participants who were stratified according to treatment regimen, patients on multiple daily injection therapy were compared with those on insulin pump therapy. Patients treated with multiple daily injections were more likely to have improved glycemic outcomes (hemoglobin A_{1c} and time in target range) and neonatal outcomes (less likely to have neonatal intensive care unit admission or neonatal hypoglycemia). Thus, initiating insulin pump therapy (Answer C) is not the best next step. Interestingly, the beneficial effect of CGM was true in both patients treated with multiple daily insulin injections and in patients treated with insulin pump therapy. These data mirror those in nonpregnant patients.

The patient in this vignette previously experienced hypoglycemia while on basal insulin (Answer A), so this would not be a preferred option without understanding her glycemic control more precisely. Indeed, some pregnant patients experience declining insulin requirements in the late first trimester. However, over the course of her pregnancy, initiation of basal insulin will most likely be necessary.

Studies of hybrid closed-loop technologies (Answer D) in pregnant patients have not yet addressed the issue of neonatal outcomes, although findings from small randomized controlled trials suggest that glycemic control is improved. However, hybrid closed-loop technology devices are not FDA approved for use in pregnancy at this time.

Educational Objective
Describe key results from the CONCEPTT trial regarding glycemic control in pregnant patients.

Reference(s)

Feig DS, Donovan LS, Corcoy R et al. Continuous glucose monitoring in pregnant women with type 1 diabetes (CONCEPTT): a multicentre international randomised controlled trial. *Lancet.* 2017;390(10110):2347-2359. PMID: 28923465

Feig DS, Corcoy R, Donovan LE, et al; CONCEPTT Collaborative Group. Pumps or multiple daily injections in pregnancy involving type 1 diabetes: a prespecified analysis of the CONCEPTT randomized trial. *Diabetes Care.* 2018;41(12):2471-2479. PMID: 30327362

49

ANSWER: D) Repeated neck ultrasonography and ultrasound-guided FNA biopsy in 6 to 12 months

The patient's neck ultrasonography demonstrates a 1.7-cm right thyroid nodule that is predominantly cystic; however, the solid component of this nodule contains clear microcalcifications. This nodule would be best classified as having a high-suspicion pattern according to the American Thyroid Association sonographic risk classification system, and FNA biopsy is indicated given the size greater than 1 cm. FNA would also be indicated according to another commonly used thyroid nodule classification system in the United States, the American College of Radiology Thyroid Imaging, Reporting, and Data System (TI-RADS), with the TR4 (moderately suspicious) risk category and size greater than 1.5 cm. Consistent with both risk classification systems, this nodule was biopsied and had benign results.

The American College of Radiology recommends that follow-up imaging with neck ultrasonography be repeated for TR4 thyroid nodules at 1, 2, 3, and 5 years. Routine ultrasonography follow-up can stop after 5 years if the appearance and size of the nodule remain stable.

The 2015 American Thyroid Association guidelines for the management of thyroid nodules and cancer estimate that the risk of malignancy for nodules classified as having a high-suspicion pattern is 70% to 90%. Subsequent studies of various patient populations worldwide have demonstrated malignancy rates between 55% and 100% (median = 72%). Because a higher risk of missed malignancy with negative FNA has been demonstrated for nodules with an American Thyroid Association high-suspicion pattern, the guidelines recommend repeated neck ultrasonography and ultrasound-guided FNA biopsy in 12 months (Answer D). No further evaluation or follow-up (Answer A) would not be recommended management for a nodule with a high-suspicion pattern or for TR4 nodules according to the American Thyroid Association or American College of Radiology, respectively.

Ultrasound-guided drainage of cyst fluid (Answer B) is also not correct. The patient has no compressive signs or symptoms such as dysphagia, dysphonia, dyspnea, or cough related to her small mixed cystic and solid thyroid nodule and thus a drainage procedure is not indicated.

CT imaging of the neck and chest (Answer E) is incorrect. Although this type of imaging study is sometimes indicated in patients with thyroid nodules, particularly if substernal goiter and signs or symptoms of tracheal and esophageal compression are present, there is no clear indication for CT imaging at this time.

Lastly, referral for right lobectomy and isthmusectomy (Answer C) is not indicated given the benign cytology results, lack of compressive symptoms, and normal thyroid function.

Educational Objective
Recommend a repeated FNA biopsy of a thyroid nodule with suspicious ultrasonography findings and 1 benign biopsy result.

Reference(s)

Brito JP, Gionfriddo MR, Al Nofal A, et al. The accuracy of thyroid nodule ultrasound to predict thyroid cancer: systematic review and meta-analysis. *J Clin Endocrinol Metab.* 2014;99(4):1253-1263. PMID: 24276450

Haugen BR, Alexander EK, Bible KC, et al. 2015 American Thyroid Association management guidelines for adult patients with thyroid nodules and differentiated thyroid cancer: the American Thyroid Association Guidelines Task Force on Thyroid Nodules and Differentiated Thyroid Cancer. *Thyroid.* 2016;26(1):1-133. PMID: 26462967

Tessler FN, Middleton WD, Grant EG, et al. ACR thyroid imaging, reporting and data system (TI-RADS): white paper of the ACR TI-RADS committee. *J Am Coll Radiol.* 2017;14(5):587-595. PMID: 28372962

50

ANSWER: B) Initiate topical minoxidil

This vignette presents a common scenario in which women previously on oral contraceptive therapy have suppressed androgen excess through pregnancy and lactation and develop symptoms after they stop breastfeeding and do not immediately restart hormonal contraception. They can develop hirsutism, androgenetic alopecia, and/or irregular menses if they have underlying polycystic ovary syndrome. In this woman with regular menses who did not have difficulty conceiving, polycystic ovary syndrome is unlikely. Additional laboratory testing to measure androstenedione and free testosterone (Answer D) could possibly confirm biochemical hyperandrogenism, but this is not necessary to do before treating the patient since an elevated DHEA-S value has been documented. Androgenetic alopecia is very distressing to patients, and initiating treatment early is important to prevent further hair loss.

Elevated DHEA-S in young women does not specifically point to the adrenal gland as the source of androgen excess, as the ovary produces 20% to 30% of DHEA, and DHEA circulating to the adrenal gland can then be sulfated in the adrenal. A much higher DHEA-S value (700-800 µg/dL [18.97-21.68 µmol/L]) would prompt further evaluation, with the first consideration being ACTH-dependent Cushing syndrome. ACTH-independent Cushing syndrome is less likely at her young age, and DHEA-S elevation would be more likely due to elevated ACTH. Therefore, CT of the adrenal glands (Answer E) is not indicated unless she develops a tumor-range DHEA-S level and further evaluation suggests ACTH-independent hypercortisolism.

Finasteride (Answer C) is FDA-approved for androgenetic alopecia in men. However, its use is off-label for androgenetic alopecia in women. There are not enough studies of either finasteride or spironolactone (Answer A) to define a consistent treatment effect in androgenetic alopecia.

Topical minoxidil (Answer B) is FDA-approved for use in women and is considered the first-line treatment of androgenetic alopecia. The specific mechanism of minoxidil's effect is not known. Since it increases hair density and decreases hair loss, it is believed to affect hair follicles by lengthening the anagen or growth phase, shortening the telogen or resting phase, and promoting the maturation of miniaturized follicles and hairs to terminal hairs. Although most studies have not found a significant difference in the effect of the 2% and 5% concentrations, many dermatologists recommend the 5% male dosing to women with androgenetic alopecia because it comes in a foam that is less drying and irritating to the skin. The recommended dosing is twice daily, but studies in women demonstrated an effect with once-daily dosing. If treatment is discontinued, symptoms can return. Because she did not have symptoms while on oral contraceptives, another option for this patient might be to restart oral contraceptives to lower androgens. This was not a treatment option listed because in a woman who has not been treated with oral contraceptives, it is not proven to treat or prevent androgenetic alopecia. Current evidence supports topical minoxidil as the first-line treatment for androgenetic alopecia.

Other treatments that have been proposed and studied include low-level laser light therapy and platelet-rich plasma injections, although not enough data conclusively support their use and they are not covered by insurance plans.

Educational Objective
Diagnose and treat androgenetic alopecia in a woman.

Reference(s)
Goodarzi MO, Carmina E, Azziz R. DHEA, DHEAS and PCOS. *J Steroid Biochem Mol Biol*. 2015;145:213-225. PMID: 25008465

Adil A, Godwin M. The effectiveness of treatments for androgenetic alopecia: a systematic review and meta-analysis. *J Am Acad Dermatol*. 2017;77(1):136-141. PMID: 28396101

van Zuuren EJ, Fedorowicz Z, Schoones J. Interventions for female pattern hair loss. *Cochrane Database Syst Rev*. 2016;2016(5):CD007628. PMID: 27225981

Martin KA, Anderson RR, Chang RJ, et al. Evaluation and treatment of hirsutism in premenopausal women: an Endocrine Society clinical practice guideline. *J Clin Endocrinol Metab*. 2018;103(4):1233-1257. PMID: 29522147

51 ANSWER: E) Perform a 1-mg overnight dexamethasone-suppression test

First and foremost, it is imperative that medication adherence is reviewed and confirmed to not be the underlying issue driving the use of large doses of insulin, particularly in the setting of continued inadequate glycemic control. In some instances, this may require contacting the pharmacy or reviewing the records to ensure that insulin prescriptions have been dispensed regularly. After medication nonadherence is ruled out, it is important to recognize that some patients with obesity and/or type 2 diabetes have an underlying metabolic condition driving the development of these disorders, particularly when patients exhibit significant insulin resistance requiring large insulin doses and/or a concentrated insulin such as U500. The presence of multiple progressive metabolic derangements or unusual features for the patient's age (eg, osteoporosis, resistant hypertension, severe insulin resistance, etc) should increase clinical suspicion and prompt further evaluation. Given this patient's metabolic profile, weight, fat distribution pattern, and insulin requirements, evaluation for hypercortisolism (Answer E) is the best next step.

There is no reason to suspect central hypothyroidism at this point, so measuring free T_4 (Answer C) is not the best next step. Certainly, the patient's slightly elevated TSH may warrant an adjustment in his levothyroxine dosage, as well as a review of the proper way to take levothyroxine (on empty stomach, waiting 30 to 60 minutes to eat, avoiding vitamins with calcium and iron for 4 hours, etc). Lastly, the slightly elevated TSH (ie, suboptimally treated primary hypothyroidism) does not explain the patient's underlying metabolic conditions and/or insulin requirements.

Another secondary disorder that can drive weight gain and hyperglycemia is acromegaly. This patient has no signs or symptoms suggestive of acromegaly. Thus, measuring IGF-1 (Answer D) is not the best next step.

Although adding an SGLT-2 inhibitor (Answer A) or GLP-1 receptor agonist (Answer B) would be a great choice to help improve glycemic control and assist with weight loss, the best step now is to investigate for hypercortisolism, particularly since the patient has morbid obesity with a few subtle features that may be consistent with hypercortisolism and suboptimally controlled diabetes in the setting of severe insulin resistance.

Educational Objective
Consider underlying metabolic disorders in a patient with suboptimally controlled type 2 diabetes mellitus and severe insulin resistance.

Reference(s)
Nieman LK, Biller BMK, Findling JW, et al. The diagnosis of Cushing's syndrome: an Endocrine Society clinical practice guideline. *J Clin Endocrinol Metab.* 2008:93(5):1526-1540. PMID: 18334580

Nieman LK. Recent updates on the diagnosis and management of Cushing's syndrome. *Endocrinol Metab (Seoul).* 2018;33(2):139-146. PMID: 29947171

Barbot M, Ceccato F, Scaroni C. Diabetes mellitus secondary to Cushing's disease. *Front Endocrinol (Lausanne).* 2018;9:284. PMID: 29915558

52 ANSWER: E) Recommend weekly oral administration of the full week's dose of levothyroxine in the clinic

Hypothyroidism is common in the general population, and daily thyroid hormone replacement therapy restores euthyroidism in most patients. Levothyroxine is one of the most commonly prescribed medications in the United States. Levothyroxine is primarily absorbed in the small intestine within the first 3 hours of ingestion. Of the administered levothyroxine dose, only 60% to 80% is absorbed. The usual dosage of oral levothyroxine is 1.6 mcg/kg per day. However, some patients remain hypothyroid despite adequate replacement. When a larger levothyroxine dosage is needed and the serum TSH level remains elevated, underlying causes should be investigated.

A persistently elevated TSH concentration may be related to either malabsorption of levothyroxine or poor regimen adherence. Poor absorption of levothyroxine can be caused by malabsorption syndromes such as celiac disease and inflammatory bowel disease or drug interference with levothyroxine absorption. Nephrotic syndrome can increase thyroid hormone excretion, leading to higher required dosage of levothyroxine. However, treatment nonadherence is the most common cause of persistent biochemical hypothyroidism. Confirming nonadherence can be difficult, as patients usually do not admit to this problem.

An absorption test can assess the absorption of levothyroxine and help distinguish between levothyroxine nonadherence vs levothyroxine malabsorption. One study investigated the absorption of levothyroxine in 23 patients using a weight-based weekly oral dose (1.6 mcg/kg body weight × 7). Free T_4 was measured at baseline and 2 hours after taking levothyroxine, and TSH was measured after 4 weeks of weekly oral levothyroxine intake. The average increase in free T_4 concentration at 2 hours was 54%. Concentrations well below this suggested levothyroxine malabsorption and values similar to this were consistent with poor adherence. In addition, the TSH level decreased from baseline in 75% of cases. Several published case reports have demonstrated that once-weekly levothyroxine therapy can identify and reduce nonadherence. In one study, observed once-weekly levothyroxine therapy with a median follow-up of 25 months demonstrated no adverse events, and 77% of patients had near normalization of TSH within 6 weeks. An earlier study showed that the mean peak free T_4 following weekly administration of levothyroxine was significantly higher than daily administration, but no cardiac toxicity was observed. A recent study published the experience of the levothyroxine absorption test from 2015 to 2018 at the Mayo Clinic. During this test, patients received a weight-based dose of levothyroxine followed by hourly measurements of total T4 and TSH levels for 6 consecutive hours. The levothyroxine dose was chosen based on a patient's BMI and age. Patients aged 18 to 65 years with a BMI less than 40 kg/m² received 1000 mcg of levothyroxine; patients aged 18 to 65 years with a BMI of 40 kg/m² or greater received 1500 mcg of levothyroxine; and patients 65 years or older received 600 mcg of levothyroxine. The percentage of levothyroxine absorption was calculated as follows:

% absorbed = [increment total T$_4$ (mcg/dL) × 10 (dL/L) / total administered levothyroxine (mcg)] × volume of distribution (L) × 100

Increment total T$_4$: peak [total T$_4$] − baseline [total T$_4$]

Volume of distribution = 0.442 × BMI

Normal absorption was characterized by calculated absorption of 60% or higher, and the investigators concluded that the 4-hour test is sufficient to determine the absorption status. Some academic settings use a weighed-based levothyroxine dose (1.6 mcg/kg body weight × 7) for the levothyroxine absorption test.

Due to the long half-life of levothyroxine, once-weekly levothyroxine replacement is an option for patients with poor adherence. The American Thyroid Association recommends weekly oral administration of the full week's dose of levothyroxine in patients in whom adherence cannot be sustained.

The patient in this vignette is a 54-year-old woman with hypothyroidism and depression, and her serum TSH levels remain elevated with low serum free T$_4$ despite increased levothyroxine dosages over the last several months. Switching her levothyroxine tablet to levothyroxine oral solution for better absorption did not change her serum TSH level much. She also reported that she takes her levothyroxine every day on an empty stomach with water and waits 2 hours before eating. In addition, she takes no medications or supplements such as calcium or iron tablets that could cause malabsorption and celiac screening was negative. She has depression and it is possible that she sometimes forgets to take her levothyroxine. As no obvious causes for levothyroxine malabsorption have been identified, she may benefit from having a levothyroxine absorption test. However, this test might not be possible in all academic institutions or private practice settings. Thus, the best option is to recommend observed once-weekly levothyroxine administration (Answer E) with measurement of the free T$_4$ level 2 hours later. A 50% increase in the free T$_4$ concentration from baseline would confirm appropriate levothyroxine absorption. Another option would be recommending observed once-weekly levothyroxine administration for 6 weeks followed by a TSH measurement at the end of 6 weeks. In this patient, the once-weekly levothyroxine dose would be approximately 875 mcg (77.1 kg × 1.6 mcg/kg × 7). Precaution should be taken in patients with coronary artery disease. If nonadherence is confirmed, the physician must discuss with the patient that persistently elevated serum TSH is due to poor regimen adherence. This patient also requires psychiatric evaluation and care.

Intravenous levothyroxine (Answer A) is used in the setting of myxedema coma in hospitalized patients and this is not routinely used in the outpatient setting. There is no indication for intravenous levothyroxine in this patient. Despite her hypothyroidism, she is not physiologically compromised. Furthermore, intravenous levothyroxine is costly. It comes in 3 vial solutions: 20 mcg/mL, 40 mcg/mL, and 100 mcg/mL. To reconstitute, one must add 5 mL of preservative-free 0.9% sodium chloride to the vial, and the resultant solution will have a final concentration of 100 mcg, 200 mcg, and 500 mcg, respectively. This reconstituted solution is stable for 4 hours and must be used immediately after reconstitution. If the reconstituted solution is not entirely used, the remaining unused solution should be discarded. In Lexicomp, the approximate costs of these 3 reconstituted solutions are listed as $110-$126, $228-$264, and $570-$633, respectively.

This patient's levothyroxine regimen was switched to an oral solution, which has a better absorption profile, and this led to no improvement in her serum TSH level. Therefore, adding liothyronine therapy (Answer C) to her current regimen or changing to desiccated thyroid (Answer B) would not be beneficial in trying to achieve better absorption.

Levothyroxine oral solution or soft gel capsule have better absorptive profiles than that of oral tablets and are less dependent on gastric PH. Thus, these formulations are better absorbed in patients with concomitant use of proton-pump inhibitors or coffee and in patients with gastric-related T4 malabsorption. Further increasing the dosage of oral solution levothyroxine to 400 mcg daily (Answer D) is not recommended, as continually increased dosages of levothyroxine have not affected her serum TSH level. Furthermore, if she suddenly decides to take the current dosage of levothyroxine, she could develop severe thyrotoxicosis and experience cardiac toxicity.

Educational Objective

Diagnose medication nonadherence in a patient with refractory hypothyroidism.

Reference(s)

Jonklass J, Bianco AC, Bauer AJ, et al; American Thyroid Association Task Force on Thyroid Hormone Replacement. Guidelines for the treatment of hypothyroidism: prepared by the American Thyroid Association Task Force on Thyroid Hormone Replacement. *Thyroid.* 2014;24(12):1670-1751. PMID: 25266247

Grebe SK, Cooke RR, Ford HC, et al. Treatment of hypothyroidism with once weekly thyroxine. *J Clin Endocrinol Metab.* 1997;82(3):870-875. PMID: 9062499

Walker JN, Shillo P, Ibbotson V, et al. A thyroxine absorption test followed by weekly thyroxine administration; a method to assess non-adherence to treatment. *Eur J Endocrinol.* 2013;168(6):913-917. PMID: 23554450

Gonzales KM, Stan MN, Morris JC, Bernet V, Castro MR. The levothyroxine absorption test; a four-year experience (2015-2018) at the Mayo Clinic. *Thyroid.* 2019;29(12):1734-1742. PMID: 31680654

Jayakumari C, Nair A, Khadar JP, et al. Efficacy and safety of once-weekly thyroxine for thyroxine-resistant hypothyroidism. *J Endocr Soc.* 2019;3(12):2184-2193. PMID: 31723717

Vita R, Saraceno G, Trimarchi F, Benvenga S. Switching levothyroxine from the tablet to the oral solution formulation corrects the impaired absorption of levothyroxine induced by proton-pump inhibitors. *J Clin Endocrinol Metab.* 2014;99(12):4481-4486. PMID: 25259910

Vita R, Saraceno G, Trimarchi F, Benvenga S. A novel formulation of L-thyroxine (L-T4) reduces the problem of L-T4 malabsorption by coffee observed with traditional tablet formulations. *Endocrine.* 2013;43(1):154-160. PMID: 22932947

53 ANSWER: A) Serum 17-hydroxyprogesterone measurement

This patient presents with typical features of virilizing congenital adrenal hyperplasia (CAH) that has been untreated for decades. The phenotype of CAH is variable and depends on residual activity of 21-hydroxylase deficiency. While classic CAH can present with salt-wasting and adrenal crises in infancy, less severe forms of CAH can escape detection because residual 21-hydroxylase activity prevents symptomatic mineralocorticoid deficiency, and latent glucocorticoid deficiency is compensated for by increased pituitary production of proopiomelanocortin, a prohormone that is cleaved into the biologically active hormones ACTH, melanocyte-stimulating hormone, and others. Sustained high concentrations of ACTH caused severe bilateral adrenal hyperplasia with increased adrenal androgen production. The elevated melanocyte-stimulating hormone results in increased melanin synthesis, causing skin hyperpigmentation. Androgen excess during growth, in the context of precocious puberty, resulted in his short stature because of premature closure of the epiphyses. The best initial diagnostic test is measurement of 17α-hydroxyprogesterone (Answer A), which is increased in patients with CAH, especially after ACTH stimulation.

A bone-marrow biopsy sample obtained after review by a hematologist showed no evidence of a hematologic malignancy contributing to polycythemia, but karyotyping done routinely as part of cytogenetic analysis revealed a 46,XX karyotype.

When questioned about an infraumbilical scar observed on physical examination, the patient recalled that he underwent surgery in childhood, presumably to repair hypospadias, and a hysterectomy with bilateral oophorectomy (no uterus or ovaries were visible on abdominal imaging). He had been treated with glucocorticoids as a young child, but was then lost to follow-up. Although not sexually active or in a relationship, he had a stable male gender identity.

Androgen excess leads to polycythemia through stimulation of erythropoiesis. Although polycythemia is a well-described risk factor for stroke, androgenic polycythemia in CAH has been reported only rarely. Androgen excess should be considered as a cause of otherwise unexplained polycythemia. Of note, the degree of polycythemia in this patient was more severe than would be expected on the basis of his serum testosterone, and it is explained by the CAH-associated production, at high concentrations, of androgenic precursors and metabolites with biologic activity at the androgen receptor.

While an elevation in hCG (Answer E) could explain the increase in serum testosterone and suppressed LH, it would not explain the marked bilateral adrenal enlargement and clinical features in this case.

There is no clinical indication to perform a pituitary-directed MRI (Answer C) or a whole-body fluorodeoxyglucose-PET (Answer B) or to measure serum estradiol (Answer D).

This patient's case highlights the harmful effects of unfettered androgen excess in individuals with untreated CAH and also serves as a reminder of the importance of a genital examination as a part of a complete physical examination.

Educational Objective
Diagnose a patient with late presentation of congenital adrenal hyperplasia and describe the complications that arise when this condition is untreated.

Reference(s)

Verma A, Lewis D, Warne G, Grossmann M. An X-traordinary stroke. *Lancet.* 2011;377(9773):1288. PMID: 21481709

Speiser PW, Arlt W, Auchus RJ, et al. Congenital adrenal hyperplasia due to steroid 21-hydroxylase deficiency: an Endocrine Society clinical practice guideline. *J Clin Endocrinol Metab.* 2018;103(11):4043-4088. PMID: 30272171

54 ANSWER: A) Increase the hydrocortisone dosage

Complete surgical resection is the only potentially curative treatment for adrenocortical carcinoma. In patients with potentially resectable stage I to III disease who are surgical candidates, complete resection is recommended as the primary treatment. The most important factors governing prognosis of adrenocortical carcinoma are disease stage and completeness of resection, but additional clues to future behavior may be provided by pathologic examination of the tumor.

The Weiss scoring system is based on 9 histopathologic features: nuclear grade, mitotic rate, atypical mitoses, clear cell component, diffuse architecture, tumor necrosis, venous invasion, sinusoidal invasion, and capsular infiltration. Several groups have also established the prognostic value of other markers of proliferation, including Ki67 expression detected with the MIB-1 antibody. Current studies are focused on identifying novel molecular markers that will more reliably predict tumor recurrence and response to adjuvant therapy.

Given the propensity for recurrence and lack of an effective treatment regimen for advanced disease, the European Society of Endocrinology clinical guidelines on adrenocortical carcinoma suggest adjuvant mitotane use in patients who are deemed to be at high risk of recurrence. This group includes those with histologically high-grade disease (as in this case, where Ki67 staining was observed in >15% of tumor cells, together with a high mitotic rate), when there is evidence of vascular and/or capsular invasion, or if there is any concern regarding tumor spillage at surgery. The role of mitotane in prolonging recurrence-free survival in patients with adrenocortical carcinoma who are considered to be at low to intermediate risk of recurrence is being addressed in the ADIUVO trial (ClinicalTrials.gov NCT00777244).

Mitotane, a derivative of the insecticide dichlorodiphenyltrichloroethane, is adrenolytic and causes atrophy and inhibition of steroidogenesis in both tumoral and normal adrenocortical tissue. Patients starting mitotane treatment are therefore at significant risk of developing hypoadrenalism. Interestingly, hypocortisolism can develop rapidly, whereas the zona glomerulosa appears to be more resistant and mineralocorticoid insufficiency rarely manifests in the early stages of treatment.

Interpreting adrenal status in patients taking mitotane is further complicated by the fact that the drug increases concentrations of corticosteroid-binding globulin, resulting in artifactually elevated serum cortisol levels, which may result in failure to recognize or confirm hypoadrenalism. In addition, mitotane exerts marked effects on cytochrome P450 enzymes with resultant increases in the metabolism of glucocorticoids (eg, cortisol, hydrocortisone, dexamethasone) and mineralocorticoids (eg, aldosterone, fludrocortisone). It is therefore routine practice to commence full, even supraphysiologic, glucocorticoid replacement therapy when mitotane treatment is initiated. The exception is for patients with endogenous Cushing syndrome due to residual cortisol-secreting adrenocortical carcinoma. Many patients eventually require a 2- or 3-fold increase in glucocorticoid replacement.

Inadequately treated adrenal insufficiency may present with features that overlap those of mitotane toxicity, and mitotane-induced adverse effects are enhanced in the presence of hypoadrenalism. Therefore, a trial of a higher glucocorticoid dosage (Answer A) is the most appropriate first step, especially if there are no other specific features of mitotane toxicity (eg, ataxia, bone marrow suppression) and plasma mitotane levels are in the therapeutic range.

If the symptoms persist despite an increase in glucocorticoid therapy, a reduction in the mitotane dosage (Answer B), or even temporary discontinuation, is indicated to see if the symptoms are alleviated.

The patient in this vignette has no specific clinical or laboratory features to indicate mineralocorticoid insufficiency, and there is no indication to begin fludrocortisone therapy (Answer C). However, it would be reasonable to measure plasma renin to ensure it is not elevated.

Mitotane may cause hypothyroidism in some patients, with low serum free T_4 and inappropriately normal TSH. Recent evidence suggests a potential direct inhibitory effect on TSH secretion. Levothyroxine therapy should therefore be considered in patients with low serum free T_4 levels and symptoms of hypothyroidism. In addition to its effects on corticosteroid-binding globulin, mitotane also increases serum concentrations of other binding proteins, including thyroxine-binding globulin, which may result in an increased levothyroxine requirement in those receiving replacement. However, in this patient, hypocortisolism must be excluded/corrected before considering a trial of levothyroxine supplementation (Answer D).

Although streptozocin (Answer E) was initially considered an adjunct or alternative to mitotane for the management of advanced adrenocortical carcinoma, other chemotherapy regimens (eg, etoposide, doxorubicin, and cisplatin) are now preferred when adjunctive/alternative approaches are indicated.

Educational Objective
Explain that mitotane therapy causes adrenal insufficiency and that higher than normal dosages of hydrocortisone are required to achieve adequate glucocorticoid replacement.

Reference(s)
Fassnacht M, Dekkers O, Else T, et al. European Society of Endocrinology clinical practice guidelines on the management of adrenocortical carcinoma in adults, in collaboration with the European Network for the Study of Adrenal Tumors. *Eur J Endocrinol*. 2018;179(4):G1-G46. PMID: 30299884

Fassnacht M, Terzolo M, Allolio B, et al; FIRM-ACT Study Group. Combination chemotherapy in advanced adrenocortical carcinoma. *N Engl J Med*. 2012;366(23):2189. PMID: 22551107

55 ANSWER: A) Roux-en-Y gastric bypass; delay pregnancy for 1 year after surgery

For many patients, bariatric surgery can be a successful and sustainable way to lose weight, with resultant improvement in both short- and long-term health outcomes. Patients who undergo bariatric surgery experience the greatest weight loss during the first postoperative year when caloric restriction is at its strictest. It can take up to 2 years for patients to reach their nadir weight following bariatric surgery. Bariatric surgery has been shown to improve fertility in women, including those with polycystic ovary syndrome.

Current guidelines recommend that women who undergo bariatric surgery defer pregnancy for at least 12 months, as nutritional deficiencies during the active weight-loss phase may affect the growth and development of the fetus. Pregnancy after both gastric bypass and sleeve gastrectomy is generally associated with favorable outcomes when compared with pregnancy in women matched for their preoperative BMI. While there is a higher risk for small-for-gestational-age infants, the risk of developing gestational diabetes and having large-for-gestational-age babies is lower in women who have had these surgeries.

Patients with gastroesophageal reflux should avoid gastric banding (Answer C) and sleeve gastrectomy (Answer B). Patients with preexisting gastroesophageal reflux who undergo sleeve gastrectomy may experience greater postoperative complications, less weight loss, and little change in reflux symptoms when compared with gastric bypass. The presence of Barrett esophagus and significant gastroesophageal symptoms are relative contraindications to undergoing sleeve gastrectomy. The best recommendation for this patient is Roux-en-Y gastric bypass and delaying pregnancy for 1 year after surgery (Answer A).

Several appetite suppressants can help with an individual's efforts at weight loss. While nonsurgical weight loss in general is known to improve fertility, there are no published data on the effectiveness of weight-loss medications in this field. All currently FDA-approved weight-loss medications, including liraglutide (Answer D) and extended-release phentermine/topiramate (Answer E), are pregnancy category X and should be avoided while attempting to become pregnant. These drugs may be considered before starting fertility treatment as long as the patient recognizes the associated risks and takes appropriate precautions to avoid pregnancy. Additionally, these drugs typically result in 5% to 10% weight loss, which may not be adequate for this particular patient.

Educational Objective
Counsel patients regarding the guidelines related to pregnancy after bariatric surgery.

Reference(s)
American College of Obstetricians and Gynecologists. ACOG practice bulletin No. 105: bariatric surgery and pregnancy. *Obstet Gynecol*. 2009;113(6):1405-1413. PMID: 19461456

Monson M, Jackson M. Pregnancy after bariatric surgery. *Clin Obstet Gynecol*. 2016;59(1):158-171. PMID: 26710306

Johansson K, Stephansson O, Neovius M. Outcomes of pregnancy after bariatric surgery. *N Engl J Med*. 2015;372(23):2267. PMID: 26039606

56

ANSWER: E) Recommend nonsteroidal antiinflammatory agents and physical therapy

The high levels of circulating GH and IGF-1 present in patients with acromegaly cause specific joint changes that increase the risk for arthropathy. Arthropathy pain (both in weight-bearing and non–weight-bearing joints) is one of the most prominent symptoms that negatively affect quality of life in patients with acromegaly. Arthropathy can result in significant deterioration of function and disability over time. Indeed, arthritic pain is one of the presenting symptoms in more than 50% of patients at the time of diagnosis.

The pathogenesis of arthropathy due to acromegaly is not well established. It is believed that there is an initial phase of cartilage hypertrophy and laxity of the periarticular ligaments, resulting in joint hypermobility. In this early phase, radiographic abnormalities include joint space widening and periarticular soft-tissue hypertrophy. However, with time, cartilage hypertrophy, scarring, and osteophytes formation occur, causing joint space narrowing. Compared with osteoarthritis in patients without acromegaly, joint spaces in patients with acromegaly tend to be more preserved. In this late phase, changes are irreversible and may become GH-independent. Acromegaly treatment has only limited effects on joint symptoms. In this stage, treatment of arthropathy should follow guidelines used for the general population. While early diagnosis and treatment of acromegaly may at least in part reverse arthropathy, most patients with acromegaly are diagnosed after the disease has been present for many years (6-8 years on average).

This patient did not have a full surgical cure. A somatostatin receptor ligand was prescribed, with subsequent normalization of age-adjusted serum IGF-1 and serum GH at target (<1.0 ng/mL [<1.0 µg/L]). Therefore, her acromegaly is considered controlled. Unfortunately, her joint pain symptoms are progressing. These should be addressed with nonsteroidal antiinflammatory agents and physical therapy (Answer E).

Radiation therapy (Answer A) is not necessary, as her acromegaly is currently controlled. Additionally, radiation may take many years to normalize GH secretion.

An increase in the lanreotide dosage (Answer B) is not necessary, as her acromegaly is controlled on the current dosage, and there is a theoretical possibility of causing GH deficiency.

A second surgery (Answer C) is unlikely to be curative given the presence of tumor in the cavernous sinus.

Finally, the addition of the GH-receptor antagonist pegvisomant (Answer D) is a reasonable strategy when the somatostatin receptor ligand fails to fully normalize serum IGF-1. Pegvisomant can also be used as a single agent when control of tumor growth is not an important issue (ie, small indolent residual adenoma far from the optic chiasm). However, no studies have shown that the addition of pegvisomant in patients whose acromegaly is controlled by a somatostatin receptor ligand have reversal of osteoarthritis symptoms.

Educational Objective
Counsel patients regarding the risk of progression of acromegaly arthropathy despite biochemical control.

Reference(s)
Giustina A, Barkan A, Beckers A, et al. A consensus on the diagnosis and treatment of acromegaly comorbidities: an update. *J Clin Endocrinol Metab.* 2020;105(4):dgz096. PMID: 31606735

Claessen KMJA, Mazziotti G, Biermasz NR, Giustina A. Bone and joint disorders in acromegaly. *Neuroendocrinology.* 2016;103(1):86-95. PMID: 25633971

Claessen KMJA, Canete AN, de Bruin PW, et al. Acromegalic arthropathy in various stages of the disease: an MRI study. *Eur J Endocrinol.* 2017;176(6):779-790. PMID: 28348071

57

ANSWER: E) Start lisinopril

Patients with diabetes mellitus are at high risk for developing atherosclerotic cardiovascular disease (ASCVD). Reducing risk factors for ASCVD is a critical component of a comprehensive treatment plan. This strategy includes control of blood pressure and lipids and use of antiplatelet agents. Initiation of therapy and management targets are dependent on a patient's pretreatment risk.

The use of an antiplatelet agent (aspirin) (Answer C) in primary prevention has to balance the benefit (reduction of ASCVD) with the risk of bleeding (often gastrointestinal). The American Diabetes Association standards of care recommend that men and women older than 50 years who have at least 1 other risk factor for ASCVD use aspirin for primary prevention. For those at intermediate risk, defined as those older than age 50 years without other risk factors or those younger than 50 years with at least 1 other risk factor, it is recommended to have a discussion about risks and benefits. For patients at low risk, defined as those younger than 50 years with no other risk factors, use of antiplatelet agents should be avoided as primary prevention. The patient in this vignette is younger than 50 years and has hypertension, so he would fall in the intermediate-risk category. Therefore, aspirin could be considered, but not without detailed discussion and it is not the best next step.

Lipid management in a patient with diabetes without history of ASCVD is dependent on age, degree of LDL-cholesterol elevation, duration of diabetes, and diabetes-related complications. For a patient who is between 40 and 79 years of age, at least moderate-intensity statin therapy is indicated. If the patient is between 20 to 39 years of age (as is the patient in this vignette), statin therapy (Answer B) is recommended if the LDL-cholesterol concentration is greater than 190 mg/dL (>4.92 mmol/L), if the patient has had long duration of diabetes (type 2 diabetes for >10 years, type 1 diabetes for >20 years), if there is evidence of microvascular disease (retinopathy, albumin-to-creatinine ratio >30, estimated glomerular filtration rate <60 mL/min per 1.73 m^2, or peripheral neuropathy), or if the patient has an ankle-to-brachial ratio less than 0.9. The patient in this vignette has had diabetes for 4 years (<10 years) and has no other features that would qualify for statin therapy.

Triglycerides are a secondary target in patients with diabetes in certain situations. If the triglyceride concentration is between 175 and 499 mg/dL (1.98-5.64 mmol/L), lifestyle changes to lower triglycerides should be recommended. If the triglyceride concentration is greater than 500 mg/dL (>5.65 mmol/L), then medication use can be considered in addition to lifestyle changes. Icosapent ethyl (Answer D) can be considered in patients with a known history of ASCVD and a triglyceride concentration between 135 and 499 mg/dL (1.53-5.64 mmol/L), with LDL cholesterol controlled on a statin. The patient in this vignette has no known history of ASCVD and has a triglyceride level less than 175 mg/dL (<1.98 mmol/L), so isocapent ethyl is not indicated.

The American Diabetes Association recommends that blood pressure be less than 140/90 mm Hg in patients with diabetes and less than 130/80 mm Hg in patients with an ASCVD risk greater than 15%. The American Heart Association recommends the goal should be less than 130/80 mm Hg in all patients with diabetes. Treatment of blood pressure reduces the risk of ASCVD. In this patient, the diastolic blood pressure is above goal regardless of the recommendation used and it should be treated. Thus, recommending no further intervention now (Answer A) is incorrect. An ACE inhibitor is a good first choice in this situation, so lisinopril (Answer E) is the best answer option.

Educational Objective
Manage cardiovascular risk reduction in an asymptomatic patient with type 2 diabetes mellitus.

Reference(s)
Arnett DK, Blumenthal RS, Albert MA, et al. 2019 ACC/AHA Guideline on the Primary Prevention of Cardiovascular Disease: Executive Summary: A Report of the American College of Cardiology/American Heart Association Task Force on Clinical Practice Guidelines. *Circulation.* 2019;140(11):e563-e595. PMID: 30879339

American Diabetes Association. 10. Cardiovascular disease and risk management: standards of medical care in Diabetes-2020. *Diabetes Care.* 2020;43(Suppl 1):S111-S134. PMID: 31862753

58 ANSWER: A) Cabozantinib

The patient has stage IV medullary thyroid carcinoma (MTC) with a serum calcitonin level that is significantly higher than before her extensive neck operation only a few months ago. In addition, the patient is experiencing new substernal chest pain and dyspnea, and chest imaging shows interval progression of hilar and mediastinal lymphadenopathy and the development of lymphangitic spread of neoplasm in the right lung. Systemic therapy should thus be initiated to manage the patient's progressive symptomatic disease. While not all practices have familiarity with systemic therapy for metastatic thyroid cancer, it is important to be aware of therapeutic options and when to consider the initiation of such therapy, and to rapidly refer patients to a center that can provide systemic therapy when indicated.

The efficacy of small molecule multikinase inhibitors (MKIs) has been demonstrated in MTC. Cabozantinib (Answer A) is a nonspecific kinase inhibitor and the second drug after vandetanib (not offered as an answer option) that was FDA approved for the treatment of advanced progressive and/or symptomatic MTC. Cabozantinib would be an appropriate initial treatment option for this patient. The EXAM trial (Efficacy of XL184 [Cabozantinib] in Advanced Medullary Thyroid Cancer), a phase 3 double-blind, placebo-controlled randomized trial of patients with advanced radiographically progressive MTC, demonstrated significant improvement in progression-free survival of patients treated with cabozantinib (11.2 months) vs placebo (4.0 months). However, adverse events (hypertension, hand-foot syndrome, nausea, diarrhea, and fatigue) were common, and dosage reductions were needed for nearly 80% of the active participants in this study.

Whereas cabozantinib and vandetanib are nonselective *RET* inhibitors that also hit multiple other targets, selpercatinib (Answer E) is a selective *RET* inhibitor that has received FDA approval for the treatment of *RET*-mutated MTC that is advanced or metastatic, as well as advanced *RET* fusion-positive nonmedullary thyroid cancer and non-small cell lung cancer. In the phase 1-2 trial, which included 55 patients with *RET*-associated MTC treated with at least 1 MKI previously, the overall response rate was 69% and 1-year progression-free survival was 82%. The response rate and progression-free survival were even higher in MKI-naïve patients. In contrast to MKIs, adverse events were low-grade (1 or 2), dosage reductions were uncommon, and treatment discontinuation due to adverse effects was rare (2%). Although selpercatinib is a promising new therapy for advanced MTC, it only demonstrates efficacy in *RET*-mutated tumors, which is not the case for this patient.

Before the availability of MKIs, cytotoxic chemotherapy was the standard of care for the treatment of metastatic MTC, but this treatment demonstrated low response rates (~20%). Following the approval of MKIs, cyclophosphamide-vincristine-dacarbazine (Answer B) would no longer be recommended as a first-line treatment.

External beam radiotherapy (EBRT) (Answer C) would not be an appropriate single modality for the treatment of this patient's progressive, symptomatic, metastatic MTC. The revised American Thyroid Association guidelines for the management of MTC published in 2015 indicate that adjuvant postoperative neck EBRT can be used for selected patients with MTC and a high likelihood of recurrence following thyroidectomy. However, no prospective trials have evaluated the outcomes with postoperative EBRT vs observation alone.

Diarrhea can occur as a complication of MTC, usually in association with large-volume metastases (liver), and it can negatively impact quality of life. Somatostatin analogues, including octreotide LAR (Answer D), may provide symptomatic improvement in some patients with diarrhea that is refractory to conservative measures. The patient described here is not experiencing diarrhea and thus treatment with octreotide LAR is not indicated. Case reports describe occasional stabilization of tumor burden in patients with metastatic MTC who are treated with somatostatin analogues, but the published evidence for using such therapies as anticancer agents in this setting is both limited and inconclusive.

Educational Objective
Manage progressive metastatic medullary thyroid carcinoma with a multikinase inhibitor.

Reference(s)
San Román Gil M, Pozas J, Molina-Cerrillo J, et al. Current and future role of tyrosine kinases inhibition in thyroid cancer: from biology to therapy. *Int J Mol Sci*. 2020;21(14):4951. PMID: 32668761

Schlumberger M, Elisei R, Müller S, Schöffski P, Brose M, Shah M, Licitra L, Krajewska J, Kreissl MC, Niederle B, Cohen EEW, Wirth L, Ali H, Clary DO, Yaron Y, Mangeshkar M, Ball D, Nelkin B, Sherman S. Overall survival analysis of EXAM, a phase III trial of cabozantinib in patients with radiographically progressive medullary thyroid carcinoma. *Ann Oncol*. 2017;28(11):2813-2819. PMID: 29045520

Schlumberger M, Jarzab B, Cabanillas ME, et al. A phase II trial of the multitargeted tyrosine kinase inhibitor lenvatinib (E7080) in advanced medullary thyroid cancer. *Clin Cancer Res*. 2016;22(1):44-53. PMID: 26311725

Wells SA Jr, Asa SL, Dralle H, et al; American Thyroid Association Guidelines Task Force on Medullary Thyroid Carcinoma. Revised American Thyroid Association guidelines for the management of medullary thyroid carcinoma. *Thyroid*. 2015;25(6):567-610. PMID: 25810047

Wirth LJ, Sherman E, Robinson B, et al. Efficacy of selpercatinib in RET-altered thyroid cancers. *N Engl J Med*. 2020;383(9):825-835. PMID: 32846061

59 ANSWER: E) Reassurance and repeated alkaline phosphatase measurement in 12 months

Elevated alkaline phosphatase is commonly encountered in clinical practice. The initial approach to such patients is centered on the attempt to delineate whether the source is hepatic or bone in origin. This generally involves measurement of γ-glutamyltransferase, which is elevated in patients with hyperphosphatasia due to an underlying liver process. Once a hepatic process is ruled out, the investigation then focuses on workup for skeletal-specific elevation of alkaline phosphatase. Differential diagnosis of hyperphosphatasia includes malignant processes such as primary or metastatic skeletal neoplasms, as well as benign processes such as osteomalacia with or without fractures. In this elderly patient, however, without referable musculoskeletal symptoms, the diagnosis is most consistent with Paget disease of bone.

Paget disease is the second most common metabolic bone disease after osteoporosis, and it affects approximately 2% to 3% of individuals in the United States who are older than 50 years. While most patients with Paget disease have no known family history of the condition, approximately 30% of individuals do have a positive family history. Moreover, current studies suggest that a first-degree relative of a patient with Paget disease is 7 times more likely to develop the disease compared with someone who has no affected relatives. Most patients with Paget disease, which may involve solitary (monostotic) or multicentric (polyostotic) foci of disease, are asymptomatic, as was this patient. However, affected individuals may present with pain at their pagetic site, which can be associated with localized swelling and cutaneous warmth. Fortunately, there is evidence that bisphosphonate therapy significantly reduces bone pain in patients with painful Paget disease, with additional evidence that intravenous zoledronic acid is superior to risedronate in relieving bone pain and reducing the risk of clinical relapse (ie, recurrence of bone pain). There is no evidence that a biochemical relapse with an increased alkaline phosphatase level necessarily predicts a painful relapse in patients treated with bisphosphonates. This certainly raises the question as to whether there is merit in treating asymptomatic patients with Paget disease with pharmacotherapy to normalize alkaline phosphatase and reduce the risk of adverse clinical outcomes, including pain, fractures, hearing loss, and referral for orthopedically indicated surgical procedures.

The PRISM and PRISM-EZ trials (Paget's Disease: Randomized Trial of Intensive vs Symptomatic Management and Paget's Disease: Randomized Trial of Intensive vs Symptomatic Management Extension with Zoledronic Acid) sought to determine whether symptomatic or intensive treatment with bisphosphonates was more effective in the short- and long-term management of Paget disease. The PRISM trial revealed that intensive bisphosphonate therapy did not reduce bone pain, fractures, or the need for orthopedic surgery compared with symptom-driven treatment in patients with Paget disease over an average of 3 years. Furthermore, long-term normalization of alkaline phosphatase over more than 7 years did not improve bone pain, improve quality of life, or reduce the need for orthopedic procedures, and may actually be associated with a higher fracture risk. Based on these results, the provision of reassurance and repeated alkaline phosphatase measurement in 12 months (Answer E) is the appropriate course for this patient. By extension, treatment with either an oral or intravenous bisphosphonate (Answers A and B) is not indicated now.

The decision to defer pharmacologic therapy may not be appropriate in certain clinical situations; for example, if there is evidence of skull or spinal column involvement or before orthopedic surgery (eg, large joint replacement in close proximity to a pagetic lesion). This is because of the vascular nature of pagetic lesions and the potential to reduce bleeding complications with treatment. While these clinical scenarios, as well as an increase in serum alkaline phosphatase more than 2 to 4 times the upper limit of normal, have been traditional considerations for pharmacotherapy in Paget disease and are current indications in the Endocrine Society guidelines, there is insufficient evidence to support this approach on a uniform basis.

Skeletal resorption markers such as C-telopeptide (Answer C) and N-telopeptide are often elevated in patients with Paget disease, corresponding to accelerated skeletal turnover that is present in this condition. They are not, however, diagnostic as an independent test, nor are they helpful in specifically predicting or confirming response to pharmacologic therapy.

Finally, this patient's biochemical and radiographic presentation is inconsistent with multiple myeloma, so serum and urine electrophoresis (Answer D) is not necessary.

Educational Objective
Explain the indications and rationale for conservative, nonpharmacologic management in a patient with asymptomatic Paget disease.

Reference(s)
Langston AL, Campbell MK, Fraser WD, MacLennan GS, Selby PL, Ralston SH; PRISM Trial Group. Randomized trial of intensive bisphosphonate treatment versus symptomatic management in Paget's disease of bone. *J Bone Miner Res.* 2010;25(1):20-31. PMID: 19580457

Tan A, Goodman K, Walker A, et al; PRISM-EZ Trial Group. Long-term randomized trial of intensive versus symptomatic management in Paget's disease of bone: The PRISM-EZ Study. *J Bone Miner Res.* 2017;32(6):1165-1173. PMID: 28176386

60 ANSWER: A) Adrenocortical carcinoma

This patient has an incidentally discovered adrenal mass, which is concerning for adrenocortical carcinoma. The radiographic characteristics of an adrenal mass are critical in evaluating whether the mass is benign or potentially malignant. Each imaging modality can provide similar and complementary information. Reassuring features that are suggestive of a benign adrenal mass include round and uniform shape, homogenous appearance, high lipid content (eg, low attenuation on unenhanced CT [<10 Hounsfield units] or loss of signal on out-of-phase sequencing on MRI), and high contrast washout on delayed contrast CT imaging (absolute washout on delayed imaging >60%, relative washout on delayed imaging >40%). Small size (generally <4 cm) is usually reassuring, but it is not a reliable feature. Lack of fluorodeoxyglucose-avidity on PET scan, if performed, is also generally reassuring.

Features that raise concern for a malignant process include larger size (>4 or 6 cm), irregular shape or contour, heterogeneous content, calcifications, low lipid content on CT or lack of signal dropout on in-phase and out-of-phase MRI imaging, poor washout on delayed contrast CT imaging, and fluorodeoxyglucose-avidity on PET scan. A benign pheochromocytoma usually has poor lipid content and poor washout on delayed contrast CT imaging, but it usually presents as a slow-growing mass with a round contour and shape and elevated metanephrines.

Although it is reassuring that this patient's adrenal mass is relatively small, round, and homogenous, the concerning features include the fact that it is new (developed within 1 year) and lacks MRI signal dropout on in-phase and out-of-phase imaging. In the context of a known germline *TP53* pathogenic variant that substantially increases the risk for adrenocortical carcinoma (Answer A), this adrenal mass is presumed to be an early detection of this malignancy. Adrenocortical carcinoma is a common malignancy in Li-Fraumeni syndrome. Adrenalectomy was performed, which revealed a high-grade stage I adrenocortical carcinoma.

This adrenal mass could certainly be a benign lipid-poor adenoma (Answer D) or pheochromocytoma (Answer E); both entities could appear similarly on MRI. However, the context of known Li-Fraumeni syndrome and rapid growth within the span of 1 year make the likelihood of adrenocortical carcinoma much higher. This adrenal mass does not have features of a typical benign lipid-rich adenoma (Answer C) or a cyst (Answer B), which can be easily recognized on CT or MRI based on fluid density.

Educational Objective
Identify the radiographic characteristics of adrenocortical carcinoma and determine the risk for adrenocortical carcinoma in patients with Li-Fraumeni syndrome.

Reference(s)
Fassnacht M, Arlt W, Bancos I, et al. Management of adrenal incidentalomas: European Society of Endocrinology clinical practice guideline in collaboration with the European Network for the Study of Adrenal Tumors. *Eur J Endocrinol*. 2016;175(2):G1-G34. PMID: 27390021

Vaidya A, Hamrahian A, Bancos I, Fleseriu M, Ghayee HK. The evaluation of incidentally discovered adrenal masses. *Endocr Pract*. 2019;25(2):178-192. PMID: 30817193

61 ANSWER: D) Medication

The patient has a pituitary macroadenoma with suprasellar extension and optic chiasmal compression, which accounts for the visual abnormalities detected by her optometrist. This is most likely to represent a clinically nonfunctioning (gonadotrope) adenoma, with modest hyperprolactinemia secondary to pituitary stalk compression.

Although the thyroid biochemistry raises the possibility of partial central hypothyroidism (low free T_4 with inappropriately normal TSH), the other laboratory results do not suggest significant pituitary dysfunction (well-preserved early morning cortisol, gonadotropins consistent with her likely postmenopausal status, IGF-1 in the upper reference range). It would be unusual for hypothyroidism to be the only manifestation of pituitary failure in the context of a pituitary adenoma prior to treatment. Therefore, hypopituitarism (Answer C) is not the most likely explanation for the abnormal thyroid function test results.

Similarly, with otherwise well-preserved anterior pituitary function, if the patient had coincidental primary hypothyroidism (Answer A), serum TSH would most likely still be elevated.

Hypercortisolism can suppress the hypothalamic-pituitary axes even in the absence of a larger tumor causing local mass effect. This is perhaps best described with reference to gonadal dysfunction in adults and growth retardation/pubertal arrest in children who have Cushing syndrome. Endogenous hypercortisolemia has also been shown to have an inhibitory action on the hypothalamic-pituitary-thyroid axis, which can result in low thyroid hormone levels. These changes revert to normal (without the need for exogenous thyroid hormone therapy) once Cushing syndrome is in remission. Although this patient is mildly overweight and has hypertension, her blood pressure is well controlled on a single agent and she does not have diabetes mellitus. Therefore, previously undiagnosed Cushing disease (Answer B) due to a pituitary macroadenoma is unlikely, although formal dynamic testing would be required to exclude this possibility.

Nonthyroidal illness (Answer E) may give rise to several different thyroid function test abnormalities, which are influenced by the timing of sample collection in relation to onset of intercurrent illness and the nature of the laboratory assays used to measure total and/or free thyroid hormone levels. One of the most commonly recognized patterns is that of apparent central hypothyroidism, most typically with low (but not suppressed) TSH, mildly low free T_3, and borderline-low/low-normal free T_4. In this patient, there is no suggestion of an intercurrent illness, and the TSH concentration is not low, both of which therefore make nonthyroidal illness (Answer E) less likely.

Whenever thyroid function test results do not appear to be consistent with the clinical picture and/or concordant with each other, the possibility of laboratory assay interference should be considered. For example, heterophilic antibody interference in the TSH assay may yield artifactually low or high results. Thyroid hormone assays may be similarly affected, although artifactual hyperthyroxinemia is more common.

However, in this case, medication (Answer D) is the most likely explanation for the finding of apparent isolated central hypothyroidism. Although the underlying mechanism is still not fully understood, carbamazepine and the related drug oxcarbazepine are well recognized to be associated with low serum free T_4 concentrations in patients taking these medications. TSH is typically normal, and the patient is clinically euthyroid. Thyroid function usually returns to normal following discontinuation of the drug. In this patient, the hyponatremia was subsequently shown to be longstanding and also attributable to carbamazepine therapy (syndrome of inappropriate antidiuretic hormone).

Educational Objective
Differentiate among different causes of apparent isolated central hypothyroidism.

Reference(s)
Xiang B, Tao R, Liu X, et al. A study of thyroid functions in patients with Cushing's syndrome: a single center experience. *Endocr Connect.* 2019;8(8):1176-1185. PMID: 31336363

Surks MI, DeFesi CR. Normal serum free thyroid hormone concentrations in patients treated with phenytoin or carbamazepine. A paradox resolved. *JAMA.* 1996;275(19):1495-1498. PMID: 8622224

62 ANSWER: C) Polycystic ovary syndrome

Congenital adrenal hyperplasia (CAH) due to 21-hydroxylase deficiency is caused by pathogenic variants in the *CYP21A2* gene. CAH is one of the most common autosomal recessive diseases. In classic CAH, more severe enzyme deficiency results in adrenal insufficiency. Female newborns often have atypical genitalia. Nonclassic CAH, which is not associated with adrenal insufficiency, is more common than classic CAH. Among white populations, the prevalence of nonclassic CAH may be as high as 1 in 1000 to 1 in 100. The prevalence varies and increases, especially in remote geographic populations. Impaired 21-hydroxylase enzyme activity leads to higher concentrations of 17-hydroxyprogesterone at baseline or with stimulation by ACTH or synthetic cosyntropin. Baseline or stimulated concentrations of 17-hydroxyprogesterone above 1000 ng/dL (>30.3 nmol/L) are diagnostic of 21-hydroxylase deficiency. In this vignette, the 17-hydroxyprogesterone levels are not consistent with nonclassic CAH due to 21-hydroxylase deficiency (Answer A). Even on low-dosage prednisone, this steroid pathway block should be evident following stimulation with standard-dose cosyntropin, so no additional testing is needed while off prednisone (Answer E).

A pattern of elevated values of 17-hydroxypregnenolone, DHEA, 17-hydroxypregnenelone/17-hydroxyprogesterone, and 17-hydroxypregnenelone/cortisol in response to cosyntropin stimulation was initially characterized as a nonclassic form of CAH due to 3β-hydroxysteroid dehydrogenase deficiency. Studies have found that results of repeated stimulation tests normalize for many of these patients once off glucocorticoid treatment and that gene sequencing identifies no abnormalities in the HSD2B1 gene in patients thought to have this diagnosis. Hyperandrogenism has been hypothesized to physiologically impair function of 3β-hydroxysteroid dehydrogenase. As in this case, a repeated cosyntropin-stimulation test did not demonstrate a potential steroid pathway block at 3β-hydroxysteroid dehydrogenase as was observed in the first test. Therefore, this patient does not have evidence for nonclassic CAH due to 3β-hydroxysteroid dehydrogenase deficiency (Answer B). It should be emphasized that diagnostic testing for this condition should not be performed because it is not considered a clinical condition or genetic condition that requires treatment any different from that used to treat other women with hyperandrogenism.

The international Rotterdam consensus criteria are used to diagnose polycystic ovary syndrome, with updated recommendations from an international evidence-based guideline from the American Society for Reproductive Medicine and European Society of Human Reproduction and Embryology. Two of three criteria must be met: (1) anovulatory cycles (interval <21 days or >35 days or fewer than 8 periods per year or day 21 luteal-phase progesterone <3 if regular menses); (2) biochemical or clinically significant evidence for androgen excess (Ferriman-Gallwey score of 4 to 6, cystic acne, androgenetic alopecia), and (3) polycystic ovarian morphology with an antral follicle count ≥20 when the transducer frequency is 8 MHz or ovarian volume ≥10 cc in an ovary with no cyst greater than 1 cm. After discontinuing the oral contraceptive pill, this patient began to have irregular menses suggestive of anovulatory cycles. She has elevated DHEA-S, which meets the criteria of androgen excess, as well as the development of hirsutism and androgenetic alopecia, so she has both biochemical and clinical evidence of androgen excess. Because she already meets 2 of the 3 criteria for polycystic ovary syndrome and the results of her hormonal evaluation have excluded other causes of oligomenorrhea such as hyperprolactinemia, thyroid disease, and nonclassic CAH, the presence of polycystic ovarian morphology is not required for the diagnosis. It is suggested that her gynecologist originally told her she did not have polycystic ovary syndrome because her ultrasound presumably did not meet criteria for polycystic ovarian morphology. However, she has polycystic ovary syndrome (Answer C) without polycystic ovarian morphology. She does not have idiopathic hirsutism (Answer D) because she has anovulatory cycles.

Educational Objective
Diagnose polycystic ovary syndrome in a woman with a history of elevated 17-hydroxypregnenolone.

Reference(s)

Pang SY, Lerner AJ, Stoner E, et al. Late-onset adrenal steroid 3 beta-hydroxysteroid dehydrogenase deficiency. I. A cause of hirsutism in pubertal and postpubertal women. *J Clin Endocrinol Metab*. 1985;60(3):428-439. PMID: 2982896

Zerah M, Rheaume E, Mani P, et al. No evidence of mutations in the genes for type I and type II 3 beta-hydroxysteroid dehydrogenase (3 beta HSD) in nonclassical 3 beta HSD deficiency. *J Clin Endocrinol Metab*. 1994;79(6):1811-1817. PMID: 7989489

Legro RS, Arslanian SA, Ehrmann DA, et al; Endocrine Society. Diagnosis and treatment of polycystic ovary syndrome: an Endocrine Society clinical practice guideline. *J Clin Endocrinol Metab*. 2013;98(12):4565-4592. PMID: 24151290

Teede HJ, Misso ML, Costello MF, et al. Recommendations from the international evidence-based guideline for the assessment and management of polycystic ovary syndrome. *Fertil Steril*. 2018;110(3):364-379. PMID: 30033227

Speiser PW, Arlt W, Auchus RJ, et al. Congenital adrenal hyperplasia due to steroid 21-hydroxylase deficiency: an Endocrine Society clinical practice guideline. *J Clin Endocrinol Metab*. 2018;103(11):4043-4088. PMID: 30272171

63 ANSWER: B) Add once-weekly subcutaneous semaglutide

Of the options listed, the best next step is to add once-weekly subcutaneous semaglutide (Answer B). Semaglutide is approved to reduce the risk of major adverse cardiovascular events (cardiovascular death, nonfatal myocardial infarction, or nonfatal stroke) in adults with type 2 diabetes mellitus and established cardiovascular disease. This approved indication is largely based on the results of the SUSTAIN-6 trial (Semaglutide and Cardiovascular Outcomes in Patients with Type 2 Diabetes).

Thus far, randomized controlled trials have failed to conclusively demonstrate that more aggressive glycemic control in patients at high risk for cardiovascular disease translates into a reduction in cardiovascular risk or mortality. While the cardiovascular outcome trials evaluating GLP-1 receptor agonists did include patients with elevated hemoglobin A_{1c} values, and improvement in hemoglobin A_{1c} was observed with the therapies being studied, it is unlikely that the observed differences in cardiovascular risk with these active medications vs comparator (placebo) groups (given in addition to other standard diabetes care) can be attributed to tighter glycemic control alone. Thus far, the differences in glycemic control (hemoglobin A_{1c}) between study arms have been 1% or less in the cardiovascular outcome trials with GLP-1 receptor agonists. These observations suggest that there may be a unique mechanism or property inherent to these particular agents that confers cardiovascular risk reduction. Accordingly, per the latest guidelines from the American Diabetes Association and the American Association of Clinical Endocrinology, the addition of a GLP-1 receptor agonist that has been shown to confer cardiovascular disease risk reduction should be considered in patients with established atherosclerotic cardiovascular disease independent of glycemic control status (baseline hemoglobin A_{1c} or individualized hemoglobin A_{1c} target).

Increasing the lisinopril dosage (Answer A) is incorrect. The patient's blood pressure is already at goal and there is no evidence that a higher degree of ACE blockade (higher lisinopril dosage) would confer additional cardiovascular disease risk reduction.

Adding ezetimibe (Answer E) to statin therapy is an effective treatment option that leads to additional LDL-cholesterol lowering. This combination therapy is recommended in situations where, with a maximal or maximally tolerated statin monotherapy treatment regimen, LDL-cholesterol targets cannot be achieved. The addition of ezetimibe leads to further cardiovascular disease risk reduction, without raising significant safety concerns. However, adding ezetimibe in this case is incorrect because the patient is already receiving high-intensity statin therapy and his LDL-cholesterol level is at goal (<70 mg/dL [<1.81 mmol/L]). The IMPROVE-IT trial (Improved Reduction of Outcomes: Vytorin Efficacy International Trial) included 18,144 patients who had been hospitalized for an acute coronary syndrome within the preceding 10 days and had LDL-cholesterol levels of 50 to 100 mg/dL (1.3-2.6 mmol/L) if they were receiving lipid-lowering therapy or 50 to 125 mg/dL (1.3-3.2 mmol/L) if they were not receiving lipid-lowering therapy. Participants were randomly assigned to the combination of simvastatin (40 mg daily) and ezetimibe (10 mg daily) or simvastatin (40 mg daily) and placebo (simvastatin monotherapy). When added to statin therapy, ezetimibe resulted in incremental lowering of LDL-cholesterol levels and improved cardiovascular outcomes. In addition, lowering LDL cholesterol to concentrations below previous targets provided additional benefit. This patient did not have a recently reported acute coronary syndrome, and his LDL-cholesterol concentration is already below 50 mg/dL (<1.30 mmol/L), so it is unclear if these results would apply.

Blockade of aldosterone receptors by spironolactone (Answer C) in addition to standard therapy has been demonstrated to substantially reduce the risk of both morbidity and death among patients with severe heart failure with reduced ejection fraction. Adding spironolactone in this case is incorrect because the patient does not have heart failure (his left ventricular ejection fraction is 50%).

The multicenter, double-blind, placebo-controlled REDUCE-IT trial (Reduction of Cardiovascular Events with Icosapent Ethyl-Intervention Trial) enrolled 8179 patients (median age at baseline, 64 years; 71% men) who had fasting triglyceride concentrations of 135 to 499 mg/dL (1.53-5.64 mmol/L) and LDL-cholesterol concentrations of 41 to 100 mg/dL (1.06-2.59 mmol/L) despite statin therapy and who had established cardiovascular disease (70%) or diabetes mellitus plus other high-risk factors (30%). The primary results demonstrated a 25% reduction in the primary endpoint of cardiovascular death, nonfatal myocardial infarction, nonfatal stroke, coronary revascularization, or unstable angina with icosapent ethyl (Answer D) vs placebo ($P < .001$).

In the REDUCE-IT cohort, 58% of participants had type 2 diabetes, with 91% prescribed at least 1 diabetes medication and 49.5% prescribed at least 2 diabetes medications. Participants with diabetes had 1.5-fold greater rates of the primary endpoint vs the placebo group. Participants assigned icosapent ethyl experienced a 7% absolute risk reduction for a first cardiovascular disease event and a 12.7% absolute reduction in risk for total events compared with those assigned placebo ($P < .001$ for both). Adding icosapent ethyl is incorrect because this patient does not have hypertriglyceridemia. Patients included in the REDUCE-IT trial had a triglyceride concentration greater than 135 mg/dL (>1.53 mmol/L). It is unclear whether icosapent ethyl is associated with reduced cardiovascular disease risk in patients with triglyceride levels less than 135 mg/dL (<1.53 mmol/L).

Educational Objective
Identify the most appropriate medication class to intensify therapy in patients with type 2 diabetes mellitus and established cardiovascular disease, according to the most recent guidelines and regardless of whether the patient's hemoglobin A_{1c} is at goal.

Reference(s)
Marso SP, Bain SC, Consoli A et al. Semaglutide and cardiovascular outcomes in patients with type 2 diabetes. *N Engl J Med.* 2016;375(19):1834-1844. PMID: 27633186

American Diabetes Association. 9. Pharmacologic approaches to glycemic treatment: standards of medical care in diabetes-2020. *Diabetes Care.* 2020;43(Suppl 1):S98-S110. PMID: 31862752

Garber AJ, Handelsman Y, Grunberger G, et al. Consensus statement by the American Association of Clinical Endocrinologists and American College of Endocrinology on the comprehensive type 2 diabetes management algorithm – 2020 executive summary. *Endocr Pract.* 2020;26(1):107-139. PMID: 32022600

Ozempic. Prescribing information. Novo Nordisk; 2020. Accessed September 2020. https://www.novo-pi.com/ozempic.pdf

Vavlukis M, Vavlukis A. Adding ezetimibe to statin therapy: latest evidence and clinical implications. *Drugs Context.* 2018;7:212534. PMID: 30023003

Bertram Pitt B, Zannad, F, Remme WJ et al. The effect of spironolactone on morbidity and mortality in patients with severe heart failure. Randomized Aldactone Evaluation Study Investigators. *N Engl J Med.* 1999;341(10):709-717. PMID: 10471456

Bhatt DL, Steg PG, Miller M, et al; REDUCE-IT Investigators. Cardiovascular risk reduction with icosapent ethyl for hypertriglyceridemia. *N Engl J Med.* 2019;380(1):11-22. PMID: 30415628

Bhatt DL, Brinton EA, Miller M. Substantial cardiovascular benefit from icosapent ethyl in patients with diabetes: REDUCE-IT DIABETES. Abstract presented at: 80th American Diabetes Association Scientific Sessions; June 12-16, 2020.

64 ANSWER: B) Secondary hyperparathyroidism

This patient has secondary hyperparathyroidism (Answer B) as a result of Roux-en-Y gastric bypass. Up to one-third of patients who undergo Roux-en-Y gastric bypass develop secondary hyperparathyroidism. The incidence is inversely related to prevailing 25-hydroxyvitamin D levels. In one study, secondary hyperparathyroidism was most prevalent in patients with a 25-hydroxyvitamin D concentration of 10 ng/mL or less (≤25.0 nmol/L) and least prevalent in those with values of 20 ng/mL or greater (≥50.0 nmol/L). Current guidelines recommend 3000 units of vitamin D daily. However, in practice, higher dosages may be required to maintain a 25-hydroxyvitamin D level of at least 30 ng/mL (≥75 nmol/L). This patient has a urinary calcium excretion that is less than the recommended threshold of 100 to 200 mg/24 h (expert opinion), and he may benefit from additional vitamin D and calcium supplementation. The total recommended calcium intake after gastric bypass surgery is 1200 to 1500 mg of elemental calcium per day through dietary sources and supplementation.

Normocalcemic primary hyperparathyroidism (Answer A) should not be diagnosed until all secondary causes of hyperparathyroidism have been assessed for and excluded. Normocalcemic primary hyperparathyroidism is often erroneously diagnosed in these patients with the unfortunate consequence of unnecessary parathyroidectomy.

Familial hypocalciuric hypercalcemia (Answer D) is caused by inactivating pathogenic variants in the gene encoding the calcium-sensing receptor. Affected patients typically present with mild hypercalcemia, elevated PTH, and low urinary calcium excretion. Although this patient's urinary calcium excretion is low, he has a normal serum calcium concentration that is not consistent with this diagnosis.

About 8% to 13% of patients develop de novo nephrolithiasis after Roux-en-Y gastric bypass, with most (94%) being calcium oxalate stones. Multiple factors contribute to this: (1) restriction of oral intake can lead to decreased urinary volumes; (2) malabsorption of fatty acids causes preferential binding of calcium over oxalate in the intestinal lumen, leading to oxalate absorption; (3) bile acid malabsorption promotes intestinal oxalate absorption by increasing intestinal mucosal permeability; and (4) decreased urinary citrate excretion after Roux-en-Y gastric bypass promotes calcium oxalate crystallization. This patient would benefit from meeting with a bariatric dietician to review nutrition and hydration goals. Additionally, he should be counseled to take calcium supplements with food to reduce enteric hyperoxaluria. Calcium phosphate nephropathy (Answer C) is not a recognized complication of Roux-en-Y gastric bypass surgery.

There is no reason to believe this patient has parathyroid carcinoma (Answer E) based on his clinical presentation and biochemical findings.

Educational Objective
Distinguish between secondary hyperparathyroidism and normocalcemic primary hyperparathyroidism in a patient who has had gastric bypass surgery.

Reference(s)
Hewitt S, Aasheim ET, Sovik TT, et al. Relationships of serum 25-hydroxyvitamin D, ionized calcium and parathyroid hormone after obesity surgery. *Clin Endocrinol (Oxf)*. 2018;88(3):372-379. PMID: 29235126

Parrott J, Frank L, Rabena R, Craggs-Dino L, Isom KA, Greiman L. American Society for Metabolic and Bariatric Surgery Integrated Health Nutritional Guidelines for the Surgical Weight Loss Patient 2016 Update: Micronutrients. *Surg Obes Relat Dis*. 2017;13(5):727-741. PMID: 28392254

65 ANSWER: E) Emtricitabine/tenofovir

Hemoglobin A_{1c} measurement is a valuable tool in the management of diabetes, but there are situations when the hemoglobin A_{1c} level may not provide an accurate assessment of glycemic control. In this case, the elevated fructosamine value is more consistent with his continuous glucose monitoring values, confirming the suspicion that his hemoglobin A_{1c} is underestimating his true level of glycemia.

Certain medications are known to alter red blood cell survival, hematopoiesis, or predominant hemoglobin type. Generally, the published literature regarding the effect of medications on hemoglobin A_{1c} is not extensive (*see table*). Nucleoside reverse transcriptase inhibitors have been shown to cause mild hemolysis that may not be associated with anemia or macrocytosis. This reduced erythrocyte survival results in falsely low hemoglobin A_{1c} levels. Thus, emtricitabine/tenofovir (Answer E) is the best explanation for the current discrepancy between mean glucose measurements on continuous glucose monitoring and the fructosamine value vs the hemoglobin A_{1c} level. Measurement of serum haptoglobin and/or lactate dehydrogenase would be reasonable to establish whether this is the cause.

Other medications associated with reduced red blood cell survival include dapsone, ribavirin, and trimethoprim/sulfamethoxazole. Hydroxyurea, an antimetabolite used to treat sickle cell disease or myeloproliferative disorders, causes a shift from HgA to HgF, resulting in lower hemoglobin A_{1c} levels.

Table. Medications That Affect Hemoglobin A_{1c}

Postulated mechanism	Falsely low hemoglobin A_{1c}	Falsely high hemoglobin A_{1c}
Increased erythrocyte destruction	Dapsone, ribavirin, antiretrovirals, trimethoprim/sulfamethoxazole	
Altered hemoglobin	Hydroxyurea	
Altered glycation	Vitamin D, vitamin E, aspirin (low-dosage)	
Assay interference		Aspirin (high-dosage), chronic opioid use

Reprinted from Unnikrishnan R, Anjana RM, Mohan V. Drugs affecting HbA$_{1c}$ levels. *Indian J Endocrinol Metab*. 2012;16(4):528-531.

Other causes of low hemoglobin A_{1c} levels would be anything that decreases glycation of hemoglobin. High dosages of vitamin C or vitamin E and long-term aspirin are reported to cause reduced glycation of hemoglobin, although the dosages of vitamin C and E typically used in supplements may not cause this problem. Since glycation of hemoglobin occurs across the red blood cell lifespan, factors that increase erythropoiesis resulting in a greater population of young erythrocytes cause low hemoglobin A_{1c}. Vitamin B_{12} supplementation and erythropoietin may cause this situation. Finally, long-term high-dosage aspirin is postulated to cause falsely elevated hemoglobin A_{1c} due to assay interference. Long-term opioid use may be associated with high hemoglobin A_{1c} levels through an unclear mechanism.

African American ancestry (Answer A) is associated with higher than expected hemoglobin A_{1c} for a given degree of glycemia. The same is true for iron deficiency anemia (Answer B) because of prolongation of red blood cell survival. While this patient has a history of iron deficiency anemia, his red blood cell indices do not indicate this to be the case currently, possibly because of his ongoing iron supplementation.

Regarding possible inaccuracy of continuous glucose monitor readings (Answer D), the published mean absolute relative difference for continuous glucose monitoring devices would not result in a glucose concentration that is consistent with the hemoglobin A_{1c} level, and the fructosamine value confirms that the continuous glucose monitoring readings are probably accurate.

Finally, acetaminophen (Answer C) may cause falsely high glucose readings on some continuous glucose monitoring devices, but this would imply substantial hypoglycemia and he reports no symptoms. Other substances found to interfere with continuous glucose monitor readings include lisinopril, albuterol, atenolol, and red wine. Practitioners should review the product safety guides and inform patients accordingly.

Educational Objective
List drugs that may cause falsely low hemoglobin A_{1c} values.

Reference(s)
Unnikrishnan R, Anjana RM, Mohan V. Drugs affecting HbA$_{1c}$ levels. *Indian J Endocrinol Metab.* 2012;16(4):528-531. PMID: 22837911

Basu A, Slama MQ, Nicholson WT, et al. Continuous glucose monitor interference with commonly prescribed medications: a pilot study. *J Diabetes Sci Technol.* 2017;11(5):936-941. PMID: 28332406

66 ANSWER: C) Zoledronic acid

The patient described in this vignette has Paget disease of bone, diagnosed incidentally during workup of left-sided hip pain. His imaging studies are consistent with Paget disease, with his left hip radiograph revealing cortical and trabecular thickening involving the entire left hemipelvis and proximal femur, and his bone scan showing increased radionuclide uptake involving the sternum, left humeral head, lumbar spine, sacrum, pelvis, hips, and proximal femurs. Physiologic excretion of urine with radiotracer within his indwelling Foley catheter is also noted. This patient's bone-specific alkaline phosphatase level is mildly elevated, and his left-sided hip pain may be mostly due to osteoarthritis. However, he is planning to have left hip surgery soon. Indications to treat asymptomatic Paget disease of bone include a serum alkaline phosphatase concentration more than 2 to 4 times the upper normal limit, pagetic changes at sites where complications could occur (eg, skull, spine, weight-bearing bones, and pagetic bone abutting a joint), planned surgery at an active pagetic site, and hypercalcemia in association with immobilization in patients with polyostotic disease. Therefore, this patient meets criteria to treat, and recommending no treatment (Answer E) is incorrect.

The primary agents for the treatment of Paget disease of bone are bisphosphonates. Studies have demonstrated more rapid, more frequent, and more sustained disease control after a single intravenous infusion of zoledronic acid compared with oral bisphosphonates, as well as superior effects on quality of life, including pain relief. In fact, the Endocrine Society clinical practice guideline on Paget disease of bone recommends a single 5-mg dose of intravenous zoledronic acid (Answer C) as the treatment of choice in patients who have no contraindication, as opposed to an oral bisphosphonate such as risedronate or alendronate (Answer B). If surgery is required in the near future, an intravenous bisphosphonate should be given 1 to 2 months before the operation if possible.

Calcitonin (Answer A) is an antiresorptive agent that is less potent than bisphosphonates and is unlikely to result in sustained clinical remission. However, it is relatively safe and is approved in its subcutaneous formulation for the treatment of patients with Paget disease who are intolerant of intravenous or oral bisphosphonates.

Denosumab (Answer D), a fully human monoclonal antibody to the receptor activator of nuclear factor kappaB ligand (RANKL), is an agent currently approved for the treatment of osteoporosis, for the prevention of skeletal-related events in patients with multiple myeloma, for patients with bone metastases from solid tumors, and for the treatment of hypercalcemia of malignancy refractory to bisphosphonate therapy. Although denosumab is not currently approved for the treatment of Paget disease, there is some evidence that it may have clinical utility for this indication. While this would be off-label use, it may be an appealing option for patients with contraindications to bisphosphonates such as those with impaired kidney function.

Educational Objective
Treat Paget disease in a patient who has surgery planned at an active pagetic site and recommend the most appropriate medication.

Reference(s)
Singer FR, Bone HG 3rd, Hosking DJ, et al; Endocrine Society. Paget's disease of bone: an Endocrine Society clinical practice guideline. *J Clin Endocrinol Metab.* 2014;99(12):4408-4422. PMID: 25406796

Reid IR, Sharma S, Kalluru R, Eagleton C. Treatment of Paget's disease of bone with denosumab: case report and literature review. *Calcif Tissue Int.* 2016;99(3):322-325. PMID: 27193832

Reid IR, Miller P, Lyles K, et al. Comparison of a single infusion of zoledronic acid with risedronate for Paget's disease. *N Engl J Med.* 2005;353(9):898-908. PMID: 16135834

Hosking D, Lyles K, Brown JP, et al. Long-term control of bone turnover in Paget's disease with zoledronic acid and risedronate. *J Bone Miner Res.* 2007;22(1):142-148. PMID: 17032148

Reid IR, Lyles K, Su G, et al. A single infusion of zoledronic acid produces sustained remissions in Paget disease: data to 6.5 years. *J Bone Miner Res.* 2011;26(9):2261-2270. PMID: 21638319

67 ANSWER: A) Levothyroxine, 100 mcg daily

The incidence of hypothyroidism in pregnancy is reported to be 0.3% to 0.5%. The fetal thyroid is unable to concentrate iodine and synthesize iodothyronine until the 10th to 12th week of gestation. Therefore, maternal thyroid hormones are crucial for growth and development of the fetus in the first trimester when it has no functional thyroid gland. Thyroid hormones cross the plasma membrane by diffusion and in some tissues via a number of thyroid hormone transporters, including members of the monocarboxylate transporter family and the organic anion transporting polypeptides, which are important to maintain the intracellular concentration of thyroid hormones. T_4 (prohormone) enters into the cell and deiodinase enzymes convert T_4 to T_3 (active hormone), which then binds to T_3 nuclear receptors. There are data supporting that maternal T_4, not maternal T_3, is the main source of T_3 in the fetal brain. Therefore, maternal T_3 is not sufficient to ensure appropriate fetal neurodevelopment.

In the setting of pregnancy, maternal hypothyroidism is defined as an elevated serum TSH concentration beyond the upper limit of the pregnancy-specific reference range. If a pregnancy-specific TSH reference range is not available, an upper reference limit of approximately 4.0 mIU/L may be used per the 2017 guidelines of the American Thyroid Association for the diagnosis and management of thyroid disease during pregnancy and the postpartum. When hypothyroidism is diagnosed during pregnancy, the treatment of choice for the management of hypothyroidism in pregnancy is synthetic levothyroxine, which is the same as in nonpregnant women. There may be some bioavailability differences among available levothyroxine formulations, and therefore it is better to continue with the same formulation and the same manufacturer when a patient with existing hypothyroidism becomes pregnant. Experts have recommended the initiation of levothyroxine in pregnant women with a new diagnosis of hypothyroidism as follows (*see table*).

Table. Initiation of Levothyroxine in Pregnant Women

TSH	Free T_4	Levothyroxine dosage
TSH >4.0 mIU/L (or above population and trimester-specific upper normal limit)	Low free T_4 (using assay method and trimester-specific reference range)	1.6 mcg/kg body weight per day
TSH >4.0 mIU/L (or above population and trimester-specific upper normal limit)	Normal free T_4	1.0 mcg/kg body weight per day

Some experts have recommended a starting dosage of 2 mcg/kg per day if overt hypothyroidism is diagnosed during pregnancy. Levothyroxine should be taken on an empty stomach in the morning, an hour before breakfast. After initiation of levothyroxine therapy, serum TSH should be measured in 4 weeks. The goal is to maintain TSH in the lower half of the trimester-specific reference range. If no trimester-specific reference range is available, TSH should be maintained below 2.5 mIU/L in the first trimester and below 3.0 mIU/L in later pregnancy. Switches between brand name or generic levothyroxine formulations should be avoided, as this could potentially result in variations in the serum TSH level. Other preparations of thyroid hormone are available, including liothyronine therapy and desiccated thyroid hormone. These medications are sometimes used in nonpregnant women with hypothyroidism, but this remains controversial.

The patient in this vignette was recently found to be pregnant and was also diagnosed with hypothyroidism. Therefore, levothyroxine should be initiated promptly. On the basis of her weight and thyroid function test results, levothyroxine, 100 mcg daily (Answer A), should be prescribed. The dosage of 50 mcg daily (Answer B) is not high enough for this pregnant patient with overt hypothyroidism. Other available thyroid hormone preparations would be incorrect. The combination of levothyroxine and liothyronine (Answer D) would not provide enough T_4 to maintain an appropriate T_3 level in the fetal brain. Desiccated thyroid (Answer E) contains more T_3 than T_4, and liothyronine (Answer C) would not be the correct treatment choice because maternal T_4, not maternal T_3, is the main source of T_3 in the fetal brain.

Educational Objective
Determine the best choice for thyroid hormone supplementation in a pregnant woman with hypothyroidism.

Reference(s)
Taylor PN, Lazarus JH. Hypothyroidism in pregnancy. *Endocrinol Metab Clin North Am.* 2019;48(3):547-556. PMID: 31345522

Alexander EK, Pearce EN, Brent GA, et al. 2017 guidelines of the American Thyroid Association for the diagnosis and management of thyroid disease during pregnancy and the postpartum. *Thyroid.* 2017;27(3):315-389. PMID: 28056690

68 ANSWER: A) Titrate semaglutide to goal dosage every 4 weeks based on nausea symptoms

Metformin, unless contraindicated, continues to be first-line therapy for treatment of type 2 diabetes. After metformin, the medical therapy choices are determined by patient factors. Most recently, the American Diabetes Association recommended both SGLT-2 inhibitors and GLP-1 receptor agonists for patients with type 2 diabetes who have established atherosclerotic cardiovascular disease or multiple cardiac risk factors, as these agents have demonstrated cardiovascular disease benefit. These recommendations came after trials that were designed to evaluate cardiovascular morbidity and mortality in patients with established atherosclerotic cardiovascular disease or patients at high risk for cardiovascular disease documented reduced composite cardiovascular disease outcomes (death, nonfatal myocardial infarction, and nonfatal stroke.) Additionally, SGLT-2 inhibitors were associated with reduced rate of hospitalization for heart failure. This same guideline highlights that once basal insulin dosages are at 0.5 units/kg, the dosage should not be further escalated and additional therapy should be added. Basal insulins at higher units/kg dosages are typically less beneficial, as they increase the risk for hypoglycemia.

In the Sustain-6 trial, the cardiovascular trial specific for the GLP-1 receptor agonist semaglutide, patients randomly assigned to semaglutide experienced fewer adverse cardiovascular outcomes compared with the control group. The average hemoglobin A_{1c} reduction was 1.4% with a baseline hemoglobin A_{1c} value of 8.7% (72 mmol/mol), and the average weight loss was 10.8 lb (4.9 kg). However, more events of diabetic retinopathy complications occurred in patients treated with semaglutide (3.0%) than in patients receiving placebo (1.8%). The absolute risk increase for diabetic retinopathy complications was larger among patients with a history of diabetic retinopathy at baseline. In those who had retinopathy complications, analysis revealed that they were more likely to have a higher hemoglobin A_{1c} level at baseline, to be taking insulin, to have proliferative retinopathy, and to have required laser or injection therapy at baseline. Those who had no retinopathy at baseline had no increased risk compared with placebo. Finally, in patients who experienced retinopathy complications, a rapid and steep decrease of approximately 2.5% in hemoglobin A_{1c} occurred. Rapid improvement in glycemic control is a known risk factor for worsening retinopathy.

In this vignette, the patient is already on insulin and metformin. Given the increased risk for hypoglycemia if the insulin dosage is increased beyond 0.5 units/kg (Answer E), this is not the correct strategy.

At first glance, with his known history of retinal disease, one might consider excluding semaglutide from his medication management. However, given his known atherosclerotic cardiovascular disease, hemoglobin A_{1c} level greater than 9.0% (>75 mmol/mol), BMI greater than 30 kg/m², preserved ejection fraction, and no known congestive heart failure, semaglutide is a good choice for his third agent. However, to minimize his risk for exacerbation of retinopathy, the goal is to avoid a rapid decline in his hemoglobin A_{1c}. Titrating semaglutide to the full dosage (Answer A) is the best next step to maximize the benefit on both glycemic control and cardiovascular disease. Nausea is a common adverse effect of semaglutide, but slow titration to the full dosage often allows patients to acclimate to the medication and minimizes risk of discontinuation. There is no need to avoid the full dosage, as the progression of retinopathy is not dosage related.

Continuing semaglutide at the current dosage of 0.25 mg weekly (Answer B) would most likely not provide the patient with the desired glycemic control. There is no proven benefit to use low-dosage therapy with both semaglutide and empagliflozin (Answer C), but there is a significant increase in cost associated with dual therapy. Pioglitazone alone (Answer D) is not the best choice given this patient's need for weight loss; weight gain is a known adverse effect of pioglitazone.

Educational Objective
Recommend a GLP-1 receptor agonist as the best therapy given a patient's hemoglobin A_{1c} level, weight, and known cardiovascular disease and appropriately counsel a patient regarding risk mitigation.

Reference(s)
American Diabetes Association. 9. Pharmacologic approaches to glycemic treatment: standards of medical care in diabetes-2020. *Diabetes Care*. 2020;43(Suppl 1):S98-S110. PMID: 31862752

Marso SP, Bain SC, Consoli A, et al. Semaglutide and cardiovascular outcomes in patients with type 2 diabetes. *N Engl J Med*. 2016;375(19):1834-1844. PMID: 27633186

Hooymans JM, Ballegooie EV, Schweitzer NM, Doorebos H, Reitsma WD, Slutter WJ. Worsening of diabetic retinopathy with strict control of blood sugar. *Lancet*. 1982;2:438. PMID: 6124825

69 ANSWER: C) IgG4-related hypophysitis

This patient has evidence of secondary hypogonadism and a history of primary hypothyroidism. His adrenal function is not yet well characterized, as his morning cortisol value is not high enough to rule out adrenal insufficiency but is not low enough to establish the diagnosis. Pituitary MRI shows diffuse, heterogeneous enlargement of the pituitary gland, without evidence of a discrete adenoma or cyst. Therefore, the most likely pathologic process is infiltrative or inflammatory disease. His clinical picture, including autoimmune pancreatitis, retroperitoneal fibrosis, and primary hypothyroidism, is most consistent with IgG4-related hypophysitis (Answer C). This entity is being recognized with increasing frequency. IgG4-related hypophysitis is most often part of systemic IgG4-related disease, which is an immune-mediated disease that is characterized by infiltration of IgG4-positive plasma cells and lymphocytes and fibrosis that can affect almost every organ system. IgG4-related disease may include autoimmune pancreatitis, Riedel thyroiditis, interstitial pneumonitis, interstitial nephritis, prostatitis, lymphadenopathy, retroperitoneal fibrosis, inflammatory aortic aneurysm, and inflammatory pseudotumor. Often, but not always, elevated serum IgG4 concentrations are present. IgG4-related hypophysitis is an uncommon manifestation of IgG4-related disease (1.7%-25% of cases of IgG4-related disease). More than half of the reports are from Japan, but it is not completely clear if this relates to actual increased prevalence or increased awareness. Contrary to lymphocytic hypophysitis, IgG4-related hypophysitis shows an older age and male prevalence (2.4:1). As in this patient, IgG4-related hypophysitis is often associated with other manifestations of IgG4-related disease (75%-90% of cases). A unique feature of IgG4-related hypophysitis is its favorable response to glucocorticoids, at least in terms of mass size.

Although amyloid deposits can be present in pituitary adenomas, pituitary amyloidosis (Answer A) is also a very rare disease, typically occurring in patients with generalized amyloidosis. The normal cardiac findings and the lack of symptoms of peripheral neuropathy make amyloidosis unlikely in this vignette.

Similarly, sarcoidosis (Answer B) is unlikely given the normal chest x-ray and absence of symptoms of diabetes insipidus.

Granulomatous hypophysitis (Answer D) is the second most common histopathologic variant of primary hypophysitis, but it presents with a striking female predominance (72%). While the diagnosis is based on pathology, this form of hypophysitis would not be high in the differential diagnosis list in this older man.

Typical lymphocytic hypophysitis (Answer E) is more common in young women (often, but not always, with temporal relation to pregnancy) and is not associated with multisystem involvement.

Educational Objective
Identify the features of IgG4-related hypophysitis.

Reference(s)

Wehbeh L, Alreddawi S, Salvatori R. Hypophysitis in the era of immune checkpoint inhibitors and immunoglobulin G4-related disease. *Expert Rev Endocrinol Metab.* 2019;14(3):167-178. PMID: 30939947

Yuen KCJ, Popovic V, Trainer PJ. New causes of hypophysitis. *Best Pract Res Clin Endocrinol Metab.* 2019;33(2):101276. PMID: 3178416

Lanzillotta M, Mancuso G, Della-Torre E. Advances in the diagnosis and management of IgG4 related disease. *BMJ.* 2020;369:m1067. PMID: 32546500

70 ANSWER: A) Initiate a phosphodiesterase type 5 inhibitor

This man presents with troublesome erectile dysfunction and a modest decrease in serum testosterone. He has multiple cardiovascular risk factors and longstanding diabetes, suggesting that his erectile dysfunction is predominantly due to neurovascular disease rather than related to his modestly reduced serum testosterone. Consistent with this notion is his preserved libido, as men with organic hypogonadism typically present with reduced libido. Instead, the modest reduction in his serum testosterone is not suggestive of hypogonadism but is typical for older men with obesity who have a significant comorbid burden. Such men generally do not have organic hypogonadism due to pituitary or testicular disease. Rather, the modest reduction in serum testosterone is due to nonspecific hypothalamic suppression caused by obesity and ill health. His clinical examination did not reveal any signs of androgen deficiency, and there were no features suggesting pituitary dysfunction or pituitary mass effect. Therefore, performing a pituitary-directed MRI (Answer D) is not indicated and would risk detecting an incidental microadenoma, which is not uncommon in this age group. Indeed, Endocrine Society guidelines recommend that in the absence of clinical suspicion, pituitary-directed MRI should only be considered (in the context of nonelevated gonadotropins) if the serum testosterone concentration is repeatedly less than 150 ng/dL (<5.2 nmol/L). Of note, functional hypothalamic suppression due to obesity or chronic disease is potentially reversible, with many studies reporting that weight loss and/or optimization of comorbidities can result in reactivation of the hypothalamic-pituitary axis, with increases in and sometimes normalization of serum testosterone.

The best initial treatment of this man's erectile dysfunction is initiation of a phosphodiesterase type 5 inhibitor (PDE5 inhibitor) (Answer A). PDE5 inhibitors are an effective therapy for erectile dysfunction and are generally considered first-line therapy in men without organic hypogonadism in conjunction with lifestyle measures, optimization of comorbidities, avoidance of medications that may exacerbate erectile dysfunction (eg, selective serotonin reuptake inhibitors, thiazide diuretics), and psychological support. This man does not take nitrates, which would be a contraindication to PDE5 inhibitor treatment. Given that he has no cardiovascular symptoms, no symptoms of congestive cardiac failure, controlled hypertension and successful revascularization, he falls into the low-risk category according to cardiovascular risk stratification criteria in men with erectile dysfunction. Therefore, there is no contraindication to PDE5 inhibitor therapy because of underlying cardiovascular risk (Answer E). Of note, erectile dysfunction is a sensitive marker of future cardiovascular events, and optimization of cardiovascular risk factors is an important part of holistic patient care.

While head-to-head clinical trials are lacking, PDE5 inhibitors tend to be more effective than testosterone treatment for middle-aged and older men who do not have organic hypogonadism. In meta-analyses, PDE5 inhibitors have been reported to increase, compared with placebo, the International Index of Erectile Function score (a standardized questionnaire for male erectile dysfunction) by about 5.7 to 7.7 points, which is well above the minimal clinically important difference of 4 points. By comparison, the most comprehensive meta-analysis of placebo-controlled randomized controlled trials in older men has reported that testosterone treatment increases the International Index of Erectile Function score more modestly, by about 3.0 points in men with a serum testosterone concentration less than 230 ng/dL (<8.0 nmol/L) and by about 1.5 points in men with a serum testosterone concentration of 230 to 346 ng/dL (8.0-12.0 nmol/L). Likewise, in the Testosterone Trials conducted in the United States that included 790 men aged 65 years or older with a baseline testosterone concentration less than 275 ng/dL (<9.5 nmol/L), testosterone treatment (dosed to maintain serum testosterone within the normal range for healthy young men) compared with placebo increased the International Index of Erectile Function score by 2.6 points. Overall, sexual effects of testosterone therapy are more pronounced on improved libido and measures of sexual activity and satisfaction other than erectile dysfunction. Consistent with this, in a subanalysis of the Testosterone Trials, increments in serum testosterone during testosterone treatment were positively associated with increases in libido and other measures of sexual satisfaction, but not with improvement of erectile dysfunction. Thus, initiating testosterone (Answer B) is incorrect.

Whether testosterone treatment has benefits for erectile dysfunction that are additive to PDE5 inhibitor treatment remains controversial. The most rigorous randomized controlled trial in this area enrolled 140 men with erectile dysfunction (mean age 55 years) and a mean serum testosterone concentration of 250 ng/dL (8.7 nmol/L). In phase 1, all men were started on PDE5 inhibitor treatment to optimize erectile dysfunction. This was associated with a large increase in the International Index of Erectile Function score of 7.7 points. In phase 2, PDE5 inhibitor treatment was continued, and the men were randomly assigned to testosterone or placebo. Testosterone treatment was not associated with further improvements in the International Index of Erectile Function score or with improvements of any other measures of sexual function. In contrast, one randomized controlled trial specifically recruited men who did not respond to PDE5 inhibitor therapy and reported that while there was no added benefit of testosterone treatment in the overall study population, in a post hoc analysis, testosterone therapy did have an added benefit in men with a serum testosterone concentration less than 300 ng/dL (<10.4 nmol/L). Given that this benefit was based on a secondary analysis, whether testosterone treatment improves erectile dysfunction when added to PDE5 inhibitor treatment requires confirmation. Irrespective of the unresolved issue of whether testosterone treatment may improve erectile dysfunction in men not responsive to PDE5 inhibitor treatment, based on existing data, there is no evidence that would support simultaneous initiation of a PDE5 inhibitor and testosterone (Answer C).

Educational Objective
Initiate appropriate therapy to improve erectile dysfunction in men with neurovascular erectile dysfunction and evaluate risks of therapy.

Reference(s)
Cunningham GR, Stephens-Shields AJ, Rosen RC, et al. Testosterone treatment and sexual function in older men with low testosterone levels. *J Clin Endocrinol Metab.* 2016;101(8):3096-3104. PMID: 27355400

Corona G, Rastrelli G, Morgenthaler A, Sforza A, Mannucci E, Maggi M. Meta-analysis of results of testosterone therapy on sexual function based on international index of erectile function scores. *Eur Urol.* 2017;72(6):1000-1011. PMID: 28434676

Spitzer M, Basaria S, Travison TG, et al. Effect of testosterone replacement on response to sildenafil citrate in men with erectile dysfunction. *Ann Int Med.* 2012;157(10):681-691. PMID: 23165659

Buvat J, Montorsi F, Maggi M, et al. Hypogonadal men nonresponders to the PDE5 inhibitor tadalafil benefit from normalization of testosterone levels with a 1% hydroalcoholic testosterone gel in the treatment of erectile dysfunction (TADTEST study). *J Sex Med.* 2011;8(1):284-293. PMID: 20704642

71 ANSWER: D) Start dexamethasone

Ectopic secretion of ACTH (ectopic ACTH syndrome) accounts for 10% to 15% of all cases of ACTH-dependent Cushing syndrome and may arise in the context of a neuroendocrine tumor (eg, bronchial, pancreatic, thymic, or gastrointestinal neuroendocrine tumor), small cell lung cancer, pheochromocytoma, or medullary thyroid carcinoma. The clinical presentation of ectopic ACTH syndrome can be highly variable, and not all affected patients manifest a typical cushingoid appearance; instead, features of the underlying disorder may predominate (eg, cachexia, wasting in small cell lung cancer). Biochemical hypercortisolism is often marked and is driven by high ACTH that is unresponsive to negative feedback. Signs of mineralocorticoid excess such as hypertension, fluid retention, and hypokalemia may be prominent (with saturation of renal 11β-hydroxysteroid dehydrogenase type 2 [11β-HSD2], allowing cortisol to act as a potent ligand at the mineralocorticoid receptor).

Control of hypercortisolism is a critical first step in the management of any patient with small cell lung cancer complicated by ectopic ACTH syndrome and is a prerequisite to allow the patient to safely undergo systemic chemotherapy. This is most readily achieved through the use of 1 or more adrenal enzyme (steroidogenesis) inhibitors. The most commonly deployed agents are:

- Ketoconazole: inhibits cholesterol side-chain cleavage enzyme, 11β-hydroxylase, and 17,20-desmolase (lyase)
- Metyrapone: inhibits 11β-hydroxylase and aldosterone synthase

Other agents that may be considered include:

- Osilodrostat: inhibits 11β-hydroxylase and aldosterone synthase and has recently been licensed for use in Cushing disease; however, there are limited data on its use in ectopic ACTH syndrome
- Mifepristone: a glucocorticoid receptor antagonist that has been used in exogenous Cushing syndrome complicated by type 2 diabetes or glucose intolerance; it may also be beneficial in acute/severe hypercortisolism. However, it also blocks the effects of exogenous glucocorticoids, which hinders treatment of associated hypocortisolism. In addition, monitoring of efficacy is largely limited to clinical assessment because levels of ACTH and cortisol remain high or increase further
- Mitotane: an adrenolytic drug that also inhibits 11β-hydroxylase and cholesterol side-chain cleavage enzyme through its toxic effects on adrenocortical cell mitochondria
- Etomidate: inhibits 11β-hydroxylase and is infused intravenously, initially with a low, nonhypnotic dose, in patients unable to take oral medication or in patients with severe hypercortisolism when rapid control is required

In this case, metyrapone was started instead of ketoconazole because of preexisting hepatic dysfunction. Although some clinicians reason that elevated liver enzymes in Cushing syndrome may be reflective of hepatic steatosis (and should therefore improve once hypercortisolism is controlled), in this case the ALT level is still higher than 3 times the upper normal limit despite several weeks of medical therapy. There is also evidence of tumor infiltration on cross-sectional imaging of the liver. Hence, even if it is judged that additional adrenal-blocking therapy is required, ketoconazole (Answer A) would not be the agent of choice in this context.

Further up-titration of metyrapone (Answer C) could be considered if the patient is judged to have persistent hypercortisolism. Total daily doses up to 6 g have been used, but there is often little additional benefit above 4 g per day, and adverse effects may be more troublesome. In particular, accumulation of precursors with potent mineralocorticoid effects (eg, 11-deoxycortisol, deoxycorticosterone) can lead to salt retention with edema, hypertension, and hypokalemia, necessitating concomitant mineralocorticoid receptor antagonist therapy, as in this case.

Mifepristone (Answer B) represents an alternative approach to control tissue hypercortisolism and may have a specific role in patients with Cushing syndrome complicated by hyperglycemia. However, not only is biochemical monitoring of disease control rendered largely impossible in patients receiving mifepristone, but hypokalemia may be markedly exacerbated. Hence, to date, mifepristone has had limited use in ectopic ACTH syndrome. In this case, glycemic control is not an immediate concern (hemoglobin A_{1c} is well controlled on metformin alone), and there is already evidence of mild hypokalemia despite treatment with spironolactone.

Importantly, the patient has recently developed fatigue, malaise, and nausea, which should alert the clinician to the possibility of hypocortisolism. At first glance, the 8-AM cortisol level appears to be reasonable; however, measurement of serum cortisol in this context may be confounded if an immunoassay is used that is susceptible to cross-reactivity with 11-deoxycortisol and other precursors. This can be a particular problem when ACTH drive to the adrenal glands is high, as in this case. Ideally, therefore, in patients receiving treatment with metyrapone, serum (and urinary) cortisol should be measured using tandem mass spectrometry. In the described clinical setting, starting replacement with dexamethasone (Answer D) would be appropriate as part of a block-and-replace strategy, while confirming the validity of the serum cortisol result (and corroborating with measurement of urine cortisol excretion). If hypercortisolism continues, the blockade can be increased while maintaining glucocorticoid replacement.

Although somatostatin analogue therapy (Answer E) may appear to be a rational choice to manage ACTH hypersecretion in patients with neuroendocrine tumors given the frequent expression of somatostatin receptor subtype 2, the effect of these agents is often partial and transient, as evidenced on somatostatin receptor scintigraphy or PET. Here, the patient's primary tumor is a small cell lung cancer and specific chemotherapy (± radiotherapy) is likely to be more effective in controlling ACTH secretion.

Educational Objective
Explain the benefits and limitations of different adrenal steroidogenesis inhibitors in the management of hypercortisolism and recognize pitfalls in monitoring disease control.

Reference(s)

Young J, Haissaguerre M, Viera-Pinto O et al. Management of endocrine disease: Cushing's syndrome due to ectopic ACTH secretion: an expert operational opinion. *Eur J Endocrinol.* 2020;182(4):R29-R58. PMID: 31999619

Monaghan PJ, Owen LJ, Trainer PJ, Brabant G, Keevil BG, Darby D. Comparison of serum cortisol measurements by immunoassay and liquid chromatography-tandem mass spectrometry in patients receiving the 11β-hydroxylase inhibitor metyrapone. *Ann Clin Biochem*, 2011;48(5):441-446. PMID: 21813575

72 ANSWER: C) Order genetic testing for pathogenic variants in the *CASR*, *AP2S1*, and *GNA11* genes

Hypercalcemia is a common reason for endocrinology consultation, with most outpatients ultimately confirmed to have primary hyperparathyroidism due, most commonly, to a single parathyroid adenoma or, less commonly, to multiple parathyroid adenomas or hyperplasia. The diagnosis is generally straightforward and based on elevated serum calcium (adjusted for albumin) in the context of an intact serum PTH level that is either frankly elevated or inappropriately in the mid to upper normal range. In addition, most patients with primary hyperparathyroidism have normal or elevated 24-hour urinary calcium excretion, the latter of which is defined as greater than 4 mg/kg per day. It is not uncommon in clinical practice to encounter patients who have borderline low or frankly low 24-hour urinary calcium excretion, the latter of which is generally defined as less than 50 mg daily. These patients represent a diagnostic challenge. Familial hypocalciuric hypercalcemia, a hereditary hypercalcemic disorder due to inactivating pathogenic variants in the calcium-sensing receptor gene (*CASR*), results in a higher calcium set point needed to suppress PTH secretion. Although *CASR* pathogenic variants are most common and cause what is termed familial hypocalciuric hypercalcemia type 1, inactivating pathogenic variants in the gene encoding G-protein subunit α 11 *GNA11* (familial hypocalciuric hypercalcemia type 2) and missense pathogenic variants in the *AP2S1* gene encoding the adaptor protein 2 sigma subunit (familial hypocalciuric hypercalcemia type 3) also occur. Familial hypocalciuric hypercalcemia is not surgically remediable by parathyroidectomy, and thus it is critical to rule out this condition to prevent inappropriate referral for either minimally invasive or open-neck exploration.

Historically, a 24-hour urinary calcium-to-creatinine excretion less than 0.01 has been considered a reasonably reliable indicator of the likely presence of familial hypocalciuric hypercalcemia. It is important to note that patients with vitamin D deficiency and accompanying secondary hyperparathyroidism can have a low 24-urinary calcium-to-creatinine ratio that corrects with vitamin D replacement into an expected range of greater than 0.02 that would be consistent with primary hyperparathyroidism. Patients who are 25-hydroxyvitamin D sufficient (>20 ng/mL [>49.9 nmol/L]) and exhibit a 24-hour urinary calcium-to-creatinine excretion ratio between 0.01 and 0.02 represent a gray area of greater uncertainty regarding the appropriate stratification. It is also important to note this patient's young age at presentation, as she would also be at a higher risk of hereditary hyperparathyroidism that could very well be amenable to successful parathyroidectomy. While a positive family history is a strong predictor of hereditary hyperparathyroidism, the most recent National Institutes of Health guidelines would support genetic evaluation of this patient based on an age of onset younger than 40 years. Current evidence supports consideration of genetic testing for individuals with a calcium-to-creatinine excretion less than 0.02, with a 98% sensitivity for detection of familial hypocalciuric hypercalcemia due to clinically significant *CASR* variants, although at a somewhat reduced specificity with a 35% rate of primary hyperparathyroidism in this patient population. Thus, based on this patient's age of onset of hypercalcemia and the rate of urinary calcium excretion, genetic testing for familial hypocalciuric hypercalcemia (Answer C) is indicated.

Given the need for genetic testing and uncertainty as to the underlying etiology of this patient's hypercalcemia, referral to endocrine surgery (Answer A) is not appropriate now.

This patient has normal bone density and no reported history of fractures. Therefore, treatment with zoledronic acid (Answer B) is inappropriate.

While there are limited data that patients with familial hypocalciuric hypercalcemia may benefit symptomatically from the use of a calcium-sensing receptor agonist, with improved energy and less musculoskeletal pain that may be related to the underlying disease, this patient is currently asymptomatic and would not benefit from the initiation of cinacalcet (Answer D).

Finally, while a thiazide challenge (Answer E) may have some utility in differentiating patients with nephrolithiasis, hypercalciuria, and hyperparathyroidism who may have resorptive hypercalciuria or renal calcium leak, there is no expected or confirmed utility in the workup of patients with hyperparathyroidism and hypocalciuria.

Educational Objective
Explain the indication for and clinical utility of genetic testing in a patient with hypercalcemia due to familial hypocalciuric hypercalcemia.

Reference(s)
Christensen SE, Nissen PH, Vestergaard P, Heickendorff L, Brixen K, Mosekilde L. Discriminative power of three indices of renal calcium excretion for the distinction between familial hypocalciuric hypercalcaemia and primary hyperparathyroidism: a follow-up study on methods. *Clin Endocrinol (Oxf)*. 2008;69(5):713-720. PMID: 18410554

Mariathasan S, Andrews KA, Thompson E, et al. Genetic testing for hereditary hyperparathyroidism and familial hypocalciuric hypercalcaemia in a large UK cohort. *Clin Endocrinol (Oxf)*. 2020;93(4):409-418. PMID: 32430905

73 ANSWER: A) Amlodipine

The guidelines from the American Heart Association and the American Diabetes Association on blood pressure control in patients with diabetes vary. The 2017 American Heart Association guidelines assume that all patients with diabetes are at high risk for cardiovascular disease and recommend starting antihypertensive therapy when blood pressure is greater than 130/80 mm Hg. Target blood pressure is less than 130/80 mm Hg. The American Diabetes Association sets an initial target of less than 140/90 mm Hg in patients who have a 10-year risk of atherosclerotic cardiovascular disease less than 15%. In those at higher risk (10-year risk >15%), the target is less than 130/80 mm Hg. Since the patient in this vignette has a blood pressure of 148/92 mm Hg, he is a candidate for antihypertensive therapy.

In most patients with diabetes and no evidence of proteinuria, an ACE inhibitor/angiotensin receptor blocker, calcium-channel blocker, or diuretic is considered an acceptable first-line agent. There is, however, racial variability in response to medications. Black patients are more likely to require more than 1 agent for hypertensive control and also have better response to diuretics (chlorthalidone) and calcium-channel blockers than to ACE inhibitors. Both diuretics and calcium-channel blockers are equally effective in lowering blood pressure and improving cardiovascular disease and stroke outcomes. Diuretics have better outcomes in heart failure. Either a diuretic or calcium-channel blocker should be the first choice in Black patients with hypertension. Therefore, amlodipine (Answer A) is correct.

If the patient had significant proteinuria, an ACE inhibitor (Answer B) would be the first choice. If the patient had a history of myocardial infarction, a β-adrenergic blocker (Answer D) might be a good option. Hydralazine (Answer C) and clonidine (Answer E) are rarely first choices in the treatment of hypertension and usually serve as add-on therapy for patients with difficult-to-control disease.

Emphasis on good blood pressure control is critical in all patients. This patient should be provided the added information of increased risk of cardiovascular risk and hypertension-associated mortality in Black patients. The 2017 American Hypertension Association hypertension guidelines note that a 2014 review showed hypertension-associated mortality in nonHispanic White men and women to be 19% and 15.3%, respectively, while in Black men and women it was 50% and 35.6%, respectively. In addition, compared with White patients, Black patients have a 1.3 times higher risk of nonfatal stroke, 1.8 times higher risk of fatal stroke, 1.5 times higher risk of heart failure, and 4.2 times higher risk of end-stage kidney disease.

Educational Objective
Consider race and ethnicity in the management of hypertension in patients with type 2 diabetes mellitus.

Reference(s)
Whelton PK, Carey RM, Aronow WS, et al. 2017 ACC/AHA/AAPA/ABC/ACPM/AGS/APhA/ASH/ASPC/NMA/PCNA guideline for the prevention, detection, evaluation, and management of high blood pressure in adults: a report of the American College of Cardiology/American Heart Association Task Force on Clinical Practice Guidelines. *J Am Coll Cardiol*. 2018;71(19):e127-e248. PMID: 29146535

American Diabetes Association. 10. Cardiovascular disease and risk management: standards of medical care in Diabetes-2020. *Diabetes Care*. 2020;43(Suppl 1):S111-S134. PMID: 31862753

74

ANSWER: A) No additional testing or treatment

Follicular thyroid carcinoma (FTC) is the second most common type of thyroid malignancy in the United States. The 2017 World Health Organization classification system divides FTC into 3 histologic subtypes: minimally invasive FTC (capsular invasion only), encapsulated angioinvasive FTC, and widely invasive FTC (grossly invasive). Risk factors for worse outcome with FTC include older age, larger tumor size, widely invasive subtype, lymph node or distant metastases, angioinvasion, and extrathyroidal extension. The 2015 American Thyroid Association guidelines consider tumors with extensive vascular invasion (≥4 vessels) to confer a high risk for structural recurrence (30% to 55%), while the risk of recurrence for minimally invasive FTC is only 2% to 3%. Patients with minimally invasive FTC and no risk factors for poor prognosis, as in the case described, have long-term survival rates that are similar to that of the general population. A nonstimulated postoperative thyroglobulin concentration less than 30 ng/mL (<30 μg/L) following hemithyroidectomy is consistent with an excellent response to therapy. Given this patient's diagnosis of minimally invasive FTC, appropriate postoperative thyroglobulin level, and excellent long-term prognosis, the most appropriate next step in her management is to recommend no additional testing or treatment now (Answer A).

Completion thyroidectomy (Answer C) or completion thyroidectomy and radioactive iodine therapy (Answer D) is not needed now given the patient's low risk for structural recurrence and excellent predicted survival. Both completion thyroidectomy and radioactive iodine therapy can be associated with significant complications, including recurrent laryngeal nerve injury and hypoparathyroidism (surgery) and sialoadenitis (radioactive iodine). Moreover, completion thyroidectomy would necessitate long-term thyroid hormone replacement, while the patient has no evidence of postoperative hypothyroidism following lobectomy and does not require supplementation with exogenous thyroid hormone at this time.

Prescribing low-dosage levothyroxine (Answer E) is incorrect. This patient has a low risk for structural recurrence and thus an initial TSH goal of 0.5 to 2.0 mIU/L (lower half of the reference range) is recommended. The patient's current TSH concentration of 1.9 mIU/L is at goal, so initiation of levothyroxine is unnecessary now.

Finally, repeating neck ultrasonography now (Answer B) is not warranted. The 2015 American Thyroid Association guidelines recommend that postoperative neck ultrasonography be performed 6 to 12 months after initial treatment of thyroid cancer. Repeating neck ultrasonography now, so soon after initial surgery, is both costly and unnecessary. In addition to neck ultrasonography, the guidelines suggest that monitoring of serum thyroglobulin can be considered in patients who undergo lobectomy for the management of differentiated thyroid cancer, in which case a biochemically incomplete response to therapy would be defined by a rising serum thyroglobulin level. However, the overall utility of this approach remains uncertain. A 2018 study by Park et al demonstrated that among patients without recurrent thyroid cancer, 92%, 61%, and 25% had a rise in serum thyroglobulin of more than 20%, 50%, and 100%, respectively. Moreover, among those with a confirmed recurrence, 26% had less than a 20% increase in serum thyroglobulin.

Educational Objective
Recommend the appropriate management of minimally invasive follicular thyroid carcinoma.

Reference(s)

Bojoga A, Koot A, Bonenkamp J, et al. The impact of the extent of surgery on the long-term outcomes of patients with low-risk differentiated non-medullary thyroid cancer: a systematic meta-analysis. *J Clin Med.* 2020;9(7):2316. PMID: 32708218

Haugen BR, Alexander EK, Bible KC, et al. 2015 American Thyroid Association management guidelines for adult patients with thyroid nodules and differentiated thyroid cancer: the American Thyroid Association Guidelines Task Force on Thyroid Nodules and Differentiated Thyroid Cancer. *Thyroid.* 2016;26(1):1-133. PMID: 26462967

Momesso DP, Vaisman F, Yang SP, et al. Dynamic risk stratification in patients with differentiated thyroid cancer treated without radioactive iodine. *J Clin Endocrinol Metab.* 2016;101(7):2692-2700. PMID: 27023446

Park S, Jeon MJ, Oh HS, et al. Changes in serum thyroglobulin levels after lobectomy in patients with low-risk papillary thyroid cancer. *Thyroid.* 2018;28(8):997-1003. PMID: 29845894

75 ANSWER: D) Liraglutide

Several FDA-approved weight-loss medications are available as adjunct therapy for patients who are already engaged in lifestyle modification. Patients are eligible if they have a BMI of 30 kg/m² or greater or a BMI of 27 kg/m² or greater plus weight-related comorbidities. The patient's specific struggle with cravings does not favor one weight-loss medication over another.

Phentermine (Answers A and B) is a sympathomimetic agent that suppresses appetite through its effects on the hypothalamus. In the United States, phentermine is only approved for short-term use; however, it remains the most widely prescribed weight-loss medication in the country in part because of its low cost and general tolerability. It is contraindicated for use in patients with uncontrolled hypertension, hyperthyroidism, or coronary artery disease. Similarly, phentermine-containing products, such as extended-release phentermine/topiramate should not be used in the setting of uncontrolled hypertension, as is the case with this patient.

Naltrexone and bupropion (Answer C) act synergistically at the level of the hypothalamus to increase concentrations of the anorexigenic compound α-MSH. While bupropion may be helpful for both weight loss and smoking cessation, naltrexone is an opioid receptor antagonist. The combination of naltrexone/bupropion can therefore decrease the efficacy of opioids such as oxycodone and should be avoided. Other contraindications to the use of combination naltrexone/bupropion are seizure disorders and uncontrolled hypertension. Patients in the drug arm of the COR-I study (Contrave Obesity Research I study) experienced a transient rise in systolic blood pressure by 1 to 2 mm Hg in the first 12 weeks of therapy. However, this was followed by a gradual reduction in blood pressure in line with weight loss.

Metformin (Answer E) does not have a primary indication for weight loss and moreover would not be recommended given this patient's degree of renal impairment.

Liraglutide (Answer D) is a GLP-1 receptor agonist that is used therapeutically for the management of weight loss and diabetes. It acts centrally at the level of the hypothalamus, as well as peripherally in the gastrointestinal tract to promote satiety. It can be used without dosage adjustment in patients with mild to moderate renal impairment. This medication is recommended with caution for patients with severe renal impairment (estimated glomerular filtration rate <30 mL/min per 1.73 m²). Therefore, in this patient with stable stage 3 chronic kidney disease, liraglutide is the most appropriate weight-loss medication. Once-weekly high-dose (2.4 mg) semaglutide, another GLP-1 receptor agonist, has also been shown to exert a beneficial effect on weight loss. The US FDA recently approved semaglutide for long-term weight management in adults with a BMI of 27 kg/m² or greater who have at least 1 weight-related comorbidity or in adults with a BMI of 30 kg/m² or greater. Similar to liraglutide, it can be used without dosage adjustment in patients with mild to moderate renal impairment.

Educational Objective
Choose the appropriate weight-loss medication in a patient with uncontrolled hypertension and kidney disease.

Reference(s)
Jensen MD, Ryan DH, Apovian CM, et al. 2013 AHA/ACC/TOS guideline for the management of overweight and obesity in adults: a report of the American College of Cardiology/American Heart Association Task Force on Practice Guidelines and The Obesity Society. *J Am Coll Cardiol.* 2014;63(25 Pt B):2985-3023. PMID: 24239920

76 ANSWER: B) Measure 24-hour urinary free cortisol

Medullary thyroid cancer (MTC) is a neuroendocrine tumor that arises from parafollicular cells (or C cells), and it accounts for 1% to 2% of thyroid cancers in the Unites States. Serum calcitonin is a tumor marker for MTC. These tumors also produce carcinoembryonic antigen. Approximately 75% of all cases are sporadic and 25% are hereditary, including multiple endocrine neoplasia type 2. At the time of diagnosis, cervical lymph node metastases are present in 70% of cases and 5% to 10% of patients have distant metastases, including liver, lung, bones, and rarely brain and skin. The most common presentation of a patient with MTC is a thyroid nodule. Affected patients can develop clinical symptoms such as diarrhea due to secretion of calcitonin. MTC can also produce other neuropeptide hormones such as ACTH, causing ectopic Cushing syndrome, and this accounts for 2% to 8% of ectopic Cushing syndrome cases. Ectopic Cushing syndrome can be present at the time of MTC diagnosis or many years after diagnosis. Patients with MTC and ectopic Cushing syndrome experience weakness, hypokalemia, hypertension, elevated glucose levels/diabetes, weight gain, and diarrhea.

In ACTH-dependent hypercortisolism, ACTH is produced by a pituitary adenoma (Cushing disease) in 80% of cases and by nonpituitary tumors in 20% of cases (eg, small cell lung cancers, bronchial cancer, thymic cancer, pancreatic carcinoid tumors, pheochromocytomas, and MTC). In a retrospective study of 1640 patients with MTC, 0.7% of patients developed ectopic ACTH secretion. MTC with ectopic Cushing syndrome has a poorer prognosis than MTC alone because of increased mortality secondary to complications of hypercortisolism.

In this vignette, the patient has metastatic MTC and presents with weakness, fatigue, bilateral leg edema, and uncontrolled hypertension despite 3 antihypertensive medications. Additionally, her laboratory results document hypokalemia and elevated glucose in addition to high serum calcitonin and carcinoembryonic antigen. These findings should raise concern for elevated serum cortisol related to ectopic ACTH production, which is causing ectopic Cushing syndrome. Therefore, the best next step is to measure cortisol in a 24-hour urine specimen (Answer B). Glucocorticoid excess in patients with ectopic Cushing syndrome exceeds the capacity of 11β-hydroxysteroid dehydrogenase type 2 to inactivate cortisol to cortisone (inactive form), which thus activates the mineralocorticoid receptors and leads to elevated blood pressure and profound hypokalemia. In a patient with MTC and ectopic Cushing syndrome, serum cortisol and ACTH levels are elevated and the high-dose dexamethasone-suppression test does not suppress cortisol.

In a patient with uncontrolled hypertension despite multiple medications, secondary causes of hypertension should be considered, including pheochromocytoma, aldosteronism, Cushing syndrome, and renal artery stenosis. However, the patient in this vignette does not have a pathogenic variant in the *RET* gene. Therefore, her uncontrolled hypertension is unlikely to be related to pheochromocytoma and measuring plasma free metanephrines (Answer D) or obtaining dedicated adrenal CT (Answer A) is unnecessary. She also underwent total thyroidectomy and did not have a hypertensive crisis.

In a patient with MTC and uncontrolled hypertension, hypokalemia, weakness, and elevated glucose, ectopic Cushing syndrome should be investigated before looking for other causes such as renal artery stenosis (Answer C) or aldosteronism (Answer E).

Educational Objective
Diagnose ectopic Cushing syndrome in a patient with metastatic medullary thyroid cancer.

Reference(s)
Wells SA Jr, Asa SL, Dralle H, et al; American Thyroid Association Guidelines Task Force on Medullary Thyroid Carcinoma. Revised American Thyroid Association guidelines for the management of medullary thyroid carcinoma. *Thyroid*. 2015;25(6):567-610. PMID: 25810047

Laboureau-Soares Barbosa S, Rodien P, Leboulleux S, et al; Groupe d'Etude des Tumeurs Endocrines. Ectopic adrenocorticotropic hormone-syndrome in medullary carcinoma of the thyroid: a retrospective analysis and review of the literature. *Thyroid*. 2005;15(6):618-623. PMID: 16029131

77 ANSWER: D) Canagliflozin

This patient has type 2 diabetes, established cardiovascular disease, chronic kidney disease, and macroalbuminuria. Canagliflozin (Answer D), an SGLT-2 inhibitor, is approved to reduce the risk of major adverse cardiovascular events in adults with type 2 diabetes and established cardiovascular disease. This agent also reduces the risk of end-stage kidney disease, cardiovascular death, and hospitalization for heart failure in adults with type 2 diabetes and diabetic nephropathy with albuminuria (>300 mg/24 h). Based on the recommendation of the data and safety monitoring committee in the CREDENCE trial (Canagliflozin and Renal Outcomes in Type 2 Diabetes and Nephropathy), the study was stopped early after a planned interim analysis. At that time, 4401 patients had undergone random assignment, with a median follow-up of 2.62 years. The relative risk of the primary outcome was 30% lower in the canagliflozin group than in the placebo group, with event rates of 43.2 and 61.2 per 1000 patient-years, respectively (hazard ratio, 0.70; 95% CI, 0.59-0.82; $P = .00001$). The relative risk of the renal-specific composite of end-stage kidney disease, a doubling of the creatinine level, or death of renal causes was lower by 34% (hazard ratio, 0.66; 95% CI, 0.53-0.81; $P < .001$), and the relative risk of end-stage kidney disease was lower by 32% (hazard ratio, 0.68; 95% CI, 0.54-0.86; $P = .002$). In addition, the CANVAS trial (Canagliflozin and Cardiovascular and Renal Events in Type 2 Diabetes) demonstrated that the rate of the primary outcome (major adverse cardiovascular events) was lower with canagliflozin than with placebo (occurring in 26.9 vs 31.5 participants per 1000 patient-years; hazard ratio, 0.86; 95% CI, 0.75-0.97; $P < .001$ for noninferiority; $P = .02$ for superiority).

Exenatide LAR (Answer A), a long-acting GLP-1 receptor agonist, did not demonstrate cardiovascular risk reduction in the EXSCEL cardiovascular outcomes trial (Effects of Once-Weekly Exenatide on Cardiovascular Outcomes in Type 2 Diabetes). Accordingly, it is not approved by the US FDA to reduce cardiovascular risk. While the addition of liraglutide, semaglutide, or dulaglutide would be a reasonable choice in this case, given they are all approved to reduce the risk of major adverse cardiovascular events in adults with type 2 diabetes mellitus and established cardiovascular disease, these agents would not confer the renal benefits also afforded by canagliflozin. Although some preliminary data suggest that GLP-1 receptor agonists may also confer renal protection, these studies were not powered appropriately to address this issue. A currently ongoing study is trying to answer this question (Effect of Semaglutide Versus Placebo on the Progression of Renal Impairment in Subjects With Type 2 Diabetes and Chronic Kidney Disease [FLOW]) and is estimated to be completed in August 2024.

Use of pioglitazone (Answer C), a PPARγ agonist, particularly in patients receiving higher insulin dosages, increases the risk of fluid retention and potentially the risk of congestive heart failure. Given this patient's insulin requirements, pioglitazone would not be the best option.

The patient's blood pressure is currently well controlled, so the addition of antihypertensive therapy (Answer E) is not indicated. In addition, combining ACE inhibitor and angiotensin-receptor blocker therapy is not recommended. The ONTARGET study (Ongoing Telmisartan Alone and in Combination with Ramipril Global Endpoint Trial) compared the ACE inhibitor ramipril, the angiotensin-receptor blocker telmisartan, and the combination of the 2 drugs in patients with vascular disease or with diabetes who were at high risk. Telmisartan was equivalent to ramipril in patients with vascular disease or high-risk diabetes and was associated with less angioedema. The combination of the 2 drugs was associated with more adverse events without an increase in benefit. For these reasons, addition of the angiotensin-receptor blocker losartan is incorrect.

Aliskiren (Answer B), a direct renin inhibitor, should not be added to the regimen of a patient treated with an ACE inhibitor or angiotensin-receptor blocker. The ALTITUDE study (Aliskiren Trial in Type 2 Diabetes Using Cardiorenal Endpoints) failed to identify a benefit of aliskiren as an adjunct to therapy with an ACE inhibitor or an angiotensin-receptor blocker and found that vs placebo, aliskiren was associated with more cases of nonfatal stroke, renal complications, hyperkalemia, and hypotension.

Educational Objective
Identify patients with type 2 diabetes and chronic kidney disease who may benefit from SGLT-2 inhibitor therapy.

Reference(s)
Perkovic V, Jardine MJ, Neal B, et al; CREDENCE Trial Investigators. Canagliflozin and renal outcomes in type 2 diabetes and nephropathy. *N Engl J Med.* 2019;380(24):2295-2306. PMID: 30990260

Neal B, Perkovic V, Mahaffey KW, et al; CANVAS Program Collaborative Group. Canagliflozin and cardiovascular and renal events in type 2 diabetes. *N Engl J Med.* 2017;377(7):644-657. PMID: 28605608

Parving H, Brenner BM, McMurray JJV et al; ALTITUDE Trial Investigators. Cardiorenal end points in a trial of aliskiren for type 2 diabetes. *N Engl J Med.* 2012;367(23):2204-2213. PMID: 23121378

ONTARGET Investigators; Yusuf S, Teo KK, et al. Telmisartan, ramipril, or both in patients at high risk for vascular events. *N Engl J Med.* 2008;358(15):1547-1559. PMID: 18378520

Holman RR, Bethel MA, Mentz RJ, et al; EXSCEL Study Group. Effects of once-weekly exenatide on cardiovascular outcomes in type 2 diabetes. *N Engl J Med.* 2017;377(13):1228-1239. PMID: 28910237

78 ANSWER: A) Observation

In specialized centers (pituitary centers of excellence), surgical remission is achieved in 80% to 90% of patients with acromegaly due to a pituitary microadenoma. However, in patients with macroadenomas, surgical cure rates are significantly lower (50% to 75%, even in experienced centers), and these figures fall further if the tumor is very large or invasive.

In patients with residual active disease following primary surgery, the choice lies between a repeated surgery, medical therapy, or radiotherapy. Reoperation, as for primary surgery, should only be undertaken in a specialized center and after full multidisciplinary evaluation. Distinguishing between residual tumor and postoperative appearances on MRI can be difficult, and the second surgery may be technically more challenging. Medical therapy is therefore often recommended to control residual disease following the primary surgery.

Cabergoline, a relatively long-acting dopamine agonist, has the advantage of being relatively inexpensive and orally administered. However, its effectiveness is modest, and its use is therefore generally limited to patients with mild disease (eg, IGF-1 <2.5 times the upper normal limit). It may also be preferred in patients with mixed somatolactotroph tumors and significant hyperprolactinemia.

First-generation somatostatin receptor ligands (eg, octreotide and lanreotide) are generally preferred as first-line adjunctive therapy in patients with persistent disease, reflecting their favorable risk-benefit profiles. The GH receptor antagonist pegvisomant is used as second-line therapy in patients who do not achieve biochemical control with maximal dosages of somatostatin receptor ligands, although some clinicians advocate it as an alternative first-line therapy. The second-generation somatostatin receptor ligand pasireotide is currently reserved for patients with more refractory/challenging disease, reflecting its tendency to cause glycemic disturbance.

The patient in this vignette has clear evidence of clinical, biochemical, and radiologic improvements following primary surgery, but the key question is whether she still has residual active disease. The finding of a raised IGF-1 level (1.4 times the upper normal limit) and the postoperative MRI appearance could both be consistent with residual tumor in the right side of the sella. However, most of the patient's symptoms have resolved, her blood pressure and glycemic control are satisfactory on minimal therapy, and the preoperative MRI shows a tumor that would be favorable for complete resection in the hands of an experienced neurosurgeon. In addition, her fasting GH concentration is less than 0.4 ng/mL, which suggests complete remission even without the requirement for an oral glucose tolerance test.

Importantly, in a subgroup of patients with acromegaly, serum GH and IGF-1 results are discordant, especially in the early postoperative period. Patients usually show controlled GH and elevated IGF-1 (as in this case), but the opposite may occur.

In this context, it is reasonable to adopt a close observation strategy (Answer A) until the picture becomes clearer. Certainly, repeated surgery (Answer C) or radiotherapy (Answer B) are not indicated at this early stage, and both run the risk of unnecessary damage to the remaining normal pituitary gland. Medical therapy in the form of cabergoline (Answer D), a somatostatin receptor ligand (Answer E), or pegvisomant would almost certainly normalize the patient's IGF-1 level, but in so doing, it may commit the patient to months or years of unnecessary treatment. On biochemical assessment 3 months later, her GH concentration was less than 0.4 ng/mL and her IGF-1 concentration was normal. No further treatment was needed.

Educational Objective
Explain how biochemical indicators of disease activity (GH and IGF-1) may be discordant following surgery, especially in the early postoperative phase.

Reference(s)
Giustina A, Barkhoudarian G, Beckers A, et al. Multidisciplinary management of acromegaly: a consensus. *Rev Endocr Metab Disord*. 2020;21(4):667-678. PMID: 32914330

Casanueva F, Barkan A, Buchfelder M, et al; Pituitary Society, Expert Group on Pituitary Tumors. Criteria for definition of pituitary tumor centers of excellence (PTCOE): a Pituitary Society statement. *Pituitary*. 2017;20(5):489-498. PMID: 28884415

79 ANSWER: E) 7 units in the morning and 7 units at bedtime

Almost 2 decades ago, the first basal insulin analogue (glargine) became available in the United States. Compared with NPH insulin, which reaches a peak between 4 to 8 hours and has a 12- to 14-hour duration of action, insulin glargine has little to no peak activity and a longer duration of action. Glargine's mean duration of action is 22 ± 4 hours. A variety of basal insulin analogues have since become available, including insulin detemir (*figure 1*). Because NPH insulin has a shorter duration of action but more of a peak, the typical practice has been to give two-thirds of the dose in the morning and one-third of the dose in the evening, as in this vignette. When converting most basal insulin analogue insulins, the total daily dose of NPH is calculated, then 80% of that dose is administered as a single dose of basal insulin. Thus, administering 10 units in the morning and 10 units at bedtime (Answer A) or 20 units at bedtime (Answer D) is incorrect, as this is too high a basal dose and would increase the risk of hypoglycemia.

Figure 1. Basal Insulin Analogues

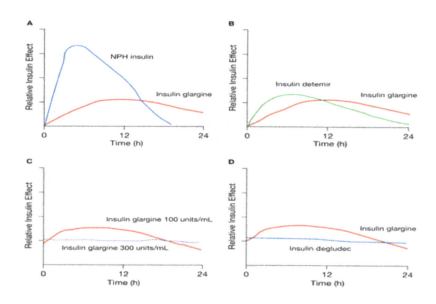

Reprinted from: https://upload.wikimedia.org/wikipedia/commons/f/f2/Insulin_short-intermediate-long_acting.svg.

However, the conversion from NPH insulin to insulin detemir requires additional consideration. Insulin detemir can last up to 24 hours and may be given twice daily or as a single dose. At higher units/kg, its duration is longer but at doses less than 0.3 units/kg, as with this patient's dose, it has a shorter duration of action and is ideally administered twice daily (*figure 2*). Thus, converting her regimen to 7 units at bedtime (Answer C) or 16 units in the morning (Answer B) is incorrect because the dose in Answer C is too low and the dose in Answer B is too high. At the dose this patient needs, it would be less likely to last 24 hours and there would be increased risk of hyperglycemia. Thus, twice-daily dosing is needed to ensure 24-hour duration.

Figure 2. Activity Profiles in Patients With Type 1 Diabetes in a 24-Hour Glucose Clamp Study

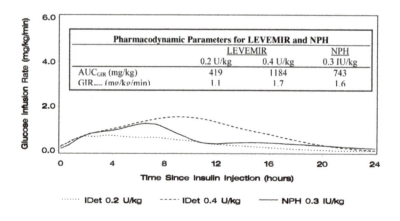

Reprinted from: Levemir. Prescribing information. Novo Nordisk; 2005. https://www.accessdata.fda.gov/drugsatfda_docs/label/2007/021536s015lbl.pdf

Finally, careful review of the patient's history demonstrates several episodes of nocturnal hypoglycemia. The glucose log shows a concentration of 202 mg/dL (11.2 mmol/L) the morning of day 2 after a bedtime glucose concentration of 122 mg/dL (6.8 mmol/L) on day 1. This could reflect another episode of nocturnal hypoglycemia, as the value of 202 mg/dL (11.2 mmol/L) could reflect a rebound high. One should also factor in a decrease in the total basal insulin dose given the repeated nocturnal hypoglycemia. Thus, 16 units in the morning is incorrect, as this dose is both too high and once-daily dosing is insufficient to last 24 hours. The best strategy is to administer

7 units in the morning and 7 units at bedtime (Answer E), as in addition to conversion at 80% and splitting the dose, there is an additional 20% decrease in total insulin in order to prevent hypoglycemia.

Fast-acting insulin analogues such as lispro are preferred over human insulins (insulin regular) because they are more similar to endogenous prandial insulin release. They absorb within 10 to 15 minutes, peak at 30 to 90 minutes, and have a shorter duration of action (4-6 hours). Conversely, human insulin absorbs in 30 to 45 minutes, peaks at 2 to 3 hours, and can last up to 8 hours. Because fasting-acting insulin analogues mirror normal physiology better than human insulin, they lessen glucose excursions with meals and decrease the risk for hypoglycemia.

Educational Objective
Convert between different types of basal insulin.

Reference(s)
Hirsch IB. Insulin analogues. *N Engl J Med.* 2005;352(2):174-183. PMID: 15647580

Levemir. Prescribing information. Novo Nordisk; 2005. Accessed September 2020. https://www.accessdata.fda.gov/drugsatfda_docs/label/2007/021536s015lbl.pdf

80 ANSWER: D) Repeat ultrasound-guided FNA of a left lateral lymph node for cytology with thyroglobulin washout

Neck ultrasonography has demonstrated a suspicious left thyroid nodule and multiple enlarged lymph nodes with cystic changes and peripheral blood flow in this patient's left central and lateral neck. Ultrasound-guided FNA of the thyroid nodule demonstrated indeterminate cytology, while FNA of a left supraclavicular lymph node was nondiagnostic (no lymph node elements). Although cystic change is common in thyroid nodules and does not increase the risk of malignancy, cystic change in lymph nodes is a highly suspicious finding that is often seen in metastatic papillary thyroid cancer. FNA of cystic lymph nodes is more likely to yield a nondiagnostic cytology result in comparison to that of noncystic lymph nodes. However, the diagnostic yield can be increased by assessing the level of thyroglobulin measured in a saline rinse of the FNA specimen. A 2019 study that assessed the detection of papillary thyroid cancer in cystic lymph nodes found that the addition of the thyroglobulin washout to cytology evaluation increased the overall sensitivity and specificity for detecting metastases from 80% and 100%, respectively (cytology alone), to 98% and 100%, respectively (combination). To best inform surgical decision-making for this patient, the most appropriate next step would be to repeat ultrasound-guided FNA of the left lateral lymph node for cytology and thyroglobulin washout (Answer D). Several studies have validated a thyroglobulin washout of 1.0 ng/mL as the optimal threshold for distinguishing malignant from benign lymph nodes. Thyroglobulin antibodies do not appear to hinder the ability to detect thyroglobulin in lymph node specimens, although they commonly cause negative interference in serum measurements.

For comparison, a normal-appearing cervical lymph node (*see image, yellow arrow*) with ellipsoid shape, hypoechoic cortex, and intact fatty hilum and a corresponding Doppler image demonstrating hilar flow are shown.

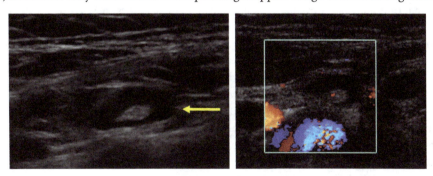

Neither referral for diagnostic left lobectomy (Answer A) nor referral for total thyroidectomy (Answer B) should be pursued as the next step in this patient's management. The appearance of this patient's left lateral cervical lymphadenopathy is highly suspicious for thyroid cancer metastasis, but a definitive pathologic diagnosis has yet to be ascertained. If the patient were to undergo thyroid surgery at this juncture, she would soon require a second surgery to address her lymph node metastases, which would increase her risk for surgical complications, particularly through reentry into the central neck. A central neck dissection is always indicated at the time of initial surgery for patients with papillary thyroid cancer and lateral lymph node metastases because more than 90% of patients also have disease in the central compartment.

Repeating ultrasound-guided FNA of the left thyroid nodule for cytology (Answer C) is incorrect. In the absence of the suspicious cervical lymphadenopathy described in this vignette, the most appropriate next step in the management of a thyroid nodule with Bethesda IV cytology is either to perform a diagnostic lobectomy or to first conduct molecular testing to supplement the malignancy risk assessment according to both the 2015 American Thyroid Association management guidelines for adult patients with thyroid nodules and differentiated thyroid cancer and the 2017 Bethesda System for Reporting Thyroid Cytopathology. Although repeating thyroid FNA for cytology evaluation can yield benign results with Bethesda III nodules (atypia of undetermined significance; follicular lesion of undetermined significance) and should be considered in this setting, another FNA for cytologic evaluation is not indicated for thyroid nodules with a Bethesda IV diagnosis.

Performing rhTSH-stimulated radioactive iodine (^{123}I) whole-body scanning (Answer E) would not provide useful diagnostic information in this patient with an intact thyroid gland. High radioactive iodine uptake by the thyroid gland will reduce the sensitivity of whole-body scanning to detect extrathyroidal disease, including lymph node or distant metastases.

Educational Objective
Describe the utility of obtaining thyroglobulin washout in the evaluation of lymph node metastasis, particularly those demonstrating cystic change.

Reference(s)
Cibas ES, Ali SZ. The 2017 Bethesda System for reporting thyroid cytopathology. *Thyroid.* 2017;27(11):1341-1346. PMID: 29091573

Grani G, Fumarola A. Thyroglobulin in lymph node fine-needle aspiration washout: a systematic review and meta-analysis of diagnostic accuracy. *J Clin Endocrinol Metab.* 2014;99(6):1970-1982. PMID: 24617715

Khadra H, Mohamed H, Al-Qurayshi Z, Sholl A, Killackey M, Kandil E. Superior detection of metastatic cystic lymphadenopathy in patients with papillary thyroid cancer by utilization of thyroglobulin washout. *Head Neck.* 2019;41(1):225-229. PMID: 30536535

Konca Degertekin C, Yalcin MM, Cerit T, et al. Lymph node fine-needle aspiration washout thyroglobulin in papillary thyroid cancer: diagnostic value and the effect of thyroglobulin antibodies. *Endocr Res.* 2016;41(4):281-289. PMID: 26905960

81 ANSWER: A) Anxiety unrelated to a functional pheochromocytoma or paraganglioma

Approximately one-third of all pheochromocytomas and paragangliomas are attributed to an inherited genetic alteration in 1 of more than a dozen identified genes. Pathogenic alterations in the *SDHB* gene are among the most commonly detected and can predispose an individual to a lifetime risk of developing pheochromocytoma, paraganglioma (including metastatic pheochromocytoma and paraganglioma), renal cell carcinoma, and gastrointestinal stromal tumors. Therefore, patients with pathogenic variants in *SDHB* are advised to undergo an imaging surveillance program to detect tumors at an early stage to allow for necessary interventions. Other genes associated with inherited pheochromocytoma and paraganglioma include *NF1, VHL, RET, SDHA, SDHC, SDHD, SDHAF2, EPAS1, TMEM127, MAX,* and *FH.*

Pheochromocytomas are tumors arising from the adrenal medulla, which may secrete catecholamines that induce adrenergic symptoms and signs such as palpitations, anxiety, sweating, pallor, and elevated blood pressure and heart rate. Paragangliomas are tumors arising from the ganglia of the autonomic nervous system, and therefore they can occur in any region from the skull base to the pelvic floor. Sympathetic paraganglia can also secrete catecholamines. Thus, this patient's hyperadrenergic symptoms should certainly raise suspicion of a new functional pheochromocytoma or paraganglioma. Importantly, 6 months earlier there was no evidence of such a tumor on imaging, and her plasma metanephrines are normal. Pheochromocytomas and paragangliomas are typically very slowly growing; thus, it would be unusual for a new functional tumor to arise and contribute to symptomology within a 6-month period.

Metanephrines are the stable and inactive metabolites of catecholamines that provide the highest sensitivity and specificity for diagnosing pheochromocytoma and paraganglioma. Further, metanephrines have a very high negative predictive value; a normal result almost certainly excludes the possibility of a functional tumor as the cause of symptoms. Metanephrine is the metabolite of epinephrine, and normetanephrine is the metabolite of norepinephrine.

Typically, pheochromocytomas and paragangliomas that induce clinical symptoms are associated with metanephrine and/or normetanephrine levels that are substantially higher than the upper limit of the reference range—usually 4 times or more (less commonly 2 or 3 times higher). Importantly, mild elevations above the upper limit of the normetanephrine reference range (<2 times) are common and are usually attributed to enhanced sympathoadrenergic tone (eg, in a state of anxiety, stress, or illness) and/or the use of catecholamine reuptake inhibitors (eg, some antidepressant medications and cocaine or methamphetamines). These mild elevations are a frequent cause of false-positive values. Mild elevations in the metanephrine fraction are a less common cause of false-positives and generally raise more concern for an epinephrine-producing pheochromocytoma.

The combination of normal imaging and metanephrines 6 months ago, plus normal metanephrine values now, strongly suggests that the symptoms are not related to a new functional pheochromocytoma or paraganglioma (Answers B, C, and D). A nonfunctional paraganglioma (Answer E) is not expected to contribute to any hyperadrenergic symptoms. This patient's symptoms resolved spontaneously over the course of several weeks and were retroactively attributed to increased stress and anxiety in her personal life (Answer A). Two years later, her routine surveillance MRI imaging and plasma metanephrines were again normal, providing further reassurance that she had no observable tumors or functional catecholamine excess.

Educational Objective
Evaluate for pheochromocytoma and paraganglioma in a patient with an *SDHB* pathogenic variant.

Reference(s)
Lenders JWM, Duh Q-Y, Eisenhofer G, et al; Endocrine Society. Pheochromocytoma and paraganglioma: an Endocrine Society clinical practice guideline. *J Clin Endocrinol Metab*. 2014;99(6):1915-1942. PMID: 24893135

Neumann HPH, Young WF Jr, Eng C. Pheochromocytoma and paraganglioma. *N Engl J Med*. 2019;381(6):552-565. PMID: 31390501

82 ANSWER: B) Basal insulin

This patient developed diabetes mellitus after treatment with pembrolizumab, an immune checkpoint inhibitor. The development of diabetes mellitus is a rare adverse event in this setting, but it may be fulminant and associated with diabetic ketoacidosis. Thus, treatment with basal insulin (Answer B) is the best next step. Indeed, this patient was found to have moderate urinary ketones at home by using her son's ketone test strips.

Restoration of antitumor immune responses by blockade of inhibitory immune receptors has become standard of care in some oncologic treatment paradigms. Specifically, this involves blockade of cytotoxic T-lymphocyte antigen-4 (CTLA-4), programmed cell death protein 1 (PD-1), or its ligand PD-L1. This unfettered immune response is associated with development of autoimmune endocrinopathies, most commonly thyroid disorders and hypophysitis. However, autoimmune diabetes mellitus has also been reported. Diabetes mellitus diagnosed in this setting has many similarities to type 1 diabetes: association with susceptible HLA genotypes, presentation with diabetic ketoacidosis, and low or undetectable C-peptide levels. Interestingly, only about 50% of persons with immune checkpoint inhibitor–associated diabetes have detectable islet-cell antibodies at the time of diagnosis, in contrast to persons with type 1 diabetes in whom islet-cell antibodies are present in 85% to 90%. Thus, their absence does not exclude this diagnosis. There are cases in which islet-cell antibodies develop over time. The frequency of islet-cell antibodies before presentation with immune checkpoint inhibitor–associated diabetes is not known. Blockade of the PD-1/PD-L1 pathway is associated with immune checkpoint inhibitor–induced diabetes. CTLA-4 inhibitor therapy is very rarely associated with diabetes.

After initiation of immune checkpoint inhibitors, onset of diabetes can occur over a wide range of time, from within a few weeks of the first cycle to 1 year after starting treatment. The mean time to diagnosis occurs at 4 to 5 cycles of chemotherapy, although it happens earlier in patients who were given a combination immune checkpoint inhibitor regimen and had antibodies to glutamic acid decarboxylase. About one-quarter of affected patients may have had previous immunotherapy. About 50% have elevated lipase levels indicating pancreatic inflammation. However, elevation of amylase and lipase without symptoms to suggest pancreatitis and without onset of diabetes has been reported in patients treated with immune checkpoint inhibitors. Finally, in terms of disease course, diabetes mellitus is almost always permanent; discontinuation of insulin is unlikely. Metformin (Answer A), a GLP-1 receptor agonist (Answer E), an SGLT-2 inhibitor (Answer D), or a sulfonylurea (Answer C) would not be the best next step because none of these medications treats the underlying defect and could incur risk for diabetic ketoacidosis.

Examples of immune checkpoint inhibitors include the following (although many more agents are in development):

PD-1: pembrolizumab, nivolumab, and cemiplimab
PD-L1: atezolizumab, avelumab, and durvalumab
CTLA-4: ipilimumab

Educational Objective
Identify the risk for diabetes mellitus in patients prescribed immune checkpoint inhibitor therapy and explain that islet-cell antibodies are negative in this setting more often than in patients with newly diagnosed type 1 diabetes.

Reference(s)
de Filette JMK, Pen JJ, Decoster L, et al. Immune checkpoint inhibitors and type 1 diabetes mellitus: a case report and systematic review. *Eur J Endocrinol.* 2019;181(3):363-374. PMID: 31330498

Quandt Z, Young A, Anderson M. Immune checkpoint inhibitor diabetes mellitus: a novel form of autoimmune diabetes. *Clin Exp Immunol.* 2020;200(2):131-140. PMID: 32027018

83 ANSWER: D) Decrease dietary oxalate intake

The patient in this vignette has recurrent kidney stones in the setting of osteoporosis and gastric bypass surgery. Gastric bypass has been linked to metabolic changes that can alter urine chemistry profiles, resulting in higher urinary oxalate, lower urinary citrate, and higher calcium oxalate supersaturation, leading to a higher risk of nephrolithiasis. This patient's kidney stones are composed primarily of calcium oxalate, which is the most common type of kidney stone. Because the risk of stone formation increases with increasing urinary oxalate, a lower intake of dietary oxalate should be recommended; thus, decreasing dietary oxalate intake (Answer D) is correct. Examples of oxalate-rich foods and beverages to avoid include beets, nuts (eg, peanuts, almonds, walnuts, cashews, pecans), peanut butter, rhubarb, spinach, sweet potatoes, wheat bran, strawberries, kiwi, soy products, chocolate/cocoa, tea, and draft beer. In addition, it is important to recognize that vitamin C is metabolized into oxalate; therefore, increasing orange juice intake (Answer E), which is a rich source of vitamin C, is incorrect. Other dietary risk factors for recurrent nephrolithiasis include higher sodium intake (which increases urinary calcium excretion) and lower fluid intake. If the urine volume is less than 2 L in 24 hours, patients should increase their fluid intake with the goal of consistently producing at least 2 L of urine per day.

Unlike a typical patient with nephrolithiasis, this patient's biochemical workup revealed hypocalciuria (as opposed to hypercalciuria) despite significant calcium and vitamin D intake. This is due to the micronutrient and fat malabsorption that occurs after bariatric surgery. Calcium deficiency is associated with metabolic bone disease and secondary hyperparathyroidism, which this patient has. Increased dietary calcium intake (which in turn decreases the absorption of dietary oxalate) is associated with a decreased risk of kidney stones. Examples of calcium-rich foods and beverages include dairy products such as cheese, yogurt, ice cream, and milk and nondairy sources such as green leafy vegetables, fortified cereals, fortified soy milk, and fortified juice. Even though calcium supplements do not appear to be effective in preventing recurrent stones (and may even slightly increase the risk), these would be required in patients with calcium malabsorption and osteoporosis. Since this patient's serum calcium and vitamin D levels are normal in the setting of hypocalciuria, secondary hyperparathyroidism, and osteoporosis, it would be incorrect to decrease his ergocalciferol dosing (Answer C) or to discontinue his calcium or calcitriol supplementation (Answers A and B). Calcium citrate is better absorbed in an achlorhydric environment such as in the stomach pouch after gastric bypass, so this is preferred to calcium carbonate, which is not as well absorbed after gastric bypass because of the decreased acidity of the gastric pouch. A suggested approach is to measure urinary calcium excretion before and approximately 1 month after starting the calcium supplement. If there is a clinically significant increase in urinary calcium excretion, then the addition of a thiazide diuretic may be useful to reduce urinary calcium excretion and to help maintain bone density.

Educational Objective
Provide appropriate counseling to a patient with osteoporosis and calcium oxalate stones after gastric bypass surgery.

Reference(s)

Upala S, Jaruvongvanich V, Sanguankeo A. Risk of nephrolithiasis, hyperoxaluria, and calcium oxalate supersaturation increased after Roux-en-Y gastric bypass surgery: a systematic review and meta-analysis. *Surg Obes Relat Dis.* 2016;12(8):1513-1521. PMID: 27396545

Heilberg IP, Goldfarb DS. Optimum nutrition for kidney stone disease. *Adv Chronic Kidney Dis.* 2013;20(2):165-174. PMID: 23439376

Jackson RD, LaCroix AZ, Gass M, et al; Women's Health Initiative Investigators. Calcium plus vitamin D supplementation and the risk of fractures [published correction in *N Engl J Med.* 2006;354(10):1102]. *N Engl J Med.* 2006;354(7):669-683. PMID: 16481635

Massey LK, Liebman M, Kynast-Gales SA. Ascorbate increases human oxaluria and kidney stone risk. *J Nutr.* 2005;135(7):1673-1677. PMID: 15987848

84 ANSWER: C) Ovarian drilling

General guidelines for total testosterone concentrations suggest a threshold of 150 to 200 ng/dL (5.2-6.9 nmol/L) to trigger further evaluation for a tumoral source, although more recent data suggest that a lower threshold of 147 ng/dL (5.1 nmol/L) is appropriate with more universal use of liquid chromatography–tandem mass spectrometry.

In this case, baseline 17-hydroxyprogesterone concentrations were not elevated or above 1000 ng/dL (>30.3 nmol/L). Therefore, this patient does not have nonclassic congenital adrenal hyperplasia for which glucocorticoids (dexamethasone [Answer E]) would be considered to lower the ACTH-stimulated increase in androgens and progesterone. In addition, the results of a low-dose dexamethasone-suppression test failed to show a decrease in total testosterone of more than 40%, so a possible tumor in the ovaries or adrenal glands has not been excluded. Therefore, further evaluation for a potential tumor and/or lateralization of testosterone secretion is necessary to consider the least invasive method to lower testosterone and improve fertility. Oral contraceptives (Answer A) would not be indicated or likely be of benefit after an abnormal result from a low-dose dexamethasone-suppression test. Further evaluation is necessary.

Combined ovarian and adrenal venous sampling (selective venous sampling) is performed to help make treatment decisions in the evaluation of women with hyperandrogenism when clinical suspicion for an androgen-producing tumor is high, pelvic ultrasonography is normal, and adrenal imaging is either normal or identifies a nodule or mass with benign features. The procedure includes selective catheterization of the ovarian and adrenal veins to demonstrate a gradient in androgen concentrations and localize the source. This procedure is technically difficult and should only be performed by a highly experienced interventional radiologist. Unstimulated testosterone concentrations with a ratio greater than 3 (ovarian or adrenal vein-to-inferior vena cava) and a ratio greater than 1.4 from 1 side to the other indicate a unilateral source. In this case, the right ovarian vein-to-inferior vena cava ratio is 22.8 and the left ovarian vein-to-inferior vena cava ratio is 32.3. Although the left ovarian vein-to-right ovarian vein ratio is 1.4, clearly both ovaries are producing significant amounts of testosterone, and left oophorectomy (Answer B) is unlikely to significantly reduce the amount of testosterone enough to improve fertility.

Although ovulation induction with either letrozole (Answer D) or clomiphene citrate would be first-line treatment of infertility in women with polycystic ovary syndrome, laparoscopic ovarian drilling (laparoscopic ovarian diathermy or electrocoagulation) (Answer C) is offered as second-line treatment after pharmacologic ovulation induction is not successful. In addition, the high testosterone concentrations must be reduced to facilitate ovulation induction, so a treatment strategy that will lower this patient's significantly elevated testosterone concentrations should be considered. Ovarian drilling replaced widely used wedge resection of the ovaries because of a lower risk of adhesions. Both strategies will help lower androgens and facilitate ovulation. Gonadotropin therapy is another second-line treatment to improve fertility with pregnancy rates comparable to those with ovarian drilling, but it has a higher risk for both ovarian hyperstimulation syndrome and multiple gestation. Ovarian drilling does carry risks due to surgery and the potential for adhesion development. Although used for years, ovarian drilling has not been standardized regarding the technique, dose of energy per puncture, number of punctures, or whether both ovaries should be treated.

Educational Objective
Diagnose and treat significantly elevated total testosterone in a woman with infertility.

Reference(s)

Levens ED, Whitcomb BW, Csokmay JM, Nieman LK. Selective venous sampling for androgen-producing ovarian pathology. *Clin Endocrinol (Oxf)*. 2009;70(4):606-614. PMID: 18721192

Sharma A, Kapoor E, Singh RJ, Chang AY, Erickson D. Diagnostic thresholds for androgen-producing tumors or pathologic hyperandrogenism in women by using total testosterone concentrations measured by liquid-chromatography-tandem mass spectrometry. *Clin Chem*. 2018;64(11):1636-1645. PMID: 30068692

Farquhar C, Brown J, Marjoribanks J. Laparoscopic drilling by diathermy or laser for ovulation induction in anovulatory polycystic ovary syndrome. *Cochrane Database Syst Rev*. 2012;(6):CD001122. PMID: 22696324

85 ANSWER: B) Following a healthy dietary pattern (emphasizing high-quality foods primarily derived from plant sources)

There continues to be great interest in ways to prevent or delay the onset of type 2 diabetes. Maintaining a healthy body weight is the most effective way to minimize the risk of developing type 2 diabetes in at-risk populations.

Several studies have examined weight-independent effects of different eating patterns, macronutrient composition, and the impact of physical activity on the long-term risk of developing type 2 diabetes. The PREDIMED-Reus study involved 400 participants at high cardiovascular risk, randomly assigned to a low-fat diet or a Mediterranean-style diet with no recommendations regarding caloric restriction or physical activity. Despite no between-group difference in weight or physical activity, the incidence of type 2 diabetes was 52% lower in the intervention group. A meta-analysis of more than 190,000 participants in prospective studies demonstrated that high adherence (vs low adherence) to a healthy dietary eating pattern reduces the risk of developing diabetes by 20%, independent of changes in body weight. A healthy dietary eating pattern is one that is rich in fruits, vegetables, whole grain, fish, and poultry and low in red meat, processed foods, sugar-sweetened beverages, and starchy foods. This was confirmed in another meta-analysis of prospective studies examining the association between plant-based diets and the risk of developing type 2 diabetes after adjusting for BMI. Thus, the best recommendation for this patient is to follow a healthy dietary pattern that emphasizes high-quality foods primarily derived from plant sources (Answer B).

Low-carbohydrate diets (Answer A) are variably described in the literature; anywhere from 20 g to 100 g of carbohydrate consumption per day has been described as a low-carbohydrate diet. The primary goal is to induce ketosis, which in turn suppresses appetite, shifts metabolic fuel oxidation from carbohydrates to fat, and promotes weight loss. Studies using low-carbohydrate diets are generally short-term and heterogeneous. In addition, reported results are not convincingly separate from the weight-loss effects of the diet, and thus it is difficult to draw firm conclusions about the utility of such a dietary plan in promoting metabolic health in an at-risk individual.

Acarbose (Answer C) is an α-glucosidase inhibitor that slows down the absorption of glucose from the gut. The STOP-NIDDM trial showed that acarbose reduced progression to type 2 diabetes by 25% in a cohort of patients with impaired fasting glucose or impaired glucose tolerance, over a period of 3 years. The average BMI of patients in this study was 30 kg/m². The patient in this vignette has a normal body weight and may not benefit from acarbose.

Data from the Finnish Diabetes Prevention study group demonstrated a reduced risk of developing type 2 diabetes, independent of changes in body weight, with 4 hours of exercise per week in a population of overweight individuals with impaired glucose tolerance. Increasing physical activity to ensure at least 20 minutes of moderate-intensity activity daily (Answer E) is unlikely to change her risk of developing type 2 diabetes. Other high-quality studies of preventing the onset of type 2 diabetes have shown physical activity to be beneficial in the setting of concurrent weight loss.

Time-restricted eating or intermittent fasting (Answer D) has been shown in the short-term to have metabolic benefit; however, long-term data are lacking.

Educational Objective
Counsel an at-risk patient on the appropriate diet to mitigate risk of developing type 2 diabetes mellitus.

References

American Diabetes Association. 3. Prevention or delay of type 2 diabetes: standards of medical care in diabetes-2020. *Diabetes Care.* 2020;43(Suppl 1):S32-S36. PMID: 31862746

Salas-Salvado J, Bullo M, Babio N, et al; PREDIMED Study Investigators. Reduction in the incidence of type 2 diabetes with the Mediterranean diet: results of the PREDIMED-Reus nutrition intervention randomized trial. *Diabetes Care.* 2011;34(1):14-19. PMID: 20929998

Esposito K, Chiodini P, Maiorino MI, Bellastella G, Panagiotakos D, Giugliano D. Which diet for prevention of type 2 diabetes? A meta-analysis of prospective studies. *Endocrine.* 2014;47(1):107-116. PMID: 24744219

Qian F, Liu G, Hu FB, Bhupathiraju SN, Sun Q. Association between plant-based dietary patterns and risk of type 2 diabetes: a systematic review and meta-analysis. *JAMA Intern Med.* 2019;179(10):1335-1344. PMID: 31329220

86 ANSWER: B) Perform plasma exchange

Thyroid storm is a rare endocrine emergency with an estimated mortality rate of 20% to 30%. In addition to underlying hyperthyroidism, a precipitating factor is required to develop thyroid storm. These precipitating factors may include infection, myocardial infarction, surgery, trauma, pregnancy, or diabetic ketoacidosis. Patients with thyroid storm have severe manifestation of thyrotoxicosis and may present with multiple organ failure. Results from thyroid function tests are consistent with hyperthyroidism (suppressed TSH and elevated thyroid hormones), and the degree of elevated thyroid hormones does not matter in thyroid storm.

The treatment goal is to decrease thyroid hormone synthesis, reduce peripheral conversion of T_4 to T_3, and address adrenergic symptoms. These goals are achieved by initiating antithyroid drugs with a higher dosage than that used to manage hyperthyroidism in a patient without thyroid storm. Methimazole and propylthiouracil are antithyroid drugs available in the United States, whereas carbimazole is an antithyroid drug used in Europe. Propylthiouracil is usually favored in the management of thyroid storm because of its additional effect of inhibiting the conversion of T_4 to T_3. Propylthiouracil is prescribed at a dosage of 200 mg every 4 hours, while methimazole is usually given at a dosage of 20 mg every 4 to 6 hours. It is important to remember that propylthiouracil received a black box warning regarding increased risks of severe liver injury and acute liver failure in June 2009 by FDA. Therefore, liver enzymes should be closely monitored while on propylthiouracil. In addition, hydrocortisone, intravenously 50 to 100 mg every 8 hours, and β-adrenergic blockers such as high-dosage propranolol, 60 to 80 mg every 4 to 6 hours, are prescribed. High-dosage propranolol manages adrenergic symptoms in addition to blocking the conversion of T_4 to T_3. Other β-adrenergic blockers do not prevent the conversion of T_4 to T_3. Steroids also reduce T_4 to T_3 conversion and can treat potentially undiagnosed adrenal insufficiency. SSKI is usually started 1 hour after the initiation of antithyroid drugs to prevent the worsening of thyrotoxicosis and is given as 5 drops every 6 to 8 hours. Other medications have been used in the management of thyroid storm such as lithium, which reduces the release of thyroid hormone to the circulation, and cholestyramine, which decreases the reabsorption of T_4 from the gut. Lithium does not have much popularity due to its narrow therapeutic index and renal adverse effects.

Plasmapheresis was first used for the treatment of thyrotoxicosis in 1970. It helps to remove higher molecular weight substances from the blood. Therapeutic plasma exchange (Answer B) is a type of plasmapheresis that removes the patient plasma and replaces it with either donor plasma, fresh frozen plasma, albumin, or colloid. Therapeutic plasma exchange is usually used when a pathogenic substance or component in the blood needs to be quickly removed. Pathogenic substances can include cryoglobulins, myeloma light chains, autoantibodies, endotoxins, cholesterol-containing lipoproteins, and protein-bound thyroid hormones.

Vascular access and a plasmapheresis machine are required to perform therapeutic plasma exchange. Therapeutic plasma exchange reduces circulating thyroid hormone by removing thyroid-binding proteins (thyroxine-binding globulin, transthyretin, and albumin) and treating refractory thyroid storm. Due to the size of these thyroid-binding proteins, dialysis cannot remove them. In addition, therapeutic plasma exchange can also remove thyroid-stimulating immunoglobulins and 5′-monodeiodase (lowers T_3 production). Thyroid hormone levels sometimes increase the day after therapeutic plasma exchange due to ongoing secretion from the thyroid. Even if thyroid hormones remain elevated, clinical improvement can be observed. Plasmapheresis has several complications, including bleeding, disseminated intravascular coagulation, hypocoagulability due to coagulation factor depletion, hypotension, hypocalcemia, infection, and transfusion reactions. However, the mortality rate of plasmapheresis is less than 1%. Even though clinical improvement has been reported a few hours after the first therapeutic plasma exchange session, failure of this treatment to control thyroid storm has also been published.

The American Society for Apheresis clinical practice guidelines recommend that therapeutic plasma exchange be individualized in the treatment of thyroid storm. Plasma exchange should be considered in patients with severe symptoms of thyroid storm in whom medical therapies have failed or have caused severe adverse effects that outweigh the benefits of treatment. Plasma exchange should be performed every day to every 3 days until clinical improvement is observed. The Japan Thyroid Association and Japan Endocrine Society have similar guidelines published in 2016. However, the Japanese guidelines recommend the use of plasma exchange for treatment of thyroid storm in the presence of acute liver failure or no clinical improvement after 1 to 2 days of optimized medical therapies.

In this vignette, the patient presented with thyroid storm and his clinical status worsened (requiring intubation) very soon after his arrival to the emergency department. The Burch and Wartofsky score was 45 or greater. Medical therapy was initiated to manage thyroid storm: propylthiouracil, propranolol, hydrocortisone, and SSKI at the appropriate dosages. Cholestyramine was also added, but his clinical status continued to deteriorate. This patient's thyroid hormone levels and clinical status improved after 3 sessions of plasma exchange (Answer B).

This patient is on high dosages of propylthiouracil and remains hyperthyroid with some improvement in free T_3 and stable liver enzymes. Propylthiouracil remains the drug of choice in patients admitted to the intensive care unit with life-threatening thyroid storm because it reduces T_4 to T_3 conversion, which is not seen with methimazole. The degree of abnormal liver enzymes in this patient also does not warrant a switch to methimazole (Answer C). His elevated liver enzymes are possibly related to hyperthyroidism rather than to propylthiouracil, as they were elevated on admission. If his liver enzymes rise considerably, switching to methimazole or discontinuing antithyroid drugs would be advised.

Propranolol, 80 mg every 4 hours, is the appropriate dosage in thyroid storm and it reduces the conversion of T_4 to T_3 (along with hydrocortisone and propylthiouracil). Therefore, a higher dosage of propranolol (Answer E) would not add further benefit. In addition, his blood pressure is also on the low side, and a higher propranolol dosage could drop it further with adverse outcomes.

Adding lithium (Answer A) might be an option, but in this patient with kidney and liver abnormalities, lithium would not be the best choice.

Thyroidectomy (Answer D) would be the best treatment option once his hyperthyroidism is controlled and his clinical status is improved. At this time, he is still critically ill and no surgery is recommended. Indeed, this patient eventually had a total thyroidectomy to treat his Graves disease and was discharged home on levothyroxine.

Educational Objective
Recommend therapeutic plasma exchange in a patient with thyroid storm.

Reference(s)
Carroll R, Matfin G. Endocrine and metabolic emergencies: thyroid storm. *Ther Adv Endocrnol Metabol*. 2010;1(3):139-145. PMID: 23148158

McGonigle AM, Tobian AAR, Zink JL, King KE. Perfect storm: therapeutic plasma exchange for a patient with thyroid storm. *J Clin Apher*. 2018;33(1):113-116. PMID: 28608527

Muller C, Perrin P, Faller B, Richter S, Chantrel F. Role of plasma exchange in the thyroid storm. *Ther Apher Dial*. 2011;5(6):522-531. PMID: 22107688

Padmanabhan A, Connelly-Smith L, Aqui N, et al. Guidelines on the use of therapeutic apheresis in clinical practice—evidence-based approach from the writing committee of the American Society for Apheresis: the eighth special issue. *J Clin Apher*. 2019;34(3):171-354. PMID: 31180581

Satoh T, Isozaki O, Suzuki A, et al. 2016 guidelines for the management of thyroid storm from The Japan Thyroid Association and Japan Endocrine Society (first edition). *Endocrine J*. 2016;63(12):1025-1064. PMID: 27746415

Burch HB, Wartofsky L. Life-threatening thyrotoxicosis. Thyroid storm. *Endocrinol Metab Clin North Am*. 1993;22(2):263-277. PMID: 8325286

87 ANSWER: D) Sulfonylurea

Based on this patient's age at diagnosis, lack of a presentation typical for type 1 diabetes, and family history, she most likely has a monogenic cause, rather than type 2 diabetes. Further, her sensitivity to sulfonylureas strongly suggests *HNF1A*- or *HNF4A*-related maturity-onset diabetes of the young (MODY). On subsequent testing, she was found to have a pathogenic variant in the *HNF1A* gene. A distinguishing feature of *HNF1A*-related MODY is glycosuria when serum glucose levels are not particularly high. Neonatal hypoglycemia and fetal macrosomia are distinguishing features of *HNF4A*-related MODY. However, both of these forms of MODY are progressive and can be associated with development of microvascular complications. Therefore, finding a good treatment regimen is important. In this situation, neither acarbose (Answer A) nor metformin (Answer C) is expected to be effective over the long-term, as neither addresses the insulin secretory defect that occurs with *HNF1A*- or *HNF4A*-related MODY.

Sulfonylureas (Answer D) are often the initial treatment of choice for patients with MODY, and many patients can maintain excellent glycemic control for decades. This patient has experienced sensitivity to sulfonylureas and mild hypoglycemia, prompting her to discontinue the medication. However, she now has hyperglycemia, indicating that she should resume treatment. Reassuringly, she has not had severe hypoglycemia. Studies suggest that *HNF1A*-related MODY is associated with defective β-cell ATP generation. Sulfonylureas, by causing membrane depolarization independent of the glucose level, bypass this defect, perhaps explaining the effectiveness and extreme sensitivity of patients with *HNF1A*-related MODY to this medication class. Disease progression occurs in up to one-third of cases, typically more than 15 years after diagnosis, and insulin (Answer E) may be required. However, this patient does not appear to have this degree of progression and would most likely experience hypoglycemia on basal insulin.

Incretin-based therapies have not been extensively studied in the treatment of MODY. The rationale for using an incretin-based treatment is that patients may have less hypoglycemia because of the glucose-dependent mechanism of action. There are case studies of DPP-4 inhibitors and GLP-1 receptor agonists as add-on treatments that suggest this medication class may be a useful adjunct to sulfonylurea treatment. Regarding use of GLP-1 receptor agonists as monotherapy (Answer B), one trial compared glimepiride with liraglutide in a 6-week crossover design in 15 participants. On balance, this trial showed that both glimepiride and liraglutide were associated with improved glycemic metrics. While glimepiride was more effective than liraglutide in controlling postprandial glucose levels, glimepiride was associated with more mild hypoglycemia. At this point, GLP-1 receptor agonist monotherapy would not be considered the first choice in this patient given the lack of long-term data and clinical experience. Furthermore, she is not overweight or obese.

Educational Objective
Diagnose maturity-onset diabetes of the young and recognize that patients with 2 of the most common causes, pathogenic variants in *HNF1A* and *HNF4A*, respond to low-dosage sulfonylurea therapy.

Reference(s)
McDonald TJ, Ellard S. Maturity onset diabetes of the young: identification and diagnosis. *Ann Clin Biochem.* 2013;50(Pt 5):403-415. PMID: 23878349

Ostoft SH, Bagger JI, Hansen T, et al. Glucose-lowering effects and low risk of hypoglycemia in patients with maturity-onset diabetes of the young when treated with a GLP-1 receptor agonist: a double-blind, randomized, crossover trial. *Diabetes Care.* 2014;37(7):1797-1805. PMID: 24929431

88 ANSWER: D) Start oral calcitriol therapy

The man in this vignette presents with postoperative hypocalcemia after parathyroidectomy. He has an inappropriately normal PTH level in the setting of persistent hypocalcemia, as well as hypomagnesemia and hypophosphatemia despite stage 3 chronic kidney disease, all of which should raise suspicion for hungry bone syndrome. Hungry bone syndrome refers to the postoperative hypocalcemia that results from reversal of the PTH-induced contribution of bone to maintenance of the serum calcium concentration after parathyroidectomy. This is caused by rapid deposition of serum calcium into demineralized bone following a drop in PTH. In addition to hypocalcemia, the decrease in bone resorption after parathyroidectomy can lead to hypophosphatemia. Low magnesium and high serum potassium levels may also be observed in hungry bone syndrome, likely reflecting increased bone influx and efflux, respectively. Since magnesium is required for PTH secretion and action, the hypomagnesemia itself can impair PTH release and also decrease the sensitivity of target organs to circulating PTH. Risk factors for developing hungry bone syndrome include skeletal manifestations of primary hyperparathyroidism (radiologic evidence of high-turnover bone disease), as well as larger volume of the resected adenoma, higher preoperative alkaline phosphatase levels, and older age. Hungry bone syndrome tends to be severe and prolonged despite normal or even elevated PTH levels.

Treatment of hungry bone syndrome is aimed at each of the electrolyte abnormalities that can occur. Repleting magnesium is an important aspect in the management of hungry bone syndrome since hypomagnesemia can contribute to the development of refractory hypocalcemia. Replenishing the depleted skeletal calcium stores is also critical, initially often intravenously, but then with oral calcium supplementation (2 to 4 g of elemental calcium daily). If the serum phosphate is normal or low, calcium should be administered between meals to maximize intestinal absorption and minimize phosphate binding, making calcium citrate the preferred preparation over calcium carbonate. Calcium carbonate is also poorly absorbed in patients taking proton-pump inhibitors or H2 blockers. This patient is already receiving 2.4 g of elemental calcium daily in the citrate formulation. Increasing his dosage from 600 to 900 mg

4 times daily (Answer A) is unlikely to improve his hypocalcemia given that higher individual doses are associated with a plateau in calcium absorption that may prevent the attainment of positive calcium balance.

Concomitant use of adequate doses of active metabolites of vitamin D is recommended in patients with hungry bone syndrome in order to increase intestinal absorption of calcium and phosphate. This makes starting oral calcitriol therapy (Answer D) the best next step in the management of this patient's hypocalcemia. In fact, calcitriol therapy should be given to all patients who are hypocalcemic following parathyroidectomy, and ideally this treatment should not be delayed. For patients on hemodialysis, most physicians recommend preoperative administration of calcitriol if they are not already being treated with a vitamin D metabolite, to be started 3 to 5 days before surgery and continued postoperatively until serum calcium has stabilized.

A preoperative replete vitamin D status is thought to be associated with decreased likelihood of severe or prolonged hungry bone syndrome, and it has generally been recommended to take supplemental vitamin D to normalize 25-hydroxyvitamin D levels. This patient's 25-hydroxyvitamin D level is already low-normal, and there is no evidence that increasing his cholecalciferol dosage (Answer B) would have any added benefit in the treatment of his hypocalcemia.

The administration of phosphate (Answer C) to correct hypophosphatemia is generally avoided in patients with hungry bone syndrome since phosphate can combine with calcium and further reduce the plasma calcium concentration. In addition, this patient has only mild hypophosphatemia, and intravenous phosphate therapy is typically reserved for patients with severe, symptomatic hypophosphatemia (serum phosphate <1.0 mg/dL [<0.3 mmol/L]) or an inability to take oral therapy. Intravenous phosphate is potentially dangerous because it can precipitate with calcium and cause hypocalcemia, renal failure, and/or arrhythmias.

Finally, there is no role for rhPTH (1-84) subcutaneous injections (Answer E) in the treatment of hungry bone syndrome.

Educational Objective
Diagnose hungry bone syndrome following parathyroidectomy and recommend appropriate treatment.

Reference(s)
Witteveen JE, van Thiel S, Romijn JA, Hamdy NAT. Hungry bone syndrome: still a challenge in the post-operative management of primary hyperparathyroidism: a systematic review of the literature. *Eur J Endocrinol*. 2013;168(3):R45-R53. PMID: 23152439

Yong TY, Li JYZ. Mediastinal parathyroid carcinoma presenting with severe skeletal manifestations. *J Bone Miner Metab*. 2010;28(5):591-594. PMID: 20237944

Cooper MS, Gittoes NJL. Diagnosis and management of hypocalcaemia. *BMJ*. 2008;336(7656):1298-1302. PMID: 18535072

89 ANSWER: C) Stop cabergoline

Dopaminergic agents are the mainstay for treating prolactinomas. Because of greater effectiveness and better tolerability, cabergoline is often preferred over bromocriptine. Neither drug has been associated with higher risk of birth defects or miscarriage. However, because pregnancy outcome data at the time of conception are available for more women treated with bromocriptine (~6000 pregnancies) than with cabergoline (~1000 pregnancies) (all showing no increase in birth defects or miscarriage), some endocrinologists prefer to use bromocriptine in women seeking conception. If a patient is not interested in conceiving, birth control should be discussed, as ovulation may restart soon after therapy is initiated.

Both bromocriptine and cabergoline are pregnancy category B drugs (animal reproduction studies have failed to demonstrate a risk to the fetus and there are no adequate and well-controlled studies in pregnant women, or animal studies have shown adverse effects, but adequate and well-controlled studies in pregnant women have failed to demonstrate a risk to the fetus in any trimester). Thus, in the setting of pregnancy, they should be used only if strictly necessary. This patient had a small intrasellar microadenoma, and after 5 months of successful dopamine agonist therapy, the adenoma has most likely shrunken. During pregnancy, estrogens stimulate the proliferation of lactotroph cells, resulting in a gradual increase in pituitary size. Prolactinomas can also enlarge during pregnancy because of high estrogen levels and/or the discontinuation of dopamine agonist therapy, but the risk of mass effect symptoms (chiasmatic compression, headaches) from a microprolactinoma is rather low (about 2.5%). Therefore, continuation of cabergoline (Answer A) or simply reducing the dosage (Answer B) cannot be justified in this vignette. Cabergoline should be stopped in this case (Answer C). Prolactin levels are generally not followed during pregnancy, and MRI (preferably without gadolinium) is obtained only if mass effect is suspected. In the unlikely scenario of mass effect, dopamine agonist therapy can be reinstated in the latter part of pregnancy.

Although breastfeeding is a physiologic stimulus for prolactin secretion, there are no data supporting the idea that breastfeeding causes prolactinoma growth. Thus, nursing is not contraindicated in women with prolactinomas.

Performing periodic visual field tests after stopping cabergoline (Answer D) is not necessary in this patient given the adenoma's small size and its intrasellar location, resulting in low risk of mass effect. The situation would be different if the patient had a macroprolactinoma, which would carry a higher risk of mass effect. In these cases, the decision of whether to continue dopamine agonist therapy during pregnancy must be considered on a case-by-case basis, taking into account the size of the adenoma and its location (intrasellar vs extrasellar). Some clinicians stop the dopaminergic agent in the first trimester and restart it in later stages of pregnancy. In patients with macroprolactinomas (or large microadenomas located close to the optic chiasm), periodic visual field tests (every trimester) would be indicated.

Finally, there is no proof that switching from cabergoline to bromocriptine after pregnancy is confirmed (Answer E) has any effect on pregnancy outcomes.

Educational Objective
Manage microprolactinomas during pregnancy.

Reference(s)
Huang W, Molitch ME. Pituitary tumors in pregnancy. *Endocrinol Metab Clin North Am.* 2019;48(3):569-581. PMID: 31345524

Glezer A, Bronstein MD. Prolactinomas in pregnancy: considerations before conception and during pregnancy. *Pituitary.* 2020;23(1):65-69. PMID: 31792668

90
ANSWER: E) Continue testosterone treatment and measure PSA in 3 months

The exact role of PSA monitoring during testosterone treatment is somewhat uncertain. While androgen-deprivation therapy is effective for established prostate cancer, there is no clear evidence that endogenous testosterone concentrations are associated with increased risk of prostate cancer, nor is there any evidence that exogenous testosterone causes de novo development of prostate cancer. However, large, long-term randomized controlled trials designed to conclusively assess prostate risks of testosterone treatment are currently lacking.

This man has true, organic hypogonadism due to testicular pathology and requires testosterone replacement for optimal health and well-being. Given that previous mumps orchitis is the likely etiology of his primary hypogonadism, determining his karyotype is not necessary. Moreover, while patients with Klinefelter syndrome may be diagnosed late in life, they rarely demonstrate spontaneous fertility and typically have very small (~5 mL), firm testes bilaterally. Age in itself is not a contraindication to testosterone replacement and should be considered in men with organic hypogonadism regardless of age. Given that the prostate gland is an androgen-sensitive organ, men with untreated organic hypogonadism tend to have lower serum PSA concentrations, and testosterone replacement has been reported to restore PSA to concentrations seen in age-matched eugonadal control patients. Indiscriminate PSA testing is not without risk. A 2005 meta-analysis reported that testosterone treatment increases the risk of having a prostate biopsy, an invasive procedure with inherent risks, by up to 1.8-fold. In some older men, prostate biopsy, triggered by a PSA increase, may lead to overdiagnosis of clinically insignificant prostate cancer. Recognizing the importance of minimizing the risks and expense of unnecessary testing, current Endocrine Society guidelines recommend discussing the benefits and risks of prostate cancer screening and monitoring men aged 55 to 69 years for whom testosterone therapy is being considered who have a life expectancy greater than 10 years. The goal is to reach a joint decision between the clinician and the patient regarding prostate evaluation. The patient in this vignette elected PSA monitoring, and he has a low baseline risk of prostate cancer (~1% risk of high-grade prostate cancer should a biopsy be performed based on the prostate risk calculator https://riskcalc.org/PCPTRC/). He has had a modest rise in PSA after 6 months of testosterone therapy, which is expected.

The Endocrine Society guidelines recommend a urologic consultation for men receiving testosterone therapy if, during the first 12 months of treatment, there is a confirmed increase (given day-to-day variability in PSA measurements) in the PSA concentration of more than 1.4 ng/mL (>1.4 μg/L) above baseline, a confirmed PSA concentration greater than 4.0 ng/mL (>4.0 μg/L), or a new prostatic abnormality detected on digital rectal examination. These recommendations are based on a systematic review that included testosterone therapy trials of both men with true (organic) hypogonadism and men with reduced testosterone concentrations due to age or chronic disease. The latter group, not being truly hypogonadal, may experience a smaller rise in PSA during treatment. An example of this can be seen in the Testosterone Trials, which recruited men without organic hypogonadism who had symptoms of androgen deficiency and a modestly reduced serum testosterone concentration less than 275 ng/dL (<9.54 nmol/L). In testosterone-treated men, PSA increases greater than 1.4 ng/dL (>1.4 μg/L) above baseline were observed in only 2.4% of participants at 3 months and in 4.7% at 12 months compared with 1.6% and 0.6%, respectively, in the placebo group.

Given that this man has a low baseline risk of significant prostate cancer and a PSA increment below the recommended cutoff for urologic assessment, referral for prostate biopsy (Answer A) or performing prostate ultrasonography (Answer D) is not indicated. Instead, the modest PSA increment represents a physiologic response to testosterone replacement. Given that this man has organic hypogonadism and, as expected, experienced marked clinical improvement with testosterone replacement, testosterone replacement should not be stopped (Answer B). His serum testosterone concentration on treatment is in the low-normal reference range and reducing the treatment dosage (Answer C) is not indicated, as this would most likely result in recurrence of some hypogonadal symptoms. Therefore, testosterone treatment should be continued, the patient should be reassured that this modest rise in PSA is expected, and PSA should be measured in 3 months (Answer E).

Educational Objective
Counsel a patient who is taking testosterone replacement therapy regarding a rise in PSA.

Reference(s)
Rastrelli G, Corona G, Vignozzi L, et al. Serum PSA as a predictor of testosterone deficiency. *J Sex Med*, 2013;10(10):2518-2528. PMID: 23859334

Calof OM, Singh AB, Lee ML, et al. Adverse events associated with testosterone replacement in middle-aged and older men: a meta-analysis of randomized, placebo-controlled trials. *J Gerontol A Biol Sci Med Sci*. 2005;60(11):1451-1457. PMID: 16339333

Bhasin S, Brito JP, Cunningham GR, et al. Testosterone therapy in men with hypogonadism: an Endocrine Society clinical practice guideline. *J Clin Endocrinol Metab*. 2018;103(5):1715-1744. PMID: 29562364

Cunningham GR, Ellenberg SS, Bhasin S, et al. Prostate-specific antigen levels during testosterone treatment of hypogonadal older men: data from a controlled trial. *J Clin Endocrinol Metab*. 2019;104(12):6238-6246. PMID: 31504596

91 ANSWER: E) Ezetimibe

When deciding whether a patient is a candidate for a cholesterol-lowering medication, it is important to remember the 4 benefit groups described in the 2018 American Heart Association/American College of Cardiology guideline on the management of blood cholesterol: (1) patients with clinical atherosclerotic cardiovascular disease, (2) patients with familial hypercholesterolemia, (3) adults with type 1 diabetes or type 2 diabetes between the ages of 40 to 75 years, and (4) adults aged 40 to 75 years without diabetes and an LDL-cholesterol concentration ≥70 mg/dL (≥1.81 mmol/L) to <190 mg/dL (<4.92 mmol/L) depending on their 10-year risk of atherosclerotic cardiovascular disease. The fourth benefit group is further divided in 4 subgroups based on the individual 10-year risk of atherosclerotic cardiovascular disease: (1) low risk <5%, (2) borderline risk 5%-7.5%, (3) intermediate risk 7.5%-20%, and (4) high risk >20%. The 10-year risk of atherosclerotic cardiovascular disease of the patient in this vignette is 16%, which puts her at intermediate risk for an event. When an individual is in this risk group, the clinician should look for risk enhancers. If present, the physician and patient should discuss the benefits and risks of starting a moderate-intensity statin with a goal LDL-cholesterol reduction of 30% to 50% or an LDL-cholesterol concentration less than 100 mg/dL (<2.59 mmol/L). This patient's risk enhancers include rheumatoid arthritis, a family history of premature heart disease, a triglyceride concentration greater than 175 mg/dL (>1.98 mmol/L), and cigarette smoking status.

Statins are first-line therapy for this type of patient. Appropriately, her primary care physician tried 3 different statins (lovastatin, simvastatin, and atorvastatin). However, the patient stopped them due to adverse effects. It is important to counsel the patient that the initial recommendation is to continue trying different statins (both lipophilic and hydrophilic), as she may be able to tolerate one of them. The only way to know whether she would tolerate the medication is to try it. The next statin she tried was rosuvastatin, which still caused myalgias even when used at different dosages and administration frequencies (the patient tried taking it 3 times a week). The next medication prescribed was pravastatin, 40 mg daily, which she is tolerating without adverse effects. One may wonder whether the next step should be to increase the pravastatin dosage to 80 mg daily before adding a second agent. However, doubling the statin dosage adds only 6% further LDL-cholesterol reduction and taking higher statin dosages increases the risk of an adverse reaction. This patient needs an additional 24% LDL-cholesterol reduction to achieve her goal LDL-cholesterol concentration.

The best option now is to add ezetimibe (Answer E). Ezetimibe is a cholesterol absorption inhibitor. It works by inhibiting the Niemann-Pick C1-like 1 protein. The recommended dosage of ezetimibe is 10 mg daily. When used as monotherapy, it lowers LDL cholesterol by about 18%; however, when added to a statin, it can lower LDL cholesterol by an additional 25%.

Evolocumab (Answer A) is a fully human monoclonal antibody against PCSK9. Blocking PCSK9 increases the recycling of LDL-cholesterol receptors, which leads to LDL-cholesterol lowering. In the United States, this agent is approved to be used in addition to diet and maximally tolerated statin therapy in adults with heterozygous familial hypercholesterolemia or with clinical atherosclerotic cardiovascular disease who require additional lowering of LDL cholesterol. This patient does not meet either indication for this medication. Evolocumab can be administered subcutaneously every 2 weeks (140 mg per dose) or every 4 weeks (420 mg per dose). In patients without familial hypercholesterolemia, it can lower LDL cholesterol by 40% to 60% and in patients with familial hypercholesterolemia, its LDL-cholesterol–lowering effect is influenced by the nature of the gene pathogenic variant and ranges from 0% to 60%. Cost is one limitation of prescribing this medication.

Bempedoic acid (Answer B) inhibits ATP citrate lyase, which is one enzyme involved in the cholesterol synthesis pathway. The prodrug must be activated to its active form by acyl-CoA synthetase-1, an enzyme present in the liver but absent in most peripheral tissues. The approved dosage of bempedoic acid is 180 mg daily, and as monotherapy it decreases LDL cholesterol by 13%. The approved indications for this medication in the United States are like those of evolocumab; therefore, it would not be an option for this patient.

Colestipol (Answer C) is a bile acid sequestrant. Its dosage ranges from 2 to 16 g daily. As monotherapy, it can lower LDL cholesterol in a dose-dependent manner by 16% to 27%. One of its adverse effects is increased triglycerides; therefore, it is not recommended when a patient's triglycerides are higher than 300 mg/dL (>3.39 mmol/L), as in this patient. If her triglycerides were normal, adding colestipol would be a reasonable option.

The mechanism by which icosapent ethyl (Answer D) lowers triglycerides and cardiovascular disease risk is not known. The recommended dosage is 2 g twice daily. This medication is approved for triglyceride lowering in patients with severe hypertriglyceridemia and for cardiovascular risk reduction in the setting of mild hypertriglyceridemia in patients who are taking maximally tolerated statin therapy with a triglyceride concentration of 150 mg/dL or higher (≥1.70 mmol/L) and either established cardiovascular disease or type 2 diabetes mellitus with 2 or more risk factors for cardiovascular disease. This patient does not have an indication for this medication. In addition, high-dosage icosapent ethyl could increase this patient's LDL cholesterol by 3%.

Educational Objective
Prescribe a second-line agent for patients with intermediate risk for atherosclerotic cardiovascular disease when their LDL-cholesterol level is not at goal.

Reference(s)
Grundy SM, Stone NJ, Bailey AL, et al. 2018 AHA/ACC/AACVPR/AAPA/ABC/ACPM/ADA/AGS/APhA/ASPC/NLA/PCNA guideline on the management of blood cholesterol: a report of the American College of Cardiology/American Heart Association Task Force on Clinical Practice Guidelines. *Circulation.* 2019;73(24):3168-3209. PMID: 30423391

Pinkosky SL, Newton RS, Day EA, et al. Liver-specific ATP-citrate lyase inhibition by bempedoic acid decreases LDL-C and attenuates atherosclerosis. *Nat Commun.* 2016;7:13457. PMID: 27892461

Vascepa. Package insert. Amarin Pharma, Inc; 2019.

92 ANSWER: D) Proceed with surgery during the second trimester of pregnancy

The most appropriate next step in the management of this pregnant woman with papillary thyroid carcinoma (PTC) with cervical lymph node metastasis is to proceed with surgery in the second trimester of pregnancy (Answer D). There is evidence to suggest that surgery in the second trimester can be safely performed and most likely poses no elevated risk to the fetus. The preferred timing of surgery during pregnancy is after organogenesis is complete but before viability. However, deferring surgery for well-differentiated thyroid cancer until after delivery (for up to 1 year after diagnosis) has been shown not to negatively affect disease-specific survival or recurrence risk. The guidance offered on this subject by the 2015 American Thyroid Association guidelines for the management of thyroid nodules and cancer is that PTC discovered early in pregnancy should be monitored with neck ultrasonography. If significant growth occurs before 24 weeks or if lymph node metastasis is detected, surgery should be considered in the second trimester.

Proceeding with surgery now (Answer C) in the first trimester of pregnancy is not recommended given the potential teratogenic risk to the fetus and increased risk of early fetal loss with any surgery in early pregnancy. Elective surgery in the third trimester should also be avoided due to a possibly higher likelihood of preterm labor.

Proceeding with surgery and radioactive iodine (^{131}I) therapy 4 weeks after delivery (Answer E) is contraindicated given the patient's desire to breastfeed her infant. Active iodide transport occurs in the lactating mammary gland and is secreted into milk. Iodine 131 will thus concentrate in the lactating breast and can be transferred to the infant. Cessation of lactation should occur at least 1 to 2 months before ^{131}I treatment to avoid excess breast exposure.

Ordering neck and chest MRI (Answer A) is not indicated as a preoperative study in this patient with PTC and nonbulky locoregional lymph node disease. Cross-sectional neck imaging with intravenous contrast, either with MRI or CT (the latter only in nonpregnant patients), is only recommended according to the 2015 American Thyroid Association guidelines as an adjunct to neck ultrasonography for patients in whom there is clinical suspicion for locally advanced disease.

Prescribing levothyroxine (Answer B) is not the most appropriate next step in this patient's management. Although subclinical hyperthyroidism does not appear to pose a risk during pregnancy, there are no studies examining the optimal degree of TSH suppression in women with thyroid cancer diagnosed during pregnancy. When the serum TSH concentration is above 2.0 mIU/L, initiation of levothyroxine to maintain TSH between 0.3 and 1.0 mIU/L can be considered as long as pregnancy-adjusted free T_4 or total T_4 remains normal. The serum TSH in this patient is below the nonpregnant reference range, although the current value is within normal limits for the first trimester of pregnancy, during which the lower limit of the reference range can decrease as much as 0.4 mIU/L. Decreased TSH values in early pregnancy result from the stimulatory effect of high concentrations of hCG on the TSH receptor. Prescribing levothyroxine to lower the serum TSH further in this patient is unnecessary and could precipitate overt hyperthyroidism, which is associated with adverse pregnancy outcomes for both the mother and fetus.

Educational Objective
Manage papillary thyroid cancer diagnosed during pregnancy.

Reference(s)
Boucek J, de Haan J, Halaska MJ, et al; International Network on Cancer, Infertility, and Pregnancy. Maternal and obstetrical outcome in 35 cases of well-differentiated thyroid carcinoma during pregnancy. *Laryngoscope.* 2018;128(6):1493-1500. PMID: 28988434

Haugen BR, Alexander EK, Bible KC, et al. 2015 American Thyroid Association management guidelines for adult patients with thyroid nodules and differentiated thyroid cancer: the American Thyroid Association Guidelines Task Force on Thyroid Nodules and Differentiated Thyroid Cancer. *Thyroid.* 2016;26(1):1-133. PMID: 26462967

Papaleontiou M, Haymart MR. Thyroid nodules and cancer during pregnancy, post-partum and preconception planning: addressing the uncertainties and challenges. *Best Pract Res Clin Endocrinol Metab.* 2020;34(4):101363. PMID: 31786102

Uruno T, Shibuya H, Kitagawa W, Nagahama M, Sugino K, Ito K. Optimal timing of surgery for differentiated thyroid cancer in pregnant women. *World J Surg.* 2014;38(3):704-708. PMID: 24248429

93 ANSWER: B) Continue pump use, but start a temporary basal rate at 75% of the usual rate the morning of the procedure

Hyperglycemia in the perioperative period has been associated with adverse outcomes, including increased rate of infection. There are limited data on improved outcomes with better glycemic control. No standardized protocols exist to guide adjustment of diabetes medications preoperatively. Hospitals may have local protocols or leave the adjustment to the discretion of individual practitioners.

When determining the need for insulin adjustment preoperatively, certain patient characteristics can be useful. The type of diabetes, a history of hypoglycemia in the fasting state, type and duration of the procedure, and ability to self-regulate insulin dosing are all important features to consider.

Patients with type 1 diabetes can be given usual doses of basal insulin preoperatively unless there is evidence of nocturnal/fasting hypoglycemia, as there was in this patient. Because he did have occasional nocturnal hypoglycemia, lowering the basal dose (by 25%) is reasonable. Thus, continuing the current regimen without decreasing the rate (Answer A) is incorrect. In patients with type 2 diabetes, the basal dose is lowered by 25% more routinely. If a patient is on NPH or mixed insulin, the dose might be 50% of the intermediate-acting component on the morning of the procedure. Since the procedure is elective, of short duration (<2 hours), and the patient is most likely to be discharged home the same day, continued use of the pump for insulin delivery at 75% of the usual rate the morning of the procedure (Answer B) is the most appropriate approach. The patient should be advised to discuss the strategy with the anesthesiologist. If the procedure is longer than expected, plans should switch to fingerstick blood glucose checks and subcutaneous insulin therapy with appropriate overlap before the pump is removed.

Discontinuation of the pump and use of an insulin drip (Answer D) is unnecessary for such a short procedure. Discontinuation of the pump and initiating subcutaneous basal insulin (Answers C and E) would be an alternative approach. However, this strategy would require more patient education regarding the timing of the basal dose, when to restart the pump, and use of subcutaneous correction insulin until the pump is restarted. In addition, a dose of 20 units of insulin glargine (Answer E) is too high since the patient has been experiencing hypoglycemia.

Educational Objective
Guide the approach to glycemic control for patients with type 1 diabetes mellitus in the perioperative period.

Reference(s)
Simha V, Shah P. Perioperative glucose control in patients with diabetes undergoing elective surgery. *JAMA*. 2019;321(4):399-400. PMID: 30615031

Duggan EW, Carlson K, Umpierrez GE. Perioperative hyperglycemia management: an update. *Anesthesiology*. 2017;126(3):547-560. PMID: 28121636

94 ANSWER: A) Initiate liraglutide

The patient in this vignette presents with nonspecific symptoms, predominantly fatigue and low mood. His serum testosterone is modestly reduced and there is no evidence of organic hypogonadism. There is no clinical evidence of a pituitary mass, and thyroid function and prolactin are normal. In the absence of clinical suspicion, Endocrine Society guidelines recommend consideration of pituitary imaging (Answer D) only if the serum testosterone concentration is repeatedly less than 150 ng/dL (<5.2 nmol/L). There is no clinical suspicion of estradiol excess and therefore no indication to measure serum estradiol (Answer E). Of note, the low-normal SHBG seen in this man is typical because low SHBG is strongly associated with (central) adiposity and insulin resistance in men.

In a recent meta-analysis of randomized controlled trials including older symptomatic men with modest age-related reductions in serum testosterone, testosterone treatment had no effect on energy or mood. Therefore, testosterone treatment would not be expected to improve this man's presenting symptoms. Furthermore, in most placebo-controlled randomized controlled trials, testosterone treatment has generally not been shown to improve diabetes control or to reduce body weight. Due to the lack of adequately designed and powered clinical trials, the long-term cardiovascular effects of testosterone treatment are not known. Of note, testosterone is FDA-approved only for men with organic hypogonadism due to medical disease of the pituitary or testicles, not for age-related reductions in testosterone as in this vignette. Moreover, this patient has a high cardiovascular risk, and the effects of testosterone treatment on major adverse cardiovascular events (MACE) remain unknown due to the lack of adequately designed and powered testosterone treatment trials. A large study to evaluate the effect of testosterone therapy on the incidence of MACE and efficacy measures in hypogonadal men (TRAVERSE), with a recruitment target of 6000 participants, is currently ongoing (estimated completion date in mid-2022). For all these reasons, testosterone treatment (Answer B) would not be the first option. This issue is somewhat controversial because high-level evidence is lacking, and some practitioners would offer a pragmatic trial of testosterone treatment to determine whether this improves his clinical symptoms.

While selective estrogen receptor modulators lead (via antagonizing estradiol-mediated negative hypothalamic-pituitary feedback) to an increase in LH and consequently serum testosterone, there are no studies reporting clinically meaningful health benefits of selective estrogen receptor modulators in older men, and long-term risks are unknown. Therefore, a selective estrogen receptor modulator (Answer C) is not indicated. To increase serum testosterone, selective estrogen receptor modulators require the presence of a principally intact hypothalamic-pituitary-testicular axis. Thus, these agents increase serum testosterone only in men with functional hypothalamic-pituitary axis suppression (eg, due to obesity, ill health), but not in men with organic hypogonadism due to structural hypothalamic or pituitary disease.

The most appropriate next step in this patient's management is to initiate liraglutide (Answer A), a long-acting GLP-1 receptor agonist. In large randomized controlled trials including men with diabetes, liraglutide has, in contrast to testosterone treatment, consistently been associated with improved hemoglobin A_{1c}, weight loss, and improved cardiovascular outcomes.

Interestingly, in an open-label trial of middle-aged men with low testosterone due to obesity that compared liraglutide with testosterone treatment, men assigned to liraglutide lost more body weight than men assigned to testosterone treatment: 17.4 vs 2.0 lb (7.9 vs 0.9 kg). Men taking liraglutide were also more likely to derive a metabolic benefit, while both groups had similar improvements in sexual function. In the liraglutide group, both LH and testosterone increased. Although the findings in this open-label study must be confirmed by a blinded randomized controlled trial, they are consistent with multiple studies reporting that in men with obesity, weight loss can reverse the obesity-associated functional suppression of the male gonadal axis.

Educational Objective
Select the most appropriate medical therapy for an older man with obesity and modestly low testosterone.

Reference(s)

Ponce OJ, Spencer-Bonilla G, Alvarez-Villalobos N, et al. The efficacy and adverse events of testosterone replacement therapy in hypogonadal men: a systematic review and meta-analysis of randomized, placebo-controlled trials. *J Clin Endocrinol Metab*. 2018 [Epub ahead of print] PMID: 29562341

Jensterle M, Podbregar A, Goricar K, Gregoric N, Janez A. Effects of liraglutide on obesity-associated functional hypogonadism in men. *Endor Connect*. 2019;8(3):195-202. PMID: 30707677

Grossmann M, Matsumoto AM. A Perspective on middle-aged and older men with functional hypogonadism: focus on holistic management. *J Clin Endocrinol Metab*. 2017;102(3):1067-1075. PMID: 28359097

95 ANSWER: E) Denosumab

Androgen-deprivation therapy (ADT) is the main therapeutic approach for men with metastatic prostate cancer. ADT increases bone turnover and decreases bone mineral density, resulting in an increased fracture risk in men with prostate cancer. In fact, osteoporotic fractures occur in up to 20% of men within 5 years of starting ADT. FRAX estimates the 10-year probability of fracture for untreated patients between ages 40 and 90 years, using femoral neck bone mineral density and clinical risk factors (including glucocorticoid exposure for more than 3 months at a prednisone dosage of 5 or more mg daily, or equivalent dosages of other glucocorticoids). However, FRAX does not account for the use of ADT, and while men receiving ADT should be considered as having secondary osteoporosis in the FRAX assessment tool, this does not confer additional risk when bone mineral density is included in the calculation.

The guidelines from the American Society of Clinical Oncology recommend starting osteoporosis therapy in patients beginning ADT who are at increased fracture risk. Consistent with guidelines from the American Society of Clinical Oncology and Cancer Care Ontario, the addition of an osteoclast inhibitor may be offered to reduce fracture risk in the setting of osteoporosis (T-scores of −2.5 or less in the femoral neck, total hip, or lumbar spine) or when the 10-year probability of hip fracture is 3% or higher or the 10-year probability of a major osteoporosis-related fracture is 20% or higher. However, the American Society of Clinical Oncology guidelines also state that the short-term bone loss associated with ADT can be rapid, and because of this, clinicians should consider treatment at a higher T-score than is recommended using FRAX or similar tools. Similarly, the European Society of Medical Oncology 2020 guidelines recommend starting therapy if the lowest T-score is less than −2.0 with no other risk factors, or if any 2 of the following risk factors are present: T-score less than −1.5, age older than 65 years, cigarette smoking, BMI less than 24 kg/m^2, family history of hip fracture, personal history of fragility fracture at an age older than 50 years, and oral glucocorticoid use for more than 6 months.

In this patient who smokes cigarettes and has low bone mineral density with a hip fracture risk of 2.8% (already near the threshold of treatment), initiating ADT is expected to put him at an even higher risk of fracture, so offering no additional therapy (Answer A) is incorrect.

When an osteoclast inhibitor is indicated for men with nonmetastatic prostate cancer who are receiving ADT, denosumab (Answer E) is the preferred agent. Guidelines from American Society of Clinical Oncology and Cancer Care Ontario, among others, recommend that men who require drug therapy to prevent bone loss and fractures receive denosumab at the dosage and schedule recommended for the treatment of osteoporosis (60 mg subcutaneously every 6 months). Unlike bisphosphonates such as alendronate (Answer B) or zoledronic acid (Answer C), denosumab is FDA-approved for this specific indication and has been shown to reduce fractures in this population, while bisphosphonates only improve bone mineral density (the bisphosphonate trials were not sufficiently powered to detect reduction in fractures). In addition, this patient has chronic kidney disease with an estimated glomerular filtration rate of 35 mL/min per 1.73 m^2. In contrast to bisphosphonates, which are renally excreted and not recommended for use in those with creatinine clearance below 30 to 35 mL/min per 1.73 m^2, denosumab is not excreted by the kidneys and can be used in patients with reduced kidney function without a dosage change. Even though bisphosphonates are not approved specifically for prevention of bone loss and fractures in men receiving ADT, these may be a reasonable (albeit off-label) alternative in cases where denosumab is not available if kidney function allows. It is important to note that the FDA warning not to use bisphosphonates in patients with an estimated glomerular filtration rate less than 30 or 35 mL/min per 1.73 m^2 is based on lack of data in this population. In fact, post hoc analyses have shown that oral bisphosphonates effectively reduce fracture risk without any negative effect on kidney function in patients with an estimated glomerular filtration rate as low as 15 mL/min per 1.73 m^2. Since approximately 50% of administered bisphosphonate is excreted unchanged by the kidneys, the oral dosage in patients who have a lower estimated glomerular filtration rate should be reduced (off-label use). It is also important to remember that denosumab may induce significant hypocalcemia in patients with renal impairment, and patients should be adequately supplemented with calcium and vitamin D while taking denosumab. Furthermore, if denosumab treatment is to be discontinued, administering an alternative therapy (typically a bisphosphonate) is recommended to prevent rapid bone loss and increased risk of vertebral fractures.

Teriparatide (Answer D), an osteoanabolic agent, would not be a good option for this patient given the theoretical concern for promoting the growth of occult, disseminated cancer cells within bone. This patient also has a mildly elevated alkaline phosphatase level, and contraindications to the use of teriparatide include history of skeletal irradiation, Paget disease of bone, or unexplained elevation in alkaline phosphatase due to potential risk of osteosarcoma.

Educational Objective
Recommend appropriate therapy in a patient with low bone density and prostate cancer who is on androgen-deprivation therapy.

Reference(s)
Bienz M, Saad F. Androgen-deprivation therapy and bone loss in prostate cancer patients: a clinical review. *Bonekey Rep.* 2015;4:716. PMID: 26131363

Shahinian VB, Kuo Y-F, Freeman JL, Goodwin JS. Risk of fracture after androgen deprivation for prostate cancer. *N Engl J Med.* 2005;352(2):154-164. PMID: 15647578

Coleman R, Hadji P, Body JJ, Aapro M, Herrstedt J; ESMO Guidelines Working Group. Bone health in cancer patients: ESMO clinical practice guidelines. *Ann Oncol.* 2014;25(Suppl 3):iii124-137. PMID: 24782453

Alibhai SMH, Zukotynski K, Walker-Dilks C, et al; Cancer Care Ontario Genitourinary Cancer Disease Site Group. *Clin Oncol (R Coll Radiol).* 2017;29(6):348-355. PMID: 28169118

Saylor PJ, Rumble RB, Tagawa S, et al. Bone health and bone-targeted therapies for prostate cancer: ASCO endorsement of a Cancer Care Ontario guideline. *J Clin Oncol.* 2020;38(15):1736-1743. PMID: 31990618

96

ANSWER: B) Recommend no treatment now; measure TSH in 12 months

Hashimoto thyroiditis (chronic autoimmune hypothyroidism) is the most common cause of hypothyroidism in iodine-sufficient areas. It is more common in women, especially older women. The thyroid gland of patients with Hashimoto thyroiditis can be enlarged (goiter) or atrophic. TPO is a key enzyme in thyroid hormone synthesis and is a major autoantigen in autoimmune thyroid disorders. Patients with Hashimoto thyroiditis have positive serum TPO antibodies. Titers of TPO antibodies correlate with the degree of lymphocytic infiltration in euthyroid patients, and they are frequently present in euthyroid patients with a prevalence of 12% to 26%. However, TPO antibodies are not routinely measured in patients with overt hypothyroidism. They are mostly measured in patients with goiter to identify the etiology and in patients with subclinical hypothyroidism and thyroiditis (painless or postpartum) to predict the likelihood of progression to overt hypothyroidism. The common pathologic feature of Hashimoto thyroiditis is lymphocytic infiltration and follicular destruction.

The usual course of Hashimoto thyroiditis is gradual loss of thyroid function. In the Wickham cohort study with 20-year follow-up, an elevated serum TSH level was predictive of progression to overt hypothyroidism. In addition, female sex, older age, and presence of TPO antibodies were associated with an increased risk of progression to overt hypothyroidism. The annual rate of progression to overt hypothyroidism was 4.3% in women with elevated TSH and TPO antibodies, 3% in women with only elevated serum TSH, and 2% in women with only elevated TPO antibodies titers. A prospective study in the United Kingdom has shown that in 5.5% of patients with subclinical hypothyroidism (elevated TSH with normal free T_4), TSH returns to the normal range after 1 year without treatment. Furthermore, in the same group, 76.7% continued to have elevated TSH and 17.8% developed low free T_4 requiring levothyroxine therapy.

This patient has a normal TSH level, elevated TPO antibodies, and family history of autoimmune disorder, but her symptoms are not specific and cannot be attributed to thyroid disease. Her annual risk of developing overt hypothyroidism is around 2%. Therefore, the best option is to repeat TSH measurement in 12 months (Answer B). If her TSH remains normal in 12 months, her TSH level should continue to be monitored over time. There is no reason to do follow-up TPO antibodies titers (Answer D) to decide whether thyroid hormone replacement therapy should be initiated.

As her TSH concentration is within the normal range and her symptoms cannot be attributed to thyroid disease, there is no indication to start levothyroxine (Answer A) or desiccated thyroid (Answer C). At this time, there is no indication to perform thyroid ultrasonography (Answer E), as this patient has only mild enlargement of her thyroid gland without palpable thyroid nodules on physical examination.

Educational Objective
Explain the effect of TPO antibodies and TSH concentration in developing overt hypothyroidism.

Reference(s)
Vanderpump MP, Tunbridge WM, French JM, et al. The incidence of thyroid disorders in the community: a twenty-year follow-up of the Whickham Survey. *Clin Endocrinol (Oxf)*. 1995;43(1):55-68. PMID: 7641412

Tunbridge WM, Evered DC, Hall R, et al. The spectrum of thyroid disease in a community: the Whickham survey. *Clin Endocrinol (Oxf)*. 1977;7(6):481-493. PMID: 598014

Prummel MF, Wiersinga WM. Thyroid peroxidase autoantibodies in euthyroid subjects. *Best Pract Res Clin Endocrinol Metab*. 2005;19(1):1-15. PMID: 15826919

Parle JV, Franklyn JA, Cross KW, Jones SC, Sheppard MC. Prevalence and follow-up of abnormal thyrotrophin (TSH) concentrations in the elderly in the United Kingdom. *Clin Endocrinol (Oxf)*. 1991;34(1)77-83. PMID: 2004476

97

ANSWER: A) Dapagliflozin

The best answer is dapagliflozin (Answer A), an SGLT-2 inhibitor that is approved to reduce the risk of cardiovascular death and hospitalization for heart failure in adults with heart failure (NYHA class II-IV) with reduced ejection fraction (HFrEF), regardless of the presence or absence of diabetes mellitus. The DAPA-HF trial (Dapagliflozin in Patients with Heart Failure and Reduced Ejection Fraction) found that among patients with HFrEF (left ventricular ejection fraction ≤40%), the risk of worsening heart failure or death of cardiovascular causes was lower among those who received dapagliflozin than among those who received placebo. In addition, the DAPA-CKD trial (Dapagliflozin in Patients with Chronic Kidney Disease) found that among patients with chronic kidney disease, the risk of the composite outcome of a sustained decline in the estimated glomerular filtration rate of at least 50%, end-stage kidney disease, or death due to renal or cardiovascular causes was lower in those who received dapagliflozin than in those who received placebo. This medication may also further lower this patient's hemoglobin A_{1c} level, which is presently greater than 7.0% (>53 mmol/mol). Given his history of HFrEF, history of diabetes, reduced glomerular filtration rate, and current hemoglobin A_{1c} level, the best option is dapagliflozin. Even if this patient's hemoglobin A_{1c} level were less than 7.0% (<53 mmol/mol) or if he did not have diabetes, dapagliflozin therapy would still be indicated because of HFrEF and chronic kidney disease.

Blockade of aldosterone receptors by spironolactone, in addition to standard therapy, has been demonstrated to substantially reduce the risk of both morbidity and death among patients with severe heart failure. The addition of eplerenone (Answer C) to optimal medical therapy has been shown to reduce morbidity and mortality among patients with acute myocardial infarction complicated by left ventricular dysfunction and heart failure. However, these medications commonly cause hyperkalemia. Given that this patient's potassium concentration is already slightly elevated, eplerenone would not be the best choice.

The multicenter, double-blind, placebo-controlled REDUCE-IT trial (Reduction of Cardiovascular Events with Icosapent Ethyl-Intervention Trial) enrolled 8179 patients (median age at baseline, 64 years; 71% men) who had fasting triglyceride concentrations of 135 to 499 mg/dL (1.53-5.64 mmol/L) and LDL-cholesterol concentrations ranging from 41 to 100 mg/dL (1.06-2.59 mmol/L) despite statin therapy and who had established cardiovascular disease (70%) or diabetes mellitus plus other high-risk factors (30%). The primary results demonstrated a 25% reduction in the primary endpoint of death due to cardiovascular disease, nonfatal myocardial infarction, nonfatal stroke, coronary revascularization, or unstable angina with icosapent ethyl (Answer D) vs placebo ($P < .001$). Within the REDUCE-IT cohort, 58% of participants had type 2 diabetes, with 91% prescribed at least 1 diabetes medication and 49.5% prescribed at least 2 diabetes medications. Participants with diabetes had a 1.5-fold higher rate of the primary endpoint vs the rate in the placebo group. Participants assigned icosapent ethyl experienced a 7% absolute risk reduction for a first cardiovascular event and a 12.7% absolute risk reduction for total events compared with those assigned placebo ($P < .001$ for both). Adding icosapent ethyl is incorrect because this patient does not have hypertriglyceridemia. Patients included in the REDUCE-IT trial had a triglyceride concentration greater than 135 mg/dL (>1.53 mmol/L). It is unclear whether icosapent ethyl is associated with reduction of cardiovascular disease risk in patients with triglyceride levels less than 135 mg/dL (<1.53 mmol/L).

Some GLP-1 receptor agonists have been reported to reduce cardiovascular disease risk. However, exenatide LAR (Answer E) is not one of them. Liraglutide, albiglutide, dulaglutide, and semaglutide have all been found to reduce cardiovascular risk in cardiovascular outcomes trials, whereas lixisenatide and exenatide LAR have not. In addition, to date, GLP-1 receptor agonist therapy has not been shown to reduce the risk of hospitalization for heart failure or to protect kidney function. Although some preliminary data suggest that GLP-1 receptor agonists may also confer renal protection, these studies were not powered appropriately to address this issue. A currently ongoing study is trying to answer this question (Effect of Semaglutide Versus Placebo on the Progression of Renal Impairment in Subjects With Type 2 Diabetes and Chronic Kidney Disease [FLOW]) and is estimated to be completed in August 2024.

Alogliptin (Answer B) would not reduce cardiovascular disease risk in this patient. In fact, it might increase the risk for hospitalization due to heart failure. The same concern exists for saxagliptin. Sitagliptin and linagliptin do not have this concern, as no data have linked either of these agents with an increased risk for hospitalization due to heart failure.

Educational Objective
Recommend the most appropriate class of type 2 diabetes medication to intensify therapy in patients with heart failure and reduced ejection fraction.

Reference(s)

McMurray JJV, Solomon SD, Inzucchi SE, et al. Dapagliflozin in patients with heart failure and reduced ejection fraction. *N Engl J Med*. 2019;381(21):1995-2008. PMID: 31535829

Holman RR, Bethel MA, Mentz RJ, et al; EXSCEL Study Group. Effects of once-weekly exenatide on cardiovascular outcomes in type 2 diabetes. *N Engl J Med*. 2017;377(13):1228-1239. PMID: 28910237

Heerspink HJL, Stefánsson BV, Correa-Rotter R, et al; DAPA-CKD Trial Committees and Investigators. Dapagliflozin in patients with chronic kidney disease. *N Engl J Med*. 2020;383(15):1436-1446. PMID: 32970396

Pitt B, Zannad, F, Remme WJ, et al. The effect of spironolactone on morbidity and mortality in patients with severe heart Failure. Randomized Aldactone Evaluation Study Investigators. *N Engl J Med.* 1999:341(10):709-717. PMID: 10471456

Pitt B, Remme W, Zannad F, et al. Eplerenone, a selective aldosterone blocker, in patients with left ventricular dysfunction after myocardial infarction. *N Engl J Med.* 2003;348(14):1309-1321. PMID: 12668699

Scirica BM, Braunwald E, Raz I, et al. Heart failure, saxagliptin, and diabetes mellitus: observations from the SAVOR-TIMI 53 randomized trial. *Circulation.* 2014;130(18):1579-1588. PMID: 25189213

Zannad F, Cannon CP, Cushman WC et al. Heart failure and mortality outcomes in patients with type 2 diabetes taking alogliptin versus placebo in EXAMINE: a multicentre, randomised, double-blind trial. *Lancet.* 2015 May 23;385(9982):2067-76. PMID: 25765696

US Food and Drug Administration. FDA Drug Safety Communication: FDA adds warnings about heart failure risk to labels of type 2 diabetes medicines containing saxagliptin and alogliptin. Available at: https://www.fda.gov/drugs/drug-safety-and-availability/fda-drug-safety-communication-fda-adds-warnings-about-heart-failure-risk-labels-type-2-diabetes. Accessed September 2020

Bhatt DL, Steg PG, Miller M, et al; REDUCE-IT Investigators. Cardiovascular risk reduction with icosapent ethyl for hypertriglyceridemia. *N Engl J Med.* 2019;380(1):11-22. PMID: 30415628

Bhatt DL, Brinton EA, Miller M. Substantial cardiovascular benefit from icosapent ethyl in patients with diabetes: REDUCE-IT DIABETES. Presented at: 80th American Diabetes Association Scientific Sessions; June 12-16, 2020.

98 ANSWER: D) Luteoma of pregnancy

Although this patient described possible mild hirsutism and acne in adolescence, more severe hirsutism, terminal hair growth, cystic acne in an androgenic pattern on the face, virilization, and deepening of the voice began during pregnancy. Total testosterone concentrations rise during normal pregnancies, but they typically range from 50 to 120 ng/dL (1.7-4.2 nmol/L), not the very high concentrations seen in this case. In addition, normal gestational hyperandrogenism is not typically associated with virilization. Since there is also a rise in SHBG during pregnancy, free testosterone concentrations are not significantly increased until the third trimester. Most women are also asymptomatic or have mild symptoms because the placental aromatase converts androgens to estrogens. A female fetus is also protected from virilization by placental aromatase. The maternal ovary is the main source of increased androgens in pregnancy, although the maternal and fetal adrenal glands might also contribute.

In this case, significantly elevated total testosterone that normalizes after pregnancy suggests 1 of 2 benign causes of gestational virilization: luteomas or theca lutein cysts. Based on the description of a large unilateral ovarian complex cystic mass, the diagnosis is most likely a luteoma (Answer D). Luteomas are not tumors but represent hyperplastic masses of large luteinized stromal cells that spontaneously resolve within a few weeks after delivery. However, they have been reported to be persistent although significantly smaller in size after 14 months of serial ultrasonography. They are more likely to be unilateral with a complex cystic appearance due to areas of hemorrhage and necrosis, with sizes reported to be anywhere from 6 to 10 cm on average and total testosterone concentrations from 2000 to 10,000 ng/dL (69.4-347.0 nmol/L). Theca lutein cysts are the other more common cause of gestational virilization; they are often bilateral and develop in the third trimester.

If she had been evaluated during pregnancy, the evaluation would have included characterizing the source to rule out a malignant tumor, as well as determining the risk for virilization of a female fetus. The onset of maternal hyperandrogenism before the 12th week of gestation could result in virilization/labial fusion and clitoromegaly of a female fetus, so testing to determine fetal sex would have been pursued. After the 12th week, clitoromegaly would still be possible. If the ovarian mass suggested the presence of a possible tumor, was a solid mass, or was associated with symptomatic mass effect or risk for torsion, further evaluation, and possibly surgery to remove the mass, would have been pursued. Since she presented postpartum and her testosterone normalized, she can be followed with serial ultrasonography of the mass to confirm resolution.

During her evaluation by reproductive endocrinology, she was told she had polycystic ovarian morphology. This does not confirm a diagnosis of polycystic ovary syndrome. It is not clear whether she met 2 of the 3 Rotterdam criteria:

(1) Evidence of androgen excess before pregnancy (clinical examination findings of moderate hirsutism [Ferriman-Gallwey score ≥8], androgenetic acne or alopecia, or biochemical results of elevated androgens above the reference range)
(2) Oligoanovulatory cycles (this patient has regular menses, so there is no evidence for anovulatory cycles, and no additional testing is mentioned as part of her assisted reproduction evaluation)

(3) Polycystic ovarian morphology (it would be important to review the ultrasound results to confirm they meet current 2018 International American Society for Reproductive Medicine/European Society for Human Reproduction and Embryology guidelines for improved transducer frequency ≥8MHz, ≥20 follicles for age >20 years [prior Rotterdam criteria used less stringent criteria of ≥12 follicles <1 cm])

Based on the data provided, it is not possible to confirm the diagnosis of polycystic ovary syndrome (Answer A). In addition, women with polycystic ovary syndrome are not at greater risk for developing virilization during pregnancy, so one cannot assume this was the cause of her worsening hirsutism and virilization during pregnancy, especially given the very high total testosterone concentrations at the time of delivery.

Idiopathic hirsutism (Answer E) is a diagnosis of exclusion, when hirsutism is not caused by another hyperandrogenic endocrine disorder. The timing of severe symptoms associated with very high total testosterone concentrations that normalized after delivery is more consistent with gestational hyperandrogenism.

An alternative tumor source outside of the ovary and adrenal gland is very unlikely cause of hyperandrogenism or virilization. In a study of 369 women with total testosterone concentrations greater than 100 ng/dL (>3.47 nmol/L) measured by liquid chromatography–tandem mass spectrometry in a 10-year period, only 96 were not excluded because of exogenous testosterone use or underlying conditions such as congenital adrenal hyperplasia, androgen insensitivity syndrome, liver failure, or pregnancy. Among 28/96 women (30%) with an identified tumor, all were either an ovarian or adrenal source with most cases ovarian in origin. Therefore, an extraovarian/extraadrenal tumor (Answer C) is highly unlikely. Also, a tumoral source would not go away after pregnancy. Similarly, a theca-cell tumor (Answer B) would be unlikely to present as hyperandrogenism only in pregnancy with normalization of total testosterone after delivery.

Educational Objective
Diagnose causes of hyperandrogenism that occur during pregnancy.

Reference(s)
Legro RS, Arslanian SA, Ehrmann DA, et al; Endocrine Society. Diagnosis and treatment of polycystic ovary syndrome: an Endocrine Society Clinical Practice Guideline. *J Clin Endocrinol Metab*. 2013;98(12):4565-4592. PMID: 24151290

Teede HJ, Misso ML, Costello MF, et al; International PCOS Network. Recommendations from the international evidence-based guideline for the assessment and management of polycystic ovary syndrome. *Fertil Steril*. 2018;110(3):364-379. PMID: 30033227

Sharma A, Kapoor E, Singh RJ, Chang AY, Erickson D. Diagnostic thresholds for androgen-producing tumors or pathologic hyperandrogenism in women by using total testosterone concentrations measured by liquid-chromatography-tandem mass spectrometry. *Clin Chem*. 2018;64(11):1636-1645. PMID: 30068692

Masarie K, Katz V, Balderston K. Pregnancy luteomas: clinical presentations and management strategies. *Obstet Gyneol Surv*. 2010;65(9):575-582. PMID: 21144088

Choi JR, Levine D, Finberg H. Luteoma of pregnancy: sonographic findings in two cases. *J Ultrasound Med*. 2000;19(12):877-881. PMID: 11127014

99 ANSWER: A) Proceed with planned mastectomy

The incidence of genetic testing has exploded in parallel with the accessibility of next-generation sequencing panels. Genetic testing is most commonly used at cancer centers and often encompasses a large array of genes. As a result, many patients are found to carry pathogenic alterations that would not have otherwise been suspected based on clinical history. In this case, this patient was found to have a pathogenic *RET* variant when undergoing genetic testing for breast cancer. *RET* pathogenic variants can cause multiple endocrine neoplasia type 2; however, this patient has no personal or family history of medullary thyroid cancer, pheochromocytoma, or hyperparathyroidism, and she has normal findings on thyroid ultrasonography and a normal calcitonin level. Her plasma normetanephrine fraction is slightly elevated above the upper normal limit and this is in the context of taking venlafaxine, a norepinephrine and catecholamine reuptake inhibitor. Given the presence of the *RET* pathogenic variant, these laboratory abnormalities raise concern for a potential pheochromocytoma.

Pheochromocytomas are tumors arising from the adrenal medulla, which may secrete catecholamines that induce adrenergic symptoms and signs such as palpitations, anxiety, sweating, pallor, and elevated blood pressure and heart rate. Paragangliomas are tumors arising from the ganglia of the autonomic nervous system, and therefore they can occur in any region from the skull base to the pelvic floor. Unlike pheochromocytomas, sympathetic paragangliomas can secrete norepinephrine and dopamine but are typically unable to synthesize epinephrine.

Metanephrines are the stable and inactive metabolites of catecholamines that provide the highest sensitivity and specificity for diagnosing pheochromocytoma and paraganglioma. Metanephrine is the metabolite of epinephrine, and normetanephrine is the metabolite of norepinephrine. Thus, from a diagnostic perspective, functional pheochromocytomas may have elevated metanephrine and/or normetanephrine fractions, whereas functional paragangliomas usually only have an elevated normetanephrine fraction. Typically, pheochromocytomas and paragangliomas that induce clinical symptoms are associated with metanephrine and/or normetanephrine levels that are substantially higher than the upper limit of the reference range—usually 4 times or more (less commonly 2 or 3 times higher). Importantly, mild elevations above the upper limit of the normetanephrine reference range (<2 times) are common and are usually attributed to enhanced sympathoadrenergic tone (eg, in a state of anxiety, stress, or illness) and/or the use of catecholamine reuptake inhibitors (eg, many antidepressant medications and cocaine or methamphetamines). These mild elevations are a frequent cause of false-positive values. Mild elevations in the metanephrine fraction are a less common cause of false-positives and generally raise more concern for an epinephrine-producing pheochromocytoma.

This patient's use of venlafaxine (a norepinephrine reuptake inhibitor) should be considered a known source of false-positive results. It is not uncommon for this medication, along with others in the same drug class, to cause 2-fold elevations in normetanephrine, and very rarely 3- to 4-fold elevations. Stopping the venlafaxine and repeating testing can be done to confirm this suspicion, but this may require up to 4 to 6 weeks of cessation, which may not be safe given the indications for this patient's venlafaxine use. In this case, abdominal imaging revealing a lipid-rich adrenal adenoma (unenhanced attenuation <10 Hounsfield units), essentially excluding the possibility of a pheochromocytoma. Symptomatic pheochromocytomas are typically 1 to 2 cm or greater in size and have a lipid-poor unenhanced attenuation on CT (>10 Hounsfield units [but usually >20 Hounsfield units]), high contrast uptake on CT with intravenous contrast, and T2 hyperintensity on MRI. The collective findings in this vignette suggest that the slight normetanephrine elevations are most likely due to venlafaxine and/or sympathoadrenergic excess and exclude the possibility of a clinically relevant pheochromocytoma.

Further imaging with an MIBG scan (Answer C), a ^{68}Ga-DOTATATE PET-CT (Answer D), or abdominal MRI (Answer E) is not necessary given the lipid-rich nature of the adrenal mass. Performing an MIBG scan may in fact reveal a false-positive result due to normal physiologic adrenal medullary uptake. α-Adrenergic blockade (Answer B) is also not necessary. The patient underwent an uncomplicated mastectomy as planned (Answer A).

Educational Objective
Interpret diagnostic test results for pheochromocytoma.

Reference(s)
Lenders JWM, Duh Q-Y, Eisenhofer G, et al; Endocrine Society. Pheochromocytoma and paraganglioma: an Endocrine Society clinical practice guideline. *J Clin Endocrinol Metab.* 2014;99(6):1915-1942. PMID: 24893135

100 ANSWER: C) Discontinue depot medroxyprogesterone

This premenopausal woman presents with abnormally low bone mineral density for her age and a recent wrist fracture. In such a scenario, secondary contributors to low bone mineral density should be considered. There are numerous causes of secondary osteoporosis, including endocrine disorders, nutritional deficiencies, medications, genetic disorders (particularly of collagen metabolism), and other miscellaneous conditions (such as immobilization and HIV). Drugs that may be associated with bone loss in premenopausal women include glucocorticoids, anticonvulsants, antidepressants, and depot medroxyprogesterone. The low dosages of medroxyprogesterone acetate (DMPA) that are typically used in combination with estrogen as part of a regimen of postmenopausal hormone therapy have no effect on the ability of estrogen to prevent bone loss. In contrast, the higher dosages of DMPA that have been used to treat gynecologic disorders or that have been given for contraception have been associated with increased bone loss, presumably due to induced estrogen deficiency. The rate of bone loss with DMPA is not linear, with the greatest loss occurring during the first 2 years of use. In 2004, the US FDA added a boxed warning recommending that DMPA be used as a long-term birth control method (eg, longer than 2 years) only if other birth control methods are inadequate. Studies involving premenopausal women treated with DMPA for up to 5 years reported that the decline in bone mineral density associated with the drug was substantially reversed after discontinuation. Therefore, the best step in this scenario is to discontinue depot medroxyprogesterone (Answer C).

There are no data supporting the use of selective estrogen receptor modulators, such as raloxifene (Answer D), or bisphosphonates, such as alendronate (Answer E), to prevent bone loss or treat low bone density in patients using DMPA.

While measuring 24-hour urinary calcium excretion (Answer B) is helpful in identifying hypocalciuria or hypercalciuria as a cause of secondary osteoporosis, this would not be the best next step in this clinical scenario. In addition, urinary calcium would be expected to be low at this time, given the patient's inadequate calcium intake and suboptimal 25-hydroxyvitamin D level. This should ideally be checked after vitamin D repletion and sufficient calcium intake (~1000 mg daily for a premenopausal woman).

Finally, there is no concern for celiac disease in this patient since she has no evidence of chronic malabsorption (specifically, no anemia). Therefore, measuring tissue transglutaminase antibodies (Answer A) is incorrect.

Educational Objective
Explain how the use of depot medroxyprogesterone may be associated with bone loss in premenopausal women.

Reference(s)
Camacho PM, Petak SM, Binkley N, et al. American Association of Clinical Endocrinologists and American College of Endocrinology clinical practice guidelines for the diagnosis and treatment of postmenopausal osteoporosis – 2016. *Endocr Pract.* 2016;22(Suppl 4):1-42. PMID: 27662240

Scholes D, LaCroix AZ, Ichikawa LE, Barlow WE, Ott SM. Injectable hormone contraception and bone density: results from a prospective study [published correction appears in Epidemiology. 2002;13(6):749]. *Epidemiology.* 2002;13(5):581-587. PMID: 12192229

Rosenberg L, Zhang Y, Constant D, et al. Bone status after cessation of use of injectable progestin contraceptives. *Contraception.* 2007;76(6):425-431. PMID: 18061699

101 ANSWER: D) Sitosterolemia

This patient has sitosterolemia (Answer D). Sitosterolemia is a rare autosomal recessive disorder characterized by increased absorption and decreased excretion of plant sterols, which leads to high levels of sitosterol and campesterol. Affected patients have a pathogenic variant in a gene encoding either ATP-binding cassette subfamily G member 5 or member 8. These proteins have a role in the transport of dietary plant sterols and cholesterol out of the enterocyte and into the bile. Patients with sitosterolemia have hematologic abnormalities such as macrothrombocytopenia and stomatocytosis (erythrocytes with a central slit instead of a circular area of pallor), and they are at increased risk for premature cardiovascular disease. On physical examination, affected patients have tendinous or tuberous xanthomas on extensor areas. Restriction of plant sterol intake is required. Foods rich in plant sterols include vegetable oils, nuts, seeds, wheat germ, and avocados. In addition to dietary modifications, ezetimibe is recommended, as it blocks absorption of plant sterols at the level of the intestinal lumen.

Familial combined hyperlipidemia (Answer A) is the most common inherited form of dyslipidemia, and it is characterized by the presence of multiple hyperlipidemias within a family (hypercholesterolemia, hypertriglyceridemia, or mixed hyperlipidemia), high levels of apolipoprotein B, and premature heart disease. The difference in lipid profiles is due to different genetic variants, degree of expression of these genes, and environmental factors that alter LDL-cholesterol and triglyceride concentrations. Familial combined hyperlipidemia usually coexists with other metabolic diseases. Pharmacologic therapy is driven by the type of lipid disorder. Patients with this condition do not have an elevated campesterol level, which rules out this diagnosis.

Familial hypobetalipoproteinemia (Answer B) is caused by pathogenic variants in the genes encoding either apolipoprotein B, microsomal triglyceride transfer protein, or PCSK9, which lead to decreased LDL-cholesterol levels. Affected patients usually have LDL-cholesterol concentrations less than 50 mg/dL (<1.30 mmol/L). The lack of production of LDL cholesterol leads to accumulation of triglycerides in the liver, which increases the risk of fatty liver. This patient's LDL-cholesterol concentration of 84 mg/dL (2.18 mmol/L) rules out this diagnosis.

Familial dysbetalipoproteinemia (Answer C) is caused by pathogenic variants in the gene encoding apolipoprotein E and is characterized by increased triglyceride-rich lipoprotein remnants due to impaired clearance. These particles promote atherosclerosis of the coronary arteries and peripheral arteries, which leads to premature cardiovascular disease. Most affected individuals are homozygous for the apolipoprotein *E2* allele; however, penetrance is incomplete and additional metabolic stressors are needed to develop this condition (eg, developing insulin resistance or obesity). Biochemically, patients present with elevated total cholesterol and triglycerides, in a 2:1 molar ratio. A pathognomonic physical examination finding is palmar crease xanthomas. Treatment starts with dietary counseling to decrease both fat and carbohydrate intake. Pharmacologic therapy with statin and fibrates is also recommended depending on the individual's lipid profile. This patient has premature heart disease; however, his lipid panel only shows mild hypertriglyceridemia, which would not be consistent with the findings in familial dysbetalipoproteinemia.

Familial hypercholesterolemia (Answer E) is a common inherited disorder characterized by elevated LDL cholesterol (in most cases >190 mg/dL [>4.92 mmol/L]) and a family history of premature heart disease. The etiology of familial hypercholesterolemia can be established in up to 70% of cases. Patients with a known defect have either a pathogenic variant or deletion in the genes encoding the following proteins: LDL receptor, apolipoprotein B_{100}, or PCSK9. Patients are classified into 2 groups depending on the number and type of pathogenic variants they inherit. Most patients with familial hypercholesterolemia have a heterozygous pathogenic variant. The prevalence of heterozygous familial hypercholesterolemia is 1 in 200 to 1 in 500 individuals. LDL-cholesterol levels are usually 2 to 3 times higher than normal (200-250 mg/dL [5.18-6.48 mmol/L]). Patients with homozygous familial hypercholesterolemia are rarely seen in clinical practice, as the prevalence is 1 in 1 million. Their LDL-cholesterol concentration is 6 times higher than normal values. Identifying all patients with familial hypercholesterolemia is important, as they have premature atherosclerotic cardiovascular disease if untreated. Characteristic physical examination findings are corneal arcus and Achilles tendon xanthomas. Given the degree of LDL-cholesterol elevation, most affected patients require combined treatment with a statin, a cholesterol absorption inhibitor, and a PCSK9 inhibitor. In some cases, they even need LDL apheresis. This patient's LDL-cholesterol concentration is 84 mg/dL (2.18 mmol/L), which is not consistent with familial hypercholesterolemia.

Educational Objective
Identify the clinical and laboratory features of a patient with sitosterolemia.

Reference(s)
Marais D. Dysbetalipop roteinemia: an extreme disorder of remnant metabolism. *Curr Opin Lipidol*. 2015;26(4):292-297. PMID: 26103610

Van Greevenbroek MMJ, Stalenhoef AFH, de Graaf J, Brouwers MCGJ. Familial combined hyperlipidemia: from molecular insights to tailored therapy. *Curr Opin Lipidol*. 2014;25(3):176-182. PMID: 24811296

Welty FK. Hypobetalipoproteinemia and abetalipoproteinemia. *Curr Opin Lipidol*. 2014;25(3):161-169. PMID: 24751931

Tada H, Nohara A, Inazu A, Sakuma N, Mabuchi H, Kawashiri MA. Sitosterolemia, hypercholesterolemia, and coronary artery disease. *J Atheroscler Thromb*. 2018;25(9):783-789. PMID: 30033951

Yoo E-G. Sitosterolemia: a review and update of pathophysiology, clinical spectrum, diagnosis and management. *Ann Pediatr Endocrinol Metab*. 2016;21(1):7-14. PMID: 27104173

102 ANSWER: B) Measure serum β-hydroxybutyrate

This patient is at risk for developing euglycemic diabetic ketoacidosis due to SGLT-2 inhibitor therapy. FDA guidelines suggest medications in this class be stopped 3 to 4 days before surgical procedures that carry an increased risk of diabetic ketoacidosis. In this case, empagliflozin was not stopped before surgery due to the urgent nature of the coronary artery bypass graft procedure. Indeed, he developed diabetic ketoacidosis on the fourth hospital day despite glucose levels ranging from 150 to 250 mg/dL (8.3-13.9 mmol/L), and this prolonged his stay in the intensive care unit.

Is there something that could have been done to evaluate his risk for diabetic ketoacidosis? Some authors suggest routine monitoring of serum β-hydroxybutyrate (Answer B) in such a clinical scenario. Interestingly, urinary ketones (Answer C) may not be present with SGLT-2 inhibitor use because their urinary excretion is limited. Therefore, among the choices to assess for possible excess ketone production, measuring serum β-hydroxybutyrate is preferred. The finding of elevated serum ketones should prompt one to consider continuation of intravenous insulin. Another contributing factor in this scenario could be inadequate nutrition and this should be evaluated. In this patient's case, oral food intake was quite poor.

This patient is not necessarily at increased risk for lactic acidosis. His metformin was stopped when he was admitted to the hospital, and recommendations suggest stopping metformin only 24 hours before surgery. Also, he does not have renal failure or heart failure. Therefore, it is not necessary to check lactic acid levels (Answer A).

At this point, his glycemic control is adequate, and it would be reasonable to continue with the plan to transition to subcutaneous insulin rather than continue the intravenous insulin drip (Answer D).

There is interesting preclinical and clinical information regarding the use of GLP-1 receptor agonist infusions in the setting of percutaneous revascularization procedures to reduce myocardial ischemia. However, it is not used in such a clinical setting yet, as sufficient clinical studies have not been performed. While initiation of GLP-1 receptor agonist treatment (Answer E) may be indicated based on its efficacy for glycemic control and cardiovascular risk reduction, now would not be the right time to start this medication, as the patient is still recovering from surgery and may not be consuming food properly.

Educational Objective
Assess the risk for normoglycemic diabetic ketoacidosis and describe the finding that urinary ketone excretion is limited in patients treated with SGLT-2 inhibitors.

Reference(s)
Thiruvenkatarajan V, Meyer EJ, Nanjappa N, Van Wijk RM, Jesudason D. *Br J Anaesth.* 2019;123(1):27-36. PMID: 31060732

van den Boom W, Schroeder RA, Manning MW, Setji TL, Fiestan GO, Dunson DB. *Diabetes Care.* 2018;41(4):782-788. PMID: 29440113

Levy N, Dhatariya K. Pre-operative optimisation of the surgical patient with diagnosed and undiagnosed diabetes: a practical review. *Anaesthesia.* 2019;74(Suppl 1):58-66. PMID: 30604420

US Food and Drug Administration. FDA Drug Safety Communication. FDA revises labels of SGLT2 inhibitors for diabetes to include warnings about too much acid in the blood and serious urinary tract infections. Available at: https://www.fda.gov/drugs/drug-safety-and-availability/fda-revises-labels-sglt2-inhibitors-diabetes-include-warnings-about-too-much-acid-blood-and-serious. Accessed March 2021.

103 ANSWER: D) Discontinue tenofovir

Osteoporosis and low-trauma fractures are a significant issue in patients who undergo solid-organ transplant and have a number of contributing factors. Perhaps most importantly, antirejection medications, including glucocorticoids, directly inhibit bone formation and can induce a rapid and robust decrease in bone mineral density, in addition to compromising skeletal integrity due to promotion of osteocyte apoptosis. Current evidence, however, suggests that the elevated fracture risk due to glucocorticoid use diminishes within 6 to 12 months of discontinuation. In addition, patients who undergo hepatic transplant appear to demonstrate a significant attenuation of fracture risk after 12 months, most likely due to a combination of glucocorticoid dosage reduction, as well as reconstitution of normal hepatic function and its attendant effects on vitamin D metabolism. In this patient who underwent remote hepatic transplant and has a history of glucocorticoid use, the occurrence of new fragility fractures should prompt one to consider alternative mechanisms of bone fragility other than osteoporosis. Indeed, this should prompt consideration of disorders that also present with low bone density by DXA scanning. Osteomalacia, which cannot be distinguished from osteoporosis on the basis of bone mineral density testing due to the presence of insufficient mineralization of skeletal matrix, should be considered in this patient.

Osteomalacia, which can result in either insufficiency or frank fractures and typically involves the weight-bearing lower extremities, is generally due to disturbances in vitamin D metabolism, hypophosphatemia, or inherited or acquired processes independent of disturbances in calcium and phosphorus metabolism. This patient has biochemical hypophosphatemia, which is even more clinically pronounced in the context of renal insufficiency given the inherent impairment in phosphorus excretion. Hypophosphatemic osteomalacia can be due to inherited or acquired processes that most typically involve increased action of FGF-23, a naturally occurring phosphaturic hormone. The condition can also be due to primary renal tubular dysfunction, most classically Fanconi syndrome that results in excessive renal loss of bicarbonate, amino acids, glucose, urea, and phosphorus (often referred to by the acronym BAGUP). This patient is on tenofovir, which is a well-established cause of acquired proximal tubular dysfunction in patients treated for HIV infection, as well as hepatitis B. Discontinuation of tenofovir in this patient (Answer D) resulted in dramatic improvement in bone mineral density at all skeletal sites and definitive healing of her proximal femoral fracture.

Distinguishing osteoporosis from osteomalacia is also critical to determine which specific bone-targeted therapies should be avoided because they could actually aggravate the underlying disease. Specifically, the use of potent bisphosphonate therapy such as zoledronic acid (Answer B) in patients with osteomalacia can further impair skeletal mineralization and aggravate bone pain, impair fracture healing, and potentially increase the risk for further fractures.

Adequate intake of and systemic levels of 25-hydroxyvitamin D are important for optimal intestinal calcium absorption and most likely for maximum benefit of antifracture therapies. Prevailing data, however, support a minimal additional benefit of vitamin D supplementation (Answer A) for patients with 25-hydroxyvitamin D levels greater than 20 ng/mL (>49.9 nmol/L).

Although hyperparathyroidism can have attendant negative skeletal consequences, this patient's modest elevation of intact PTH is most likely due to stage 3 chronic kidney disease. Available data do not demonstrate an antifracture benefit of treatment with calcium-sensing receptor agonists such as cinacalcet (Answer C).

Finally, although calcineurin inhibitors may contribute to an increase in fracture risk in patients following solid-organ transplant, the skeletal effect is minor compared with that observed with glucocorticoids. Furthermore, these agents are indispensable in the antirejection management of these patients, so discontinuing tacrolimus (Answer E) is incorrect.

Educational Objective
Identify tenofovir as a cause of hypophosphatemic osteomalacia and hip fracture in a patient treated for chronic hepatitis B.

Reference(s)
Moon NH, Shin WC, Do MU, Cho HJ, Suh KT. An uncommon case of bilateral pathologic hip fractures: antiviral drug-induced osteomalacia in a patient with hepatitis B. *Hip Pelvis.* 2018;30(2):109-114. PMID: 29896460

Biver E, Calmy A, Rizzoli R. Bone health in HIV and hepatitis B or C infections. *Ther Adv Musculoskelet Dis.* 2017;9(1):22-34. PMID: 28101146

104 ANSWER: C) Perform pituitary-directed MRI

This case has many clues suggesting the presence of organic hypogonadism, and there is a high index of suspicion for central pathology (hypothalamic-pituitary). The patient is relatively young, his BMI is not in the obese range, and he has a low comorbid burden. Further, he has typical clinical symptoms and signs (gynecomastia, borderline-low testicular size) suggestive of androgen deficiency. His mild anemia, while nonspecific, is consistent with androgen deficiency. His serum testosterone is frankly low and his LH is inappropriately low-normal, indicating a central pathology, and his mildly raised prolactin level is consistent with a pituitary stalk effect. His free T_4 is borderline-low with a normal TSH concentration, suggesting possible secondary hypothyroidism. Therefore, the best next step in this patient's management is to perform a pituitary-directed MRI (Answer C) and to assess other pituitary endocrine axes as appropriate.

Given that the clinical and biochemical diagnosis of hypogonadism is clear-cut, free testosterone measurement (Answer A) would not add any clinically useful information. Free testosterone measurements (usually calculated from total testosterone, SHBG, and albumin) may occasionally be helpful if the serum total testosterone concentration is borderline or SHBG abnormalities are suspected, but not all authorities agree on this issue.

His hypogonadism should not be dismissed as being functional (ie, a consequence of older age and obesity) and is therefore not expected to resolve with lifestyle changes, such as weight loss. While referral to an exercise physiologist for lifestyle measures (Answer E) may be part of holistic care, it is not the best next step.

Importantly, testosterone treatment (Answer D) should never be started before diagnostic workup is complete and a clear diagnosis has been made. Failure to do so may lead to missing important underlying pathologies, such as a pituitary tumor. Also, exogenous testosterone treatment suppresses the hypothalamic-pituitary-testicular axis even in healthy men, and once testosterone has been initiated, accurate evaluation for an underlying etiology is virtually impossible. Of note, testosterone treatment compromises fertility and should not be started in men desiring paternity in the near future.

This patient's low libido should resolve with testosterone replacement. Should erectile dysfunction (not reported by the patient) be an issue after restoration of eugonadism with testosterone replacement, a phosphodiesterase type 5 inhibitor (Answer B) might be effective, but it is not the best next step.

This patient's pituitary MRI showed a pituitary macroadenoma not abutting the optic chiasm. After neurosurgical consultation, he elected monitoring rather than immediate surgery. He had no desire for paternity, so testosterone treatment was commenced, which led to marked improvements in libido and energy. He was able to lose more weight, and metabolic syndrome and mild anemia resolved.

Educational Objective
Diagnose secondary hypogonadism on the basis of clinical clues and avoid attributing low testosterone to overweight/metabolic syndrome without considering other causes.

Reference(s)
Basaria S. Male hypogonadism. *Lancet.* 2014;383(9924):1250-1263. PMID: 24119423

Bhasin S, Brito JP, Cunningham GR, et al. Testosterone therapy in men with hypogonadism: an Endocrine Society clinical practice guideline. *J Clin Endocrinol Metab.* 2018;103(5):1715-1744. PMID: 29562364

105 ANSWER: B) Add dulaglutide

Since the ACCORD trial (Action to Control Cardiovascular Risk in Diabetes trial) reported increased mortality associated with hypoglycemia when attempting to achieve tighter hemoglobin A_{1c} goals, there has been a movement to personalize hemoglobin A_{1c} goals based on risk. The hemoglobin A_{1c} goal may be higher in patients who are older, have a longer duration of diabetes, have renal disease, or have other comorbidities that increase the likelihood of hypoglycemia.

In this vignette, one first must determine the patient's hemoglobin A_{1c} goal. He is younger with recently diagnosed diabetes and an estimated glomerular filtration rate greater than 60 mL/min per 1.73 m². Thus, a hemoglobin A_{1c} target less than 7.0% (<53 mmol/mol), or even less than 6.5% (<48 mmol/mol), would be appropriate for him based on current guidelines.

Continuing current therapy (Answer A) is incorrect, as adding additional agents would be recommended since he has not reached his glycemic target after 6 months of treatment. Increasing the metformin dosage (Answer C) would also be incorrect, as recent meta-analysis of metformin showed a small decrease in hemoglobin A_{1c} on monotherapy (on average, only 1.12% [95% CI, 0.92-1.32; P = .00001; I^2, 80.2%]). In the higher-dosage arms, there was an additional reduction in hemoglobin A_{1c} of 0.26% (95% CI, 0.14-0.38; P = .0001; I^2, 55.5%). Thus, this patient would be unlikely to reach his hemoglobin A_{1c} goal by maximizing the metformin dosage.

Furthermore, potential interactions with other medications should be considered. Recent reports have noted an increased risk for lactic acidosis with concomitant use of tenofovir and metformin. This risk increases with increasing dosage and when creatinine clearance is less than 50 mL/min per 1.73 m², as tenofovir accumulates because of reduced elimination by the kidneys. However, this patient's estimated glomerular filtration rate is currently greater than 60 mL/min per 1.73 m². There is no clear indication to stop metformin (Answers D and E), as it has been effective in improving his glycemic control, and his renal function is sufficient to minimize the risk of lactic acidosis despite tenofovir therapy. In addition, monotherapy with dulaglutide or sitagliptin would be unlikely to achieve this patient's hemoglobin A_{1c} target of less than 7.0% (<53 mmol/mol). Generally, patients with diabetes who have suboptimal glycemic control require added therapy, not substitute therapy. Thus, the best strategy at this point would be to add dulaglutide (Answer B) for dual therapy. Intensification of therapy is recommended not only for glycemic control but also for weight, potential renal, and cardiovascular benefits. The REWIND trial (Dulaglutide and Cardiovascular Outcomes in Type 2 Diabetes), a double-blind, randomized placebo-controlled trial, demonstrated that dulaglutide led to cardiovascular event reduction in patients with a prior cardiovascular event, as well as acted as primary prevention in those with cardiovascular risk factors. This patient is at risk for cardiovascular disease given his age and history of hypertension. Also, HIV is an independent risk factor for myocardial infarction and other cardiovascular disease.

Educational Objective
Intensify diabetes therapy considering drug interactions and glycemic goals.

Reference(s)
ACCORD Study Group, Buse JB, Bigger JT, et al. Action to Control Cardiovascular Risk in Diabetes (ACCORD) trial: design and methods. *Am J Cardiol.* 2007;99(12A):21i-33i. PMID: 17599422

Hirst JA, Farmer AJ, Ali R, Roberts NW, Stevens RJ. Quantifying the effect of metformin treatment and dose on glycemic control. *Diabetes Care.* 2012;35(2):446-454. PMID: 22275444

Biktarvy. Prescribing information. Gilead Sciences; 2018. Accessed September 2020. https://www.accessdata.fda.gov/drugsatfda_docs/label/2018/210251s000lbl.pdf

Gerstein HC, Colhoun HM, Dagenais GR, et al; REWIND Investigators. Dulaglutide and cardiovascular outcomes in type 2 diabetes (REWIND): a double-blind, randomised placebo-controlled trial. *Lancet.* 2019;394(10193):121-130. PMID: 31189511

Freiberg MS, Chang CC, Kuller LH, et al. HIV infection and the risk of acute myocardial infarction. *JAMA Intern Med.* 2013;173(8):614-622. PMID: 23459863

106 ANSWER: C) Refer to an otolaryngologist

Thyroidectomy is recommended in the management of several conditions, including large goiter with compressive symptoms, multinodular goiter, toxic nodular goiter, Graves disease, and thyroid nodule biopsy-proven thyroid cancer. Despite being a safe procedure, it carries some risk of complications, the most common of which are hypocalcemia due to postsurgical hypoparathyroidism, hoarseness or voice change due to recurrent laryngeal nerve injury, hematoma or seroma, or infection. Horner syndrome or chyle leak can also be seen. These complications are reduced if an experienced surgeon performs the thyroid surgery. In a study including 16,954 patients with total thyroidectomy from 1998 to 2009 with half of patients having thyroid cancer, the surgeon volume threshold of more than 25 total thyroidectomies per year was associated with improved patient outcomes and fewer complications.

Postsurgical hypoparathyroidism is easily diagnosed because affected patients experience symptoms of hypocalcemia such as tingling and numbness around their lips, mouth, hands, and feet. These patients need calcium supplementation and some may require calcitriol. The hypoparathyroidism can be transient or permanent (persistent low calcium 6 to 9 months after thyroid surgery). The risk of permanent hypoparathyroidism is estimated to be 2% to 3% if the procedure is performed by an experienced surgeon.

The recurrent laryngeal nerve innervates all of the intrinsic muscles of the larynx with the exception of the cricothyroid muscle, which is innervated by the superior laryngeal nerve. Recurrent laryngeal nerve injury can happen during thyroidectomy, parathyroidectomy, or endotracheal intubation. Tumors can also cause recurrent laryngeal nerve injury. Types of recurrent laryngeal nerve injury include traction, compression, sharp, or thermal injury, with traction injury being the most common. Injury causes vocal fold paralysis, and affected patients present with hoarseness, changes in vocal pitch, noisy breathing, cough, globus sensation, and dysphagia. The injury can be unilateral or bilateral. Bilateral injury causes respiratory distress with stridor and the patient often needs emergent reintubation or tracheostomy. The incidence of vocal fold paralysis after thyroidectomy is underestimated in the literature, and it has been reported to be 2.3% to 26% in different studies. Such patients are at increased risk for aspiration pneumonia. Injury to the superior laryngeal nerve is more difficult to recognize, and it results in voice weakness or fatigue, as well as changes to both quality and pitch of the voice. Any of these symptoms that persist beyond 48 hours after thyroid surgery should raise concern for possible vocal cord motion abnormalities, and patients should be referred promptly for direct laryngoscopy. Transient hoarseness that resolves within 24 to 48 hours after thyroid surgery is usually related to vocal cord edema caused by endotracheal intubation.

Another complication is Horner syndrome, which is caused by interruption of the sympathetic pathway that supplies the neck, eyes, and head. Symptoms include miosis, ptosis, and anhidrosis. This complication is very rare (0.2% after thyroidectomy) and it is mostly associated with lateral neck dissection.

Patients with vocal fold paralysis after thyroid surgery should undergo laryngoscopy, voice therapy, and counseling. Some of these patients might need medialization of the paralyzed vocal fold to improve swallowing and phonation. Different techniques are available for vocal fold medialization:

(1) Medialization thyroplasty: involves making an external incision to place an implant that permanently moves the affected vocal cord medially
(2) Injection laryngoplasty: the affected vocal cord is injected with a material (eg, collagen, hyaluronic acid, calcium hydroxyapatite, fat, or Teflon) that fills the vocal cord and moves it medially
(3) Arytenoid adduction: involves placing a permanent suture through the muscular portion of the arytenoid cartilage, pulling the affected vocal cord medial to correct vocal cord paralysis

In this vignette, the patient had total thyroidectomy with bilateral central neck dissection for biopsy-proven papillary thyroid carcinoma. Following thyroid surgery, he noticed hoarseness and intermittent cough that were still present at his follow-up appointment 10 days after surgery. These symptoms suggest an injury to the recurrent laryngeal nerve. It is important to recognize the vocal fold paralysis early, as treatment can improve symptoms and decrease morbidity such as aspiration pneumonia. Thus, reassessing in 3 months (Answer B) or recommending no immediate intervention (Answer E) is incorrect. Laryngoscopy should be performed by an experienced otolaryngologist (Answer C) to establish the diagnosis of vocal fold paralysis.

His intermittent cough is also most likely related to recurrent laryngeal nerve injury, and referral to a pulmonologist (Answer D) is not indicated at this time.

His TSH concentration is slightly elevated, and his levothyroxine dosage should be further increased to shift the TSH concentration in the desired range based on his risk for thyroid cancer recurrence. Once the levothyroxine dosage is adjusted, TSH should be measured 4 to 6 weeks later. Measuring TSH in 6 months (Answer A) is not an appropriate timeframe for monitoring TSH levels in this setting.

Educational Objective
Suspect recurrent laryngeal nerve injury after total thyroidectomy.

Reference(s)
Haugen BR, Alexander EK, Bible KC, et al. 2015 American Thyroid Association management guidelines for adult patients with thyroid nodules and differentiated thyroid cancer: the American Thyroid Association Guidelines Task Force on Thyroid Nodules and Differentiated Thyroid Cancer. *Thyroid.* 2016;26(1):1-133. PMID: 26462967

Adam MA, Thomas S, Youngwirth L, et al. Is there a minimum number of thyroidectomies a surgeon should perform to optimize patient outcomes? *Ann Surg.* 2017;265(2):402-407. PMID: 28059969

Chandrasekhar SS, Randolph GW, Seidman MD, et al; American Academy of Otolaryngology-Head and Neck Surgery. Clinical practice guideline: improving voice outcomes after thyroid surgery. *Otolaryngol Head Neck Surg.* 2013;148(6S):S1-S37. PMID: 23733893

107 ANSWER: A) Pantoprazole, 40 mg daily

Laparoscopic sleeve gastrectomy is the most commonly performed bariatric surgery in the United States. Its popularity is owed to its simplicity, short operating time, and lower risk of short- and long-term adverse events when compared with Roux-en-Y gastric bypass.

New-onset symptomatic gastroesophageal reflux is a common complication after sleeve gastrectomy, occurring in 10% to 20% of patients. Symptoms of gastroesophageal reflux may worsen in patients with preexisting reflux symptoms or a known hiatal hernia. In many bariatric centers, these conditions are relative contraindications to pursuing sleeve gastrectomy. Symptoms of gastroesophageal reflux typically become more common as time elapses since surgery, possibly due to the development of de novo hiatal hernias from increased pressure within the sleeve over years.

Patients presenting with classic reflux symptoms should be started on proton-pump inhibitor therapy (Answer A) as first-line treatment. If symptoms do not improve or continue to worsen despite high-dosage proton-pump inhibitor therapy, further diagnostic studies are warranted. Such studies include an upper gastrointestinal endoscopy (Answer B) and barium esophagography (Answer C). In rare circumstances, patients with severe gastroesophageal reflux after sleeve gastrectomy require revision of their current anatomy to Roux-en-Y gastric bypass.

Symptomatic gallstone disease is most likely to occur in the first year after surgery and is most strongly associated with the degree of weight loss achieved. Thus, abdominal ultrasonography to screen for gallstones (Answer E) is not the best next step now. In a retrospective study comparing Roux-en-Y gastric bypass, sleeve gastrectomy, and adjustable gastric banding, the rate of symptomatic gallstone disease was 9.5%, 3.8%, and 2.6%, respectively, with mean time to symptom development of 10.2 months. There are currently no consensus guidelines on the role of prophylactic cholecystectomy, intraoperative ultrasonography, or the use of ursodeoxycholic acid prophylaxis postoperatively. This patient is unlikely to have developed gallstones this far out from surgery, and thus treatment with ursodeoxycholic acid (Answer D) is incorrect.

Educational Objective
Identify gastroesophageal reflux as a common complication in a patient who has had sleeve gastrectomy.

Reference(s)
Arterburn DE, Telem DA, Kushner RF, Courcoulas AP. Benefits and risks of bariatric surgery in adults a review. *JAMA.* 2020;324(9):879-887. PMID: 32870301

Himpens J, Dobbeleir J, Peeters G. Long-term results of laparoscopic sleeve gastrectomy for obesity. *Ann Surg.* 2010;252(2):319-324. PMID: 20622654

DuPree CE, Blair K, Steele SR, Martin MJ. Laparoscopic sleeve gastrectomy in patients with preexisting gastroesophageal reflux disease: a national analysis. *JAMA Surg.* 2014;149(4):328-334. PMID: 24500799

108

ANSWER: A) Transient osteoporosis

Hip pain is a common presenting concern, most likely secondary only to low back pain in terms of frequency of musculoskeletal complaints. Delineation of the nature and location of the hip area discomfort is paramount to accurately diagnosing the underlying etiology. The acute onset of the condition, combined with the absence of characteristic history and physical examination findings, argues against the presence of a chronic inflammatory condition such as rheumatoid arthritis (Answer E). Additionally, there is no history of fever or corroborative hematology findings to suggest the presence of septic arthritis (Answer C). The examination findings strongly suggest involvement of the hip joint with or without involvement of the proximal femur, and do not support involvement of the proximal posterior lateral femur, which would be consistent with subtrochanteric bursitis (Answer B).

The most likely diagnosis based on this patient's presentation is transient osteoporosis of the hip (Answer A). Transient osteoporosis of the hip is a relatively poorly understood condition that presents subacutely with intense discomfort in the hip region that is exacerbated by weightbearing. In addition, the condition typically affects individuals in the fourth to sixth decades of life and affects men more often than women, although the condition has been described in pregnant women. The condition appears to result in relatively diffuse edema of the femoral head and neck regions, although the underlying precipitating factor or factors have not been well characterized. Nonetheless, several associated clinical findings have been described in these patients, including low bone density, vitamin D deficiency, cigarette smoking, alcohol overuse, and glucocorticoids. There is certainly overlap between transient osteoporosis of the hip and avascular necrosis of the hip (Answer D) in terms of associated clinical risk factors, including glucocorticoid use, alcohol overuse, and cigarette smoking. Nonetheless, the presentation of avascular necrosis is typically more insidious and less acute than that of transient osteoporosis of the hip. The radiographic findings in avascular necrosis are distinct from transient osteoporosis of the hip, in that the former typically has evidence for femoral head deformity or collapse and subchondral lucency (crescent sign) seen on MRI.

Recovery from transient osteoporosis of the hip occurs with resolution of edema and hypervascularity, which is accompanied by reduction in pain and improvement in radiographic imaging. Treatment generally involves bisphosphonates (oral or intravenous) that have been shown to shorten recovery time (~2-3 months vs ~6 months with conservative therapy such as rest, restricted weightbearing, and analgesics), although these results have been observed only in small nonrandomized studies and case-control series. Core decompression of the proximal femur is not helpful in transient osteoporosis of the hip, whereas it may be considered in patients with avascular necrosis of the hip. Potential complications of transient osteoporosis of the hip include subchondral, femoral neck, or subcapital fractures, although fractures are more commonly reported in pregnant women. Transient osteoporosis of the hip typically resolves without recurrence, although additional involvement in the distal part of the affected extremity can occur in patients with a similar but distinct condition called regional migratory osteoporosis, which can also present with painful focal skeletal lesions.

Educational Objective
Diagnose transient osteoporosis of the hip.

Reference(s)
Asadipooya K, Graves L, Greene LW. Transient osteoporosis of the hip: review of the literature. *Osteoporos Int*. 2017;28(6):1805-1816. PMID: 28314897

Cano-Marquina A, Tarín JJ, García-Pérez MÁ, Cano A. Transient regional osteoporosis. *Maturitas*. 2014;77(4):324-329. PMID: 24582491

109

ANSWER: A) Measure venous plasma glucose

The first step in the evaluation and management of hypoglycemia is to document the Whipple triad, which consists of the following: (1) symptoms of hypoglycemia, (2) hypoglycemia (blood glucose concentration <50 mg/dL [<2.78 mmol/L]), and (3) relief of symptoms following ingestion of glucose. This patient had no symptoms at the time of her low fingerstick point-of-care glucose values. Accordingly, this should have been the first sign that the low glucose values being recorded were not true hypoglycemia. Also, the observation that her fingerstick point-of-care glucose values did not rise despite supplemental glucose and intramuscular glucagon provides further evidence that perhaps the fingerstick readings were inaccurate.

The patient has a history of peripheral arterial disease and has undergone a below-the-knee amputation of her left leg. Her current hospital admission for abdominal pain and history of weight loss, lack of appetite, and abdominal pain that worsens with prandial intake should raise suspicion for mesenteric ischemia. Thus, the fingerstick point-of-care glucose readings are most likely pseudohypoglycemia (ie, attributed to poor perfusion secondary to severe peripheral arterial disease). The pseudohypoglycemia may result from increased glucose extraction by the tissues because of low capillary flow and increased glucose transit time. Such a phenomenon has also been described in patients with vasculitis, systemic sclerosis (previously known as scleroderma), Raynaud phenomenon, and shock (hypotension). Thus, the best next step is to measure venous glucose (Answer A) using a standard glucose assay to confirm pseudohypoglycemia as the etiology of the low fingerstick point-of-care readings.

Administering octreotide (Answer B) or initiating an intravenous infusion of dextrose-containing fluids (Answer D) is incorrect because each option is a therapy for actual hypoglycemia, which this patient does not have.

Ordering a sulfonylurea panel (Answer C) is incorrect, in part, because this patient does not have confirmed hypoglycemia and because the sulfonylurea panel is only a qualitative test. It simply confirms that a recent ingestion has occurred. Hypoglycemic drugs are detected by liquid chromatography–tandem mass spectrometry if the drug concentration is greater than the limit of detection (cutoff). The presence of hypoglycemic drug(s) indicates a recent ingestion.

Lastly, measuring C-peptide (Answer E) is incorrect because this patient does not have confirmed hypoglycemia. When confirmed hypoglycemia is documented, plasma C-peptide is measured to determine whether the level of insulin secretion is inappropriate for the low glucose value. It would be of little value in this patient with pseudohypoglycemia.

Educational Objective
Select the correct diagnostic approach to hypoglycemia (to document the Whipple triad) and identify circumstances in which low point-of-care glucose values may be artifactual or artificial in nature.

Reference(s)
Garingarao CJ, Buenaluz-Sedurante M, Jimeno CA. Accuracy of point-of-care blood glucose measurements in critically ill patients in shock. *J Diabetes Sci Technol*. 2014;8(5):937-944. PMID: 25172876

Matthews J, Mashayekhi M, Hendrickson C. Pseudohypoglycemia in severe peripheral artery disease report and literature review. *Endocr Pract*. 2019;(Suppl 1):159-160.

El Khoury M, Yousuf F, Martin V, Cohen RM. Pseudohypoglycemia: a cause for unreliable finger-stick glucose measurements. *Endocr Pract*. 2008;14(3):337-339. PMID: 18463040

Bishay RH, Suryawanshi A. Artifactual hypoglycaemia in systemic sclerosis and Raynaud's phenomenon: a clinical case report and short review. *Case Rep Endocrinol*. 2016;2016:7390927. PMID: 28116181

110 ANSWER: D) Very high ACTH

After a recent diagnosis of Hashimoto thyroiditis and treatment initiation with levothyroxine, this patient developed progressive fatigue, weight loss, and syncope. Although undertreatment or overtreatment with levothyroxine (very high free T_4 [Answer A] or very high TSH [Answer B]) are potential nonspecific considerations for the ongoing symptomatology, the presentation with syncope, hypotension, hyponatremia, and hyperkalemia should raise concerns for autoimmune primary adrenal insufficiency (also termed Addison disease).

Primary adrenal insufficiency is most commonly caused by autoimmune destruction of adrenocortical cells resulting in hypocortisolemia, increased ACTH production (Answer D), hypoaldosteronism, and increased renin secretion. The deficiencies of cortisol and aldosterone result in renal sodium wasting, hypovolemia, hypotension, excess water reabsorption resulting in hyponatremia, and hyperkalemia. The clinical manifestations include progressive fatigue, weight loss, nausea, hyperpigmentation of the skin and mucous membranes, salt craving, orthostasis, and many more. Autoimmune primary adrenal insufficiency can occur in concert with other autoimmune endocrinopathies and disorders, most commonly Hashimoto thyroiditis, but also celiac disease, hypoparathyroidism, type 1 diabetes, and premature ovarian insufficiency. For this reason, these patients should be followed annually to assess for signs, symptoms, and early laboratory evidence of other associated autoimmune conditions and endocrinopathies. In this case, it is likely that the patient had concomitant hypothyroidism and adrenal insufficiency. Once treatment with levothyroxine was initiated, an increase in metabolism and renal clearance most likely precipitated clinical cortisol insufficiency and an adrenal crisis.

This patient's renin levels are expected to be very high, not low (Answer C). Thyroid-stimulating antibodies are not a part of the pathophysiology of Hashimoto thyroiditis or Addison disease. However, Graves disease is an autoimmune hyperthyroidism mediated by thyroid-stimulating immunoglobulins (Answer E), which can occur in individuals with autoimmune endocrinopathies.

Educational Objective
Diagnose Addison disease.

Reference(s)
Bancos I, Hahner S, Tomlinson J, Arlt W. Diagnosis and management of adrenal insufficiency. *Lancet Diabetes Endocrinol.* 2015;3(3):216-226. PMID: 25098712

111 ANSWER: D) Switch to a combined oral contraceptive with a higher dose of estrogen

Combined oral contraceptives (COCs) most commonly contain ethinyl estradiol, which is a potent synthetic estrogen with a long half-life that is not detectable by estradiol assays. COCs suppress the hypothalamic-pituitary-ovarian axis, which, in part, is how they prevent pregnancy. As a result, circulating FSH and estradiol levels are low or suppressed. Therefore, pituitary MRI (Answer A) is not indicated.

Lower-dosage COCs contain 10 to 20 mcg estrogen, while higher dosages range from 30 to 35 mcg. Although lower-dosage COCs were developed to potentially decrease the risk for adverse events such as venous thrombosis, there is no evidence demonstrating decreased risk to date with lower estrogen dosages. Women might decide to start with lower-dosage estrogen because of concerns for other potential adverse effects. With any COC, spotting or light bleeding can occur intermittently during the active pills in the first 3 to 6 months and then spontaneously resolve. As the endometrium transitions under the suppressive effects of the progestin to a thin endometrium, it might become more friable until the estrogen component stabilizes it. Therefore, this patient should be reassured that the spotting is not a sign of a uterine abnormality. Pelvic ultrasonography (Answer B) is not necessary unless heavier bleeding or new pelvic pain develops.

Counseling about different progestins includes discussion of more antiandrogenic progestins or androgenicity, although there are no trial data to support differences in effect when used for hirsutism or acne. Guidelines recommend considering norethindrone or levonorgestrel or norgestimate in women with obesity and in women older than 39 years because of lower relative risk for venous thrombosis. Progestin-only pills are used for contraception when a woman prefers not to use estrogens or when estrogens might be contraindicated. Since irregular bleeding is more common with progestin-only pills (Answer E) than with COCs, it would not be the recommended alternative for irregular bleeding or spotting.

A Cochrane review of 21 trials found higher rates of irregular bleeding with low-dosage estrogen COCs than with higher-dosage estrogen COCs. Although different progestins were used in the studies reviewed, there was not enough evidence to conclude that it was the progestins rather than the lower dosages of estrogen. Therefore, it would be better first to switch to a COC with a higher dosage of estrogen (Answer D) than a different progestin (Answer C), although that could be considered as the next step if spotting continues.

Educational Objective
Evaluate and treat irregular bleeding that develops on oral contraceptives.

Reference(s)
Martin KA, Anderson RR, Chang RJ, et al. Evaluation and treatment of hirsutism in premenopausal women: an Endocrine Society clinical practice guideline. *J Clin Endocrinol Metab.* 2018;103(4):1-25. PMID: 29522147

Hoopes AJ, Simmons KB, Godfrey EM, Sucato GS. 2016 updates to US medical eligibility criteria for contraceptive use and selected practice recommendations for contraceptive use: highlights for adolescent patients. *J Pediatr Adolesc Gynecol.* 2017;30(2):149-155. PMID: 28167141

Gallo MF, Nanda K, Grimes DA, Lopez LM, Schulz KF. 20 ug versus >20 ug estrogen combined oral contraceptives for contraception. *Cochrane Database Syst Rev.* 2013;2013(8):CD003989. PMID: 23904209

112 ANSWER: D) Add semaglutide

Olanzapine is a second-generation antipsychotic drug used in the treatment of schizophrenia and other mental health disorders. Second-generation antipsychotic agents have a dual blocking effect on the dopamine D2 receptor and 5-hydroxytryptamine 2 (5-HT$_2$) receptor. First-generation antipsychotic agents such as haloperidol, also known as neuroleptic agents, block only the dopamine 2 receptor. First-generation antipsychotic agents have a significant risk of causing extrapyramidal adverse effects and tardive dyskinesia, which currently limits their use. Typical antipsychotic drugs, although associated with increased weight, are less associated with insulin resistance, while second-generation antipsychotic drugs such as olanzapine and have been associated with weight gain, metabolic syndrome, and insulin resistance (independent of weight gain).

Consideration of the metabolic effects of medications and treatment choices can be further discussed with this patient's psychiatrist after her psychiatric disease has stabilized. Of the atypical antipsychotic drugs, olanzapine and clozapine have been most associated with negative metabolic effects, followed by risperidone, quetiapine, and ziprasidone. Although aripiprazole is traditionally considered metabolically "neutral," there have been reports of increased risk of developing diabetes or worsening diabetes control with this medication. A personalized treatment plan developed in conjunction with her psychiatrist is needed, and changes to her regimen should not be made without consulting her mental health specialist.

Considering her recent hospitalization, adding phentermine/topiramate (Answer C), a medication that can potentially increase anxiety and cause mood issues, is also not the best choice. Topiramate alone has been shown in small case series to lessen weight gain in patients on antipsychotic medications, but it would probably not significantly improve her glycemic control.

Lifestyle modifications such as limiting carbohydrates and/or following a low-fat diet tailored to patient preference with a nutritionist would be a good adjunct to medication therapy, but given that her fasting blood glucose concentrations have risen to greater than 150 mg/dL (>8.3 mmol/L), use of a second diabetes medication is indicated. Thus, recommending no changes and evaluating in 3 months (Answer A) is inadequate, since the likelihood of weight gain and further deterioration of glycemic control is high.

Adding additional therapy is indicated now, based on her recent blood glucose readings and the likelihood of deteriorating glycemic control worsened by her new medications. When considering the options, adding semaglutide (Answer D) is the best course of action, as it could lead to weight loss and decrease cardiovascular risks, although cardiovascular benefit has not been studied in patients younger than 50 years. There is increasing, albeit limited, data on the use of GLP-1 receptor agonists to combat the negative effects of atypical antipsychotic agents. In contrast, glimepiride (Answer E) or basal insulin (Answer B) could lead to further weight gain.

Educational Objective
Explain the increased risk for worsening hyperglycemia with atypical antipsychotic agents and the need for early medication escalation.

Reference(s)

Henderson DC, Vincenzi B, Andrea NV, Ulloa M, Copeland PM. Pathophysiological mechanisms of increased cardiometabolic risk in people with schizophrenia and other severe mental illnesses. *Lancet Psychiatry.* 2015;2(5):452-464. PMID: 26360288

Teff KL, Rickels MR, Grudziak J, et al. Antipsychotic-induced insulin resistance and postprandial hormonal dysregulation independent of weight gain or psychiatric disease. *Diabetes.* 2013;62:3232-3240. PMID: 23835329

Siskind D, Hahn M, Correll CU, et al. Glucagon-like peptide-1 receptor agonists for antipsychotic-associated cardio-metabolic risk factors: a systematic review and individual participant data meta-analysis. *Diabetes Obes Metab.* 2019;21(2):293-302. PMID: 30187620

Ko Y-H, Joe S-H, Jung I-K, Kim S-H. Topiramate as an adjuvant treatment with atypical antipsychotics in schizophrenic patients experiencing weight gain. *Clin Neuropharmacol.* 2005;28(4):169-175. PMID: 16062095

113 ANSWER: A) Atorvastatin

This patient's history of type 2 diabetes mellitus makes him a candidate for LDL-cholesterol–lowering therapy to prevent atherosclerotic cardiovascular events. What makes him different from most patients is his elevated liver enzymes and history of cirrhosis. The question is whether statin therapy is an option for him.

When statins appeared on the market, routine liver function tests were recommended because of the concern for hepatotoxicity, as they are metabolized in the liver and interact with the cytochrome P450 pathway. In 2012, the FDA changed the safety label of statins by removing the need for routine periodic monitoring of liver enzymes and recommending that they are checked before starting therapy and as clinically indicated thereafter. The main reason for the change was that the available evidence showed that irreversible liver damage from statins was rare and most likely idiosyncratic. No randomized controlled clinical trials support measuring liver enzymes before starting statin therapy. However, the consensus of a liver expert panel is that baseline values should be obtained for the purpose of comparison in the event that elevated values are documented in the future.

For patients with AST or ALT elevations in the setting of statin use, the recommended action depends on how high these values are. When the levels of AST or ALT are greater than 3 times the upper normal limit, the recommendation is to repeat the measurement. If results of the repeated tests are unchanged or higher, the statin should be stopped until further evaluation is completed. For patients who have an AST or ALT elevation less than 3 times the upper normal limit, the recommendation is to measure bilirubin and creatine kinase. If both bilirubin and creatine kinase levels are normal, the patient most likely has nonalcoholic fatty liver disease and statin therapy can be continued. If there is an elevation in indirect bilirubin that is not new and the creatine kinase level is normal, the patient may have Gilbert syndrome or nonalcoholic fatty liver disease and statin therapy can be continued. If the patient has a new elevation of bilirubin, the statin should be stopped until further workup is completed.

Liver-specific conditions that are contraindications for statins include decompensated cirrhosis and acute liver failure. A history of compensated cirrhosis, such as that described in this vignette, chronic hepatitis B, chronic hepatitis C, liver transplant, primary biliary cirrhosis, and autoimmune hepatitis are not contraindications for statin use. When patients are being treated with antivirals for hepatitis C or hepatitis B, it is important to verify that there are no drug interactions between the statin and the antiretroviral. The best recommendation for this patient is atorvastatin (Answer A).

There is little evidence regarding the use of nonstatin LDL-cholesterol–lowering therapies in patients with underlying liver disease. Ezetimibe (Answer B) can be used in patients with mild hepatic insufficiency, but it is not recommended in patients with moderate or severe disease. Both bempedoic acid (Answer C) and alirocumab (Answer E) can be used in patients with mild or moderate hepatic impairment (Child-Pugh A or B). However, neither has been studied in patients with severe hepatic impairment. Colesevelam (Answer D) is a bile acid sequestrant. This medication is not absorbed from the gastrointestinal tract and therefore it can be used in patients with hepatic impairment. Even though colesevelam is a reasonable option, it would not be this patient's best option, as it has less LDL-cholesterol–lowering potency, there is less evidence regarding its ability to prevent cardiovascular disease and it can further raise his triglycerides.

Educational Objective
Explain the indications and contraindications of statins for patients with different stages of liver disease.

Reference(s)
Bays H, Cohen DE, Chalasani N, Harrison SA, The National Lipid Association's Statin Safety Task Force. An assessment by the Statin Liver Safety Task Force: 2014 update. *J Clin Lipidol.* 2014;8(Suppl 3):S47-S57. PMID: 24793441

Adhyaru BB, Jacobson TA. Safety and efficacy of statin therapy. *Nat Rev Cardiol.* 2018;15(12):757-769. PMID: 30375494

Zetia. Package insert. Merck & Co., Inc; 2012.

Nexletol. Package insert. Esperion Therapeutics, Inc; 2020.

Praluent. Package insert. Regeneron Pharmaceuticals, Inc; 2020.

114

ANSWER: B) Recommend a nutrition consult for low-fat, low-fiber, small particle size foods

The syndrome of gastroparesis is thought to be caused by hyperglycemia, autonomic neuropathy, and inflammation of the neuroenteric system. Classically, symptoms include early satiety, postprandial fullness, nausea, vomiting, bloating, and upper abdominal discomfort. Symptoms wax and wane in about one-third of cases. Weight loss occurs in half of affected patients and is likely due to reduced caloric intake.

This patient has upper gastrointestinal symptoms, delayed gastric emptying on scintigraphy, and absence of gastric outlet obstruction on upper endoscopy, which establishes the diagnosis of gastroparesis. Interestingly, up to 60% of patients with diabetes who have delayed gastric emptying are asymptomatic, and the presence of symptoms alone cannot predict whether a patient may have delayed, rapid, or normal gastric emptying. Thus, testing to establish the diagnosis is important. Only symptoms of early satiety and the feeling of fullness are associated with delayed gastric emptying.

Assessment of gastric emptying is often done noninvasively by scintigraphy, stable isotope breath test, and motility assessment using wireless pressure and a pH capsule. Relevant medical societies recommend a 4-hour test for gastric-emptying scintigraphy. Patients should consume a standardized meal that contains 255 kcal, with 72% carbohydrate, 24% protein, 2% fat, and 2% fiber. For this meal, delayed gastric emptying is defined as greater than 60% retention at 2 hours and/or greater than 10% at 4 hours. Moderate to severe delayed gastric emptying has been defined as greater than 20% retention at 4 hours.

Small studies in both healthy patients and in those with type 1 diabetes suggest that hyperglycemia (blood glucose 288-342 mg/dL [16-19 mmol/L]) at the time of the test is associated with both decreased antral motility and delayed gastric emptying. Guidelines suggest that gastric emptying should not be evaluated when a patient has severe hyperglycemia (>275 mg/dL [>15.3 mmol/L]). Some authors note that fasting hyperglycemia before gastric-emptying studies is not associated with a delay in gastric emptying and that in patients with type 2 diabetes, hyperglycemia may cause more rapid gastric emptying. Given that this patient did not report severe hyperglycemia and her symptoms are consistent with those often associated with delayed gastric emptying, repeating the gastric-emptying study (Answer A) is not necessary. However, if glucose levels were above 275 mg/dL (>15.3 mmol/L) at the time of the gastric-emptying study, then the results may be falsely positive and should therefore be repeated.

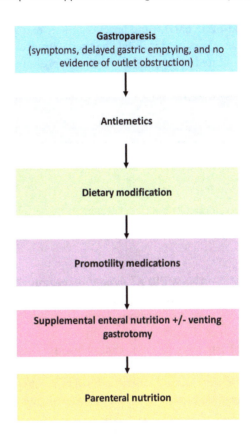

Figure. Step-Wise Approach to Management of Gastroparesis

Adapted from Bharucha AE, Kudva YC, Prichard DO. Diabetic gastroparesis. Endocr Rev. 2019;40(5):1318-1352.

Small studies in patients with diabetes, including at least 1 randomized controlled trial, indicate that following a low-fat, low-fiber, small particle size diet (Answer B) is associated with improved symptoms compared with following a standard diabetes diet. This approach is based primarily on gastric-emptying physiology that shows 2-mm–sized particles or smaller are needed to exit the stomach and that lipids in the small intestine delay gastric emptying. Unfortunately, data from the gastroparesis consortium study of the National Institute of Diabetes and Digestive and Kidney Diseases suggest that few patients follow these recommendations for dietary modification to relieve gastroparesis symptoms and a larger percentage also do not take adequate supplements to reduce nutritional deficiencies. These findings highlight care gaps that should be addressed by practitioners.

While improved glycemic control is associated with improved microvascular outcomes in general, few data suggest the same is the case for upper gastrointestinal symptoms in patients with type 1 diabetes. Studies in persons with type 2 diabetes do not suggest that improved glycemic control improves delayed gastric emptying. Thus, while improved glycemic control targeting a hemoglobin A_{1c} level less than 7.0% (<53 mmol/mol) (Answer C) is a desirable goal, it may not improve her symptoms.

Metoclopramide (Answer D) reduces nausea and vomiting by central dopamine receptor antagonism and by increasing foregut mobility by peripheral cholinergic agonism. Most randomized controlled studies, although small, suggest that symptoms are improved with metoclopramide. Interestingly, a strong correlation with improved gastric emptying has not been observed. Unfortunately, up to one-third of patients experience adverse effects: hyperprolactinemia with impotence, galactorrhea, amenorrhea, and extrapyramidal symptoms including tardive dyskinesia. In practice, this agent is often used even before firmly establishing a diagnosis. However, given the adverse effects, metoclopramide would be less desirable in a woman of reproductive age. Another antidopaminergic agent that is as effective as metoclopramide and may be more acceptable is domperidone, as it does not cross the blood-brain barrier and produces fewer extrapyramidal adverse effects. However, there are concerns about its cardiac effects, and it should be used with caution in patients with liver or cardiac disease. Domperidone is contraindicated in patients on other QT-prolonging medications.

The macrolide antibiotic erythromycin (Answer E) acts as a motilin receptor agonist and has been shown to improve symptoms of gastroparesis, but studies are very small and of short duration, making this a third-choice option.

Educational Objective
Explain the pathophysiology and diagnostic workup of gastroparesis and recommend appropriate treatment strategies.

Reference(s)
Bharucha AE, Kudva YC, Prichard DO. Diabetic gastroparesis. *Endocr Rev.* 2019;40(5):1318-1352. PMID: 31081877

115 ANSWER: A) Type V osteogenesis imperfecta

This premenopausal woman presents with abnormally low bone mineral density and a recent right hip fragility fracture; therefore, secondary contributors to osteoporosis should be considered. Her history of excess fractures since childhood, abnormally low bone mineral density, short stature, scoliosis, bone deformities, and family history of osteoporosis are all clinical features that should raise suspicion for osteogenesis imperfecta (OI), a group of disorders characterized by fragile bones with recurrent fractures. There are many different subtypes of OI based on genetic and clinical characteristics. The most common type is mild OI (type I), in which patients typically have blue-gray discoloration of the sclerae. Hearing loss is present in approximately 50% of cases. Individuals with this type of OI can live a normal lifespan. Type II is a severe perinatal form that often leads to death in the first year of life. Persons with type III OI are typically severely affected and have many fractures starting very early in life. Many have deformities and need to use a wheelchair; they often have a somewhat shortened life expectancy. Type IV is a moderate type of OI where affected patients often need braces or crutches to walk; life expectancy is normal or near-normal. About 90% of individuals with OI fit into one of the types I through IV, all of which are caused by dominant pathogenic variants in the genes encoding either the α1 or α2 chains of type I collagen. Type V OI (Answer A) is moderate in severity and characterized by the absence of blue sclerae, propensity for hyperplastic callus formation, calcification of the forearm interosseous membrane, radial-head dislocation, and osteoporosis. It is a dominantly inherited OI subtype due to a recurrent pathogenic variant in the 5′ untranslated region of the interferon-induced transmembrane protein 5 gene (*IFITM5*) located on chromosome 11p15.5. This patient's age, history, and physical examination findings are most consistent with type V OI. Although not approved for this indication, bisphosphonates are the mainstay of pharmacologic therapy for fracture prevention for most forms of OI.

Idiopathic juvenile osteoporosis (Answer B) is a nonhereditary form of transient, isolated childhood osteoporosis that occurs in prepubertal, previously healthy children. Idiopathic juvenile osteoporosis has no known cause and is diagnosed when other causes of juvenile osteoporosis, including primary diseases or medical therapies known to cause bone loss, are excluded. This rare form of osteoporosis typically occurs just before the onset of puberty, with an average age of onset of 7 years. Most children with this condition experience complete recovery of bone tissue.

Juvenile Paget disease (Answer C), also known as hereditary hyperphosphatasia, is a rare condition mainly caused by pathogenic variants in the tumor necrosis factor receptor superfamily member 11B gene (*TNFRSF11B*) that encodes osteoprotegerin, leading to generalized acceleration of skeletal turnover. It is an autosomal recessive disorder in which patients have increased serum alkaline phosphatase. This distinguishes it from OI, in which alkaline phosphatase is usually normal; however, elevated levels of serum alkaline phosphatase have been reported in some patients with type VI OI.

Hereditary resistance to vitamin D (Answer D) is caused by end-organ resistance to 1,25-dihydroxyvitamin D most often because of loss-of-function pathogenic variants in the gene encoding the vitamin D receptor (*VDR*). The typical laboratory abnormalities in this scenario include hypocalcemia, hypophosphatemia, high serum PTH levels, and high serum 1,25-dihyroxyvitamin D levels. This patient's laboratory workup is normal, which is not consistent with such a diagnosis.

Finally, hypophosphatasia (Answer E) is a rare, autosomal disorder caused by a deficiency of tissue nonspecific alkaline phosphatase and characterized by abnormal mineralization of bone and dental tissues. Patients with hypophosphatasia have decreased serum concentrations of alkaline phosphatase, which this patient does not have.

Educational Objective
Recognize the clinical manifestations of type V osteogenesis imperfecta in a patient presenting with recurrent factures.

Reference(s)
Camacho PM, Petak SM, Binkley N, et al. American Association of Clinical Endocrinologists and American College of Endocrinology clinical practice guidelines for the diagnosis and treatment of postmenopausal osteoporosis – 2016. *Endocr Pract.* 2016;22(Suppl 4):1-42. PMID: 27662240

Forlino A, Marini JC. Osteogenesis imperfecta. *Lancet.* 2016;387(10028):1657-1671. PMID: 26542481

Cho T-J, Lee K-E, Lee S-K, et al. A single recurrent mutation in the 5'-UTR of IFITM5 causes osteogenesis imperfecta type V. *Am J Hum Genet.* 2012;91(2):343-348. PMID: 22863190

Smith R. Idiopathic juvenile osteoporosis: experience of twenty-one patients. *Br J Rheumatol.* 1995;34(1):68-77. PMID: 7881843

Polyzos SA, Cundy T, Mantzoros CS. Juvenile Paget disease. *Metabolism.* 2018;80:15-26. PMID: 29080812

Tournis S, Dede AD. Osteogenesis imperfecta – a clinical update. *Metabolism.* 2018;80:27-37. PMID: 28625337

116 ANSWER: D) Skeletal survey

The pituitary stalk connects the hypothalamus to the pituitary gland and has an anterior component (pars tuberalis) and posterior component (pars infundibularis) that contain the axons of supraoptic and paraventricular neurons that end in the posterior pituitary, where they release oxytocin and vasopressin into the bloodstream. While stalk thickening is sometimes obvious on MRI, it can also be subtle, as the normal width of the pituitary stalk is still debated. Stalk thickening changes depend on the level at which it is measured, but most experts use 3.5 or 4 mm as a cutoff. Lesions of the pituitary stalk can be divided in 3 large groups: congenital, inflammatory, and neoplastic. The most important differential diagnosis is between inflammatory and neoplastic disease. The most common inflammatory diseases in the pituitary stalk are forms of hypophysitis, sarcoidosis, and granulomatosis with polyangiitis (previously known as Wegener granulomatosis). The most common neoplastic diseases are Langerhans cell histiocytosis (LCH), germinoma, lymphoma, and metastatic disease (although LCH is considered inflammatory by some investigators). Erdheim-Chester disease is rare. In general, cases with the following findings are more likely due to nonneoplastic lesions: presence of diabetes insipidus, absence of extrasellar involvement, female sex, more limited stalk thickness (<5.3 mm), and limited number of anterior pituitary hormone deficits.

A tissue diagnosis is ideal, but pituitary biopsy (Answer A) is associated with significant operative risk. Hence, the initial evaluation should rely on a less-invasive test than a biopsy. Given this patient's age and male sex, the 2 most likely diagnoses are germinoma and LCH. Because LCH involves the bones in about 60% of cases and typically causes only limited anterior pituitary failure (this patient has only hypogonadism), it is a possible diagnosis here. A skeletal survey (Answer D) is a safe and inexpensive first diagnostic step in this case. Recently, whole-body MRI has been proposed as an alternative and more sensitive (but obviously more expensive) means to detect bone lesions compared with skeletal survey, and it could be considered if the skeletal survey is normal. A confirmatory bone biopsy (if necessary) would certainly be safer than a pituitary stalk biopsy. In patients with skin lesions, skin biopsy may unveil LCH. As mentioned, stalk biopsy would be considered only at a later stage if a presumptive diagnosis cannot be established and the concern for malignancy is high. PET-CT of the brain (Answer B) would not help in the differential diagnosis of such a small lesion.

"Pure" germinomas and mature teratomas generally do not cause significant elevation of α-fetoprotein and β-hCG levels in both cerebrospinal fluid and serum, but serum and (more frequently) cerebrospinal fluid β-hCG and α-fetoprotein may be high in nongerminomatous germ-cell tumors such as yolk sac tumors, embryonic-cell carcinomas, and immature teratomas. Therefore, a lumbar puncture (Answer C) is certainly part of the armamentarium used in the differential diagnosis of pituitary stalk lesions, but not as a first test.

Finally, ^{68}Ga DOTATATE scan (Answer E) is a type of functional imaging in which a radioisotope-labeled somatostatin analogue peptide binds to somatostatin receptors. This is useful in identifying the location of neuroendocrine tumors, but it does not help in the differential diagnosis of pituitary stalk thickening.

Educational Objective
Construct the differential diagnosis for pituitary stalk thickening.

Reference(s)
Devuyst F, Kazakou P, Balériaux D, et al. Central diabetes insipidus and pituitary stalk thickening in adults: distinction of neoplastic from non-neoplastic lesions. *Eur J Endocrinol.* 2020;181(3):95-105. PMID: 32530258

Salvatori R. The differential diagnosis of pituitary stalk thickening. *Endocr Pract.* 2019;25(6):616-618. PMID: 31242126

Aricò M, Girschikofsky M, Généreau T, et al. Langerhans cell histiocytosis in adults. Report from the International Registry of the Histiocyte Society. *Eur J Cancer.* 2003;39(16):2341-2348. PMID: 14556926

Kim JR, Yoon HM, Jung AY, Cho YA, Seo JJ, Lee JS. Comparison of whole-body MRI, bone scan, and radiographic skeletal survey for lesion detection and risk stratification of Langerhans cell histiocytosis. *Sci Rep.* 2019;22;9(1):317. PMID: 30670752

117 ANSWER: E) Hepatitis B series

Review of vaccination status should be included in a comprehensive evaluation of patients with diabetes. Vaccination can reduce hospitalization from common infections such as influenza and pneumococcal pneumonia. The decision to vaccinate is often based on patient age and the presence of comorbidities. The Centers for Disease Control and the American Diabetes Association have guidelines on vaccine recommendations for patients with diabetes.

In this 61-year-old man with type 2 diabetes, annual influenza vaccination is recommended, but not the live attenuated form (Answer C). The live attenuated form is not recommended in persons older than 50 years). Tetanus-diphtheria booster (Td or Tdap) (Answer B) is recommended every 10 years in all adults. Since this man received a booster 6 years ago, he is not currently due for this vaccine. In most patients with diabetes, a single dose of the pneumococcal polysaccharide (PPSV23) vaccine (Answer A) is recommended between the ages of 19 and 64 years with an additional dose at age 65 years. If the patient has already received a dose before age 65 years, the second dose given after age 65 years should be at least 5 years after the previous dose. This man received a dose 6 years ago, so when he turns 65 in 4 years he can receive the vaccination, as it will have been 10 years since the previous dose. In special circumstances, such as elderly patients in nursing homes, or immunocompromised persons with diabetes, the PCV13 vaccine can be considered. Hepatitis A vaccination (Answer D) is not routinely recommended as part of the vaccine schedule for patients with diabetes, but the hepatitis B vaccine series (Answer E) is recommended. In patients with diabetes between the ages of 18 and 59 years, 2 or 3 doses of the hepatitis B vaccine can be administered. In patients older than 60 years, a 3-dose regimen is recommended.

Other vaccines that should be considered for this patient are the measles, mumps, and rubella (MMR) vaccine (if he has not received it yet) and the zoster vaccine (2-dose recombinant zoster vaccination is preferred).

Table. Age-Based Schedule of Recommended Vaccinations for Adults

Vaccine	Age 18-64 years	Age 65 years and older
Influenza	Yes, annually (for persons older than 50 years, inactivated [IIV] or recombinant vaccine [RIV4] recommended)	Yes, annually (inactivated [IIV] or recombinant vaccine (RIV4) recommended)
Tetanus	For persons older than age 11 years: first dose Tdap, repeat every 10 years (can be Td or Tdap)	Repeat every 10 years (can be Td or Tdap)
MMR (measles, mumps, rubella)	May need 1 or 2 doses (if born in 1957 or later)	No
Varicella	2 doses (if born in 1980 or later) until age 45 years	No
Zoster recombinant	2 doses for those 50 years or older	2 doses if not received between age 50 and 64 years
HPV (human papillomavirus)	2-3 doses in those younger than 27 years	No
Pneumococcal polysaccharide (PPSV23)	Not recommended based simply on age.	1 dose at age 65 years or older (if patient has received vaccine prior to age 65 years, can get second dose after age 65. Interval between doses must be 5 years or more)

As noted above, in addition to the age-based schedule, the hepatitis B vaccine series is recommended for persons with diabetes mellitus.

Educational Objective
Make recommendations regarding both age-related and disease-specific vaccinations for a patient with type 2 diabetes mellitus.

Reference(s)
American Diabetes Association. 4. Comprehensive medical evaluation and assessment of comorbidities: standards of medical care in diabetes-2020. *Diabetes Care.* 2020;43(Suppl 1):S37-S47. PMID: 31862747

Centers for Disease Control and Prevention. Immunization schedules. Recommended adult immunization schedule for ages 19 years or older, United State, 2020. Available at: www.cdc.gov/vaccines/schedules/hcp/imz/adult.html. Accessed for verification December 2020.

118 ANSWER: A) Calculate polyethylene glycol (PEG)-precipitable TSH

The most common cause of high serum TSH with normal free T_4 is subclinical hypothyroidism. However, assay interference in the measurement of TSH should always be considered, particularly when there is a mismatch between the patient's laboratory test results and clinical findings. Although largely asymptomatic initially, after initiation of weight-based levothyroxine, the described patient developed new clinical findings suggestive of thyrotoxicosis (heat intolerance, diaphoresis, brisk reflexes, tremor), while his TSH remained markedly elevated (40.0 mIU/L). Moreover, the patient's serum TSH level did not decrease as expected following the initiation of levothyroxine, while his measured free T_4 levels rose proportionately after levothyroxine was started. This suggests that the measured free T_4 value is likely accurate and thus measurement of free T_4 by equilibrium dialysis (Answer B) is not the most appropriate management to recommend next.

Heterophile antibodies are capable of causing positive or negative interference in common laboratory tests, including serum TSH measurement. The most common type of heterophile antibodies are human antimouse antibodies (HAMA), which occur in up to 10% of the general population. Heterophile antibodies have been ruled out in this patient by repeating the serum TSH measurement in a heterophile-blocking tube and demonstrating a similar TSH result. Thus, alternative explanations for the abnormal, but likely spurious, TSH result should be considered, including the presence of macro-TSH. Macro-TSH is a macromolecule formed between TSH and anti-TSH immunoglobulins (usually IgG) that is cleared more slowly by the kidneys in comparison to the clearance of monomeric TSH. However, the immunoreactivity of the TSH complex may be preserved, leading to spuriously elevated TSH measurements. Although uncommon, occurring in only 0.8% of patients with subclinical hypothyroidism, macro-TSH appears to affect most commercially available TSH assays. The initial steps to confirm the presence of macro-TSH are to rule out HAMA interference, as has already been done in this case, and to calculate polyethylene glycol (PEG)-precipitable TSH (Answer A). PEG at a final concentration of 12.5% precipitates γ-globulins. Macro-TSH can be strongly suspected when the patient's sample shows increased ratios of PEG-precipitable TSH and HAMA interference has been excluded. The diagnosis can ultimately be confirmed with gel filtration chromatography. Coordination with the laboratory to complete testing is often required.

Performing pituitary MRI with and without contrast (Answer C) is not indicated in this patient with suspected assay interference in the measurement of serum TSH. Despite his serum TSH level being significantly elevated (26.0 mIU/L) on confirmatory testing before starting levothyroxine treatment, his measured free T_4 remained in the lower half of the reference range (1.1 ng/dL [14.2 pmol/L]) and at that time he had no signs or symptoms of hyperthyroidism. Collectively, these findings do not support the diagnosis of thyrotrope adenoma (TSHoma) and thus pituitary imaging is not needed. Functioning thyrotrope adenomas are typically associated with inappropriately normal or mildly elevated serum TSH levels in the setting of thyroid hormone excess. A retrospective series that included 32 thyrotrope adenomas at a single center demonstrated a median TSH concentration of 4.3 mIU/L (range, 1.2-6.9 mIU/L) among patients with functioning TSHomas.

Neither increasing the levothyroxine dosage (Answer D) nor changing the levothyroxine tablets to oral solution (Answer E) is warranted. The patient already has signs and symptoms suggestive of thyrotoxicosis on his current levothyroxine dosage and the measured free T_4 level is indicative of thyroid hormone excess. Further escalation of his dosage would only lead to worsening of his hyperthyroid symptoms.

Educational Objective
Recognize macro-TSH as a rare cause of elevated serum TSH.

Reference(s)
Favresse J, Burlacu M-C, Maiter D, Gruson D. Interferences with thyroid function immunoassays: clinical implications and detection algorithm. *Endocr Rev.* 2018;39(5):830-850. PMID: 29982406

Hattori N, Ishihara T, Shimatsu A. Variability in the detection of macro TSH in different immunoassay systems. *Eur J Endocrinol.* 2016;174(1):9-15. PMID: 26438715

Loh TP, Kao SL, Halsall DJ, et al. Macro-thyrotropin: a case report and review of literature. *J Clin Endocrinol Metab.* 2012;97(6):1823-1828. PMID: 22466337.

Palonco Santos C, Sandouk Z, Yogi-Morren D, et al. TSH-staining pituitary adenomas: rare, silent, and plurihoromonal. *Endocr Pract.* 2018;24(6):580-588. PMID: 29949434

119 ANSWER: A) Left cortical-sparing laparoscopic adrenalectomy

This patient has multiple endocrine neoplasia type 2A and a history of prophylactic thyroidectomy. He now presents with a new lipid-poor left adrenal mass, new hypertension, and modestly elevated metanephrines, but no overt hyperadrenergic or episodic symptoms. Collectively, these findings strongly suggest that he has a left adrenal pheochromocytoma.

Metanephrines are the stable and inactive metabolites of catecholamines that provide the highest sensitivity and specificity for diagnosing pheochromocytoma and paraganglioma. Further, metanephrines have a very high negative predictive value; a normal result almost certainly excludes the possibility of a functional tumor as the cause of symptoms. Metanephrine is the metabolite of epinephrine, and normetanephrine is the metabolite of norepinephrine. Typically, pheochromocytomas and paragangliomas that induce clinical symptoms are associated with metanephrine and/or normetanephrine levels that are substantially higher than the upper limit of the reference range—usually 4 times or more (less commonly 2 or 3 times higher). However, in patients with an inherited predisposition for pheochromocytoma who are undergoing routine surveillance testing (such as this patient with known multiple endocrine neoplasia type 2A), new and modest elevations in metanephrines can be diagnostic for an early pheochromocytoma.

The radiographic characteristics of a pheochromocytoma include poor lipid content, high contrast uptake, and poor contrast washout. On CT, this is usually characterized by a high unenhanced attenuation (>10 Hounsfield units [but often >20 Hounsfield units]), a very high postcontrast attenuation, and poor washout after a 15-minute delay (absolute washout <60%, relative washout <40%). Of note, pheochromocytomas may occasionally have high washout characteristics. On MRI, pheochromocytomas usually display T2 hyperintensity.

The radiographic and biochemical features in this patient with multiple endocrine neoplasia type 2A are strongly indicative of an early and presymptomatic pheochromocytoma. Therefore, surgery is the treatment of choice. Laparoscopic adrenalectomy, not open adrenalectomy (Answer D), performed by an experienced surgeon after preoperative adrenergic blockade, is the preferred option to minimize morbidity and expedite recovery. Although a total left adrenalectomy (Answer C) could be performed, the preference is a left cortical-sparing adrenalectomy (Answer A) because this patient has a high risk of developing a contralateral right-sided pheochromocytoma in the future. Therefore, preserving the adrenal cortex to lower the likelihood of lifelong primary adrenal insufficiency is preferred over total laparoscopic adrenalectomy. Although bilateral adrenalectomy (Answers B and E) could eliminate the future risk of developing a pheochromocytoma, it unnecessarily increases the risk of complications and the likelihood of primary adrenal insufficiency. Recent studies have shown that with modern surgical technique and experience, cortical-sparing adrenalectomy is a safe and reliable option, especially for patients with inherited syndromes predisposing them to recurrent and bilateral pheochromocytoma. Although cortical-sparing adrenalectomy does carry a small risk for recurrent ipsilateral pheochromocytoma, presumptively due to incomplete medullary resection, this risk does not appear to be associated with decreased survival.

Educational Objective
Recommend the best surgical approach to pheochromocytoma in patients with multiple endocrine neoplasia type 2.

Reference(s)
Neumann HPH, Tsoy U, Bancos I, et al; International Bilateral-Pheochromocytoma-Registry Group. Comparison of pheochromocytoma-specific morbidity and mortality among adults with bilateral pheochromocytomas undergoing total adrenalectomy vs cortical-sparing adrenalectomy. *JAMA Netw Open.* 2019;2(8):e198898. PMID: 31397861

120 ANSWER: B) Two bedtime salivary cortisol measurements

Diagnosing Cushing syndrome is often challenging, as the features that differentiate Cushing syndrome from non–hypercortisolism-related obesity depression, hypertension, diabetes, and osteoporosis (easy bruising, facial plethora, proximal myopathy and >1-cm wide reddish-purple striae) may present only in more severe cases. Because establishing the diagnosis of Cushing syndrome is difficult on clinical grounds, the interpretation of biochemical tests is very important for the endocrinologist. For initial testing, 1 of the following tests is recommended (based on its suitability for a given patient): (1) urinary free cortisol (at least 2 measurements); (2) late-night salivary cortisol (2 measurements); (3) 1-mg overnight dexamethasone-suppression test; (4) longer low-dose dexamethasone-suppression test (2 mg/day for 48 h). All of these tests have caveats and can have false positivity or negativity.

An additional challenge is the entity known as pseudo-Cushing syndrome. Some investigators prefer to call this condition "physiologic/nonneoplastic hypercortisolism." In this condition, patients display the signs, symptoms, and abnormal hormone levels seen in Cushing syndrome without having an ACTH- or cortisol-secreting tumor. Pseudo-Cushing syndrome can be idiopathic or caused by stress, severe illness, intense chronic exercise, alcoholism, obesity, pregnancy, suboptimally controlled diabetes mellitus, major depression, malnutrition, and anorexia nervosa (although the last 2 conditions are very obviously distinguished from Cushing syndrome). Sometimes the distinction between Cushing syndrome and pseudo-Cushing syndrome is very difficult and a more cumbersome test is needed (combination of 48-hour dexamethasone-suppression test followed [2 hours after the last dexamethasone dose] by corticotropin-releasing hormone stimulation, also known as a dexamethasone–corticotropin-releasing hormone test).

Endocrinologists must be aware of the potential pitfalls of the tests ordered in the workup of Cushing syndrome. The currently recommended serum cortisol cutoff after 1 mg of dexamethasone is 1.8 μg/dL (49.7 nmol/L). Therefore, this patient's test result was abnormal. Dexamethasone is metabolized primarily by hepatic CYP3A4 and therefore enzyme-inducing anticonvulsant drugs (such as carbamazepine which was included in this patient's medication list) are known to enhance dexamethasone clearance. As a consequence, dexamethasone may not reach serum levels that suppress ACTH secretion, causing a false-positive result. Other anticonvulsant drugs that have this effect are phenytoin and phenobarbital. A similar effect is caused by rifampin and pioglitazone. For this reason, the Endocrine Society guidelines advise against using dexamethasone-suppression tests in patients taking anticonvulsant drugs.

Measuring simultaneous serum cortisol and dexamethasone levels is always advisable when performing a dexamethasone-suppression test, as fast dexamethasone metabolism occasionally occurs in patients not taking anticonvulsant drugs. Patients may also make mistakes in the timing of dexamethasone ingestion, or even forget to take it. Another potential source of a false-positive result when measuring serum cortisol after dexamethasone is seen in women who are on oral estrogen preparations, either for birth control or replacement. In this case, the first-pass effect through the liver causes an increase in serum cortisol-binding globulin, the main carrier of serum cortisol, resulting in an increase in serum cortisol measurement, which may fail to suppress despite reaching appropriate dexamethasone levels.

Urinary free cortisol is not a highly specific test, and it can be mildly to moderately elevated in the absence of Cushing syndrome. Additionally, cases have been reported of falsely elevated 24-hour urinary free cortisol levels due to interference with carbamazepine when measured with high-performance liquid chromatography.

The patient in this vignette does not yet have an established diagnosis of Cushing syndrome, and therefore the correct answer is to measure bedtime salivary cortisol (Answer B), which is not influenced by carbamazepine. Salivary cortisol measurement has its own limitations, including variability, particularly in patients with milder forms of Cushing syndrome in whom more than 2 collections may be needed to detect an abnormal value. When collecting saliva samples, patients should be instructed not to drink, eat, brush their teeth, or smoke for 30 minutes before collections. Not using steroid cream for 24 hours before collection is also important to avoid false-positive results due to contamination. Finally, when interpreting the results, one must keep in mind that normal levels may be higher in elderly male patients with diabetes.

Imaging of the pituitary (Answer A) or adrenal glands (Answer C) is incorrect, as imaging is indicated only after a biochemical diagnosis of Cushing syndrome is established (pituitary imaging in the case of ACTH-dependent Cushing syndrome and adrenal imaging in the case of ACTH-independent Cushing syndrome).

Although the composition of over-the-counter supplements is never clear, there are currently no reports of interference with cortisol dynamic testing from "prostate health supplements" as listed in the stem. While stopping supplements during Cushing syndrome workup is never a bad idea, stopping the prostate health supplement (Answer D) is not the best next step. Furthermore, this answer does not include stopping carbamazepine.

Finally, a 2-day dexamethasone-suppression test (Answer E) would have the same limitations as the overnight test in a patient taking carbamazepine.

Educational Objective
Identify possible pitfalls of Cushing syndrome workup in patients taking anticonvulsant drugs.

Reference(s)

Nieman LK, Biller BMK, Findling JW, et al. The diagnosis of Cushing's syndrome: an Endocrine Society clinical practice guideline. *J Clin Endocrinol Metab.* 2008;93(5):1526-1540. PMID: 18334580

Findling JW, Raff H. Diagnosis of endocrine disease: differentiation of pathologic/neoplastic hypercortisolism (Cushing's syndrome) from physiologic/non-neoplastic hypercortisolism (formerly known as pseudo-Cushing's syndrome). *Eur J Endocrinol.* 2017;176(5):R205-R216. PMID: 28179447

Sandouk Z, Johnston P, Bunch D, Wang S, Bena J, Hamrahian A, Kennedy L. Variability of late-night salivary cortisol in Cushing disease: a prospective study. *J Clin Endocrinol Metab.* 2018;103(3):983-990. PMID: 29329418

ENDOCRINE SELF-ASSESSMENT PROGRAM 2022

Part III

This question-mapping index groups question topics according to the 8 umbrella sections of ESAP (Adrenal, Bone-Calcium, Diabetes, Lipids-Obesity, Pituitary, Reproduction [Female], Reproduction [Male], and Thyroid). Relevant **question numbers** follow each topic.

ADRENAL

Addison disease: **110**
Adrenal incidentaloma: **3, 22**
Adrenal insufficiency: **110**
Adrenocortical carcinoma: **54, 60**
Catecholamine-secreting tumors: **22, 81, 99, 119**
Congenital adrenal hyperplasia: **43**
Cushing syndrome: **71**
Ectopic ACTH syndrome: **71**
Hypercortisolism: **71**
Hyperkalemia: **14, 34**
Hypertension: **14, 34**
Hypogonadism: **43**
Infertility: **43**
Li-Fraumeni syndrome: **60**
Mitotane: **54**
Multiple endocrine neoplasia type 2A: **119**
Nonfunctioning adrenal adenoma: **3**
Paraganglioma: **81**
Pheochromocytoma: **22, 81, 99, 119**
Primary aldosteronism: **14, 34**
RET gene: **99**
SDHB gene: **81**

CALCIUM-BONE

Alkaline phosphatase: **59**
Androgen-deprivation therapy: **95**
AP2S1 gene: **72**
CASR gene: **72**
Bisphosphonates: **8, 15, 18**
Bisphosphonate holiday: **15**
Denosumab: **5, 18, 95**
Depot medroxyprogesterone: **100**
Dual-energy x-ray absorptiometry: **25**
Familial hypocalciuric hypercalcemia: **72**
Glucocorticoid therapy: **18**
GNA11 gene: **72**
Hungry bone syndrome: **88**
Hypercalcemia: **35, 39, 46, 72**
Hyperparathyroidism, primary: **35, 39, 46, 88**
Hypocalcemia: **88**
Hypophosphatemic osteomalacia: **103**
Lithium: **35**
Nephrolithiasis: **83**
Osteogenesis imperfecta: **115**
Osteonecrosis of the jaw: **5**
Osteoporosis: **5, 8, 15, 18, 25, 83, 95, 100**
Osteoporosis, transient: **108**
Paget disease: **59, 66**
Romosozumab: **25**
Tenofovir: **103**
Vertebral fracture: **8**

DIABETES

Antipsychotic drugs: **112**
Bariatric surgery: **20**
Cardiovascular risk: **57, 63, 73, 77, 97, 105**
Chronic kidney disease: **77**
Continuous glucose monitoring: **17, 48, 65**
C-peptide: **17**
Cystic fibrosis–related diabetes mellitus: **48**
Diabetic ketoacidosis: **33, 41, 102**
Enteral nutrition: **28**
Gastroparesis: **114**
GLP-1 receptor agonists: **63, 68, 105**
GAD antibodies: **26**
HNF1A gene: **1**
Hemoglobin A_{1c}: **65**
Hospitalized patients: **28, 93**
Hypercortisolism: **51**
Hyperglycemia: **1, 28**
Hypertension: **57, 73**
Hypoglycemia: **20, 36, 109**
Hypoglycemia, postbariatric: **20**
Immune checkpoint inhibitors: **82**
Immunization: **117**
Insulin pump therapy: **17, 93**
Insulin therapy: **6, 17, 28, 65, 79, 82, 93**
Insulinoma: **36**
Latent autoimmune diabetes in adults: **26**
Maturity-onset diabetes of the young: **87**
Monogenic diabetes: **1, 87**
Neuropathy: **12**
Nonalcoholic fatty liver disease: **10**
Pioglitazone: **10**
SGLT-2 inhibitors: **33, 77, 97, 102**
Sulfonylureas: **87**
Thiazolidinediones: **10**
Type 1 diabetes mellitus: **17, 65, 79, 82, 93, 114**
Type 2 diabetes mellitus: **6, 10, 12, 26, 28, 33, 51, 57, 63, 68, 73, 77, 97, 102, 105, 109, 112, 117**
Whipple triad: **20, 36, 109**

LIPIDS-OBESITY

Bariatric surgery: **31, 45, 64, 107**
Bempedoic acid: **4**
Cardiovascular risk: **91, 113**
Chronic kidney disease: **23**
Cyclosporine: **16**
Diabetes mellitus, prevention: **85**
Ezetimibe: **91**
Familial chylomicronemia syndrome: **45**
Fibrates: **23**
Gastroesophageal reflux: **107**
Hypercholesterolemia: **4, 16, 91, 113**
Hyperparathyroidism: **64**
Hypertriglyceridemia: **23, 45**
Infertility: **55**
Iron deficiency: **31**
Lipoprotein lipase deficiency: **45**
Liraglutide: **75**
Liver disease: **113**
Medication-related weight gain: **11**
Nephrolithiasis: **64**
Obesity: **31, 55, 75**
Obesity, pharmacotherapy: **75**
Pancreatitis: **45**
Pregnancy: **55**
Sitosterolemia: **101**
Statin therapy: **113**

PITUITARY

Acromegaly: **56, 78**
Adrenal insufficiency: **21**
Arthropathy: **56**
Corticotrope tumor: **2**

Cushing disease: **120**
Diabetes insipidus: **116**
Dopamine agonist therapy: **40, 89**
Glucagon-stimulation test: **47**
Hypercortisolism: **120**
Hyperprolactinemia: **40, 61, 89**
Hypogonadism: **69**
Hypopituitarism: **47**
IgG4-related hypophysitis: **69**
Langerhans cell histiocytosis: **116**
Macroadenoma: **2, 40, 61**
Microadenoma: **89**
Pituitary stalk compression: **61**
Pituitary stalk thickening: **116**
Pregnancy: **89**
Prolactinoma: **40, 89**
Salivary cortisol: **120**
Skull base radiation: **47**
Thyrotoxicosis: **30**
Thyrotropinoma: **30**

REPRODUCTION, FEMALE
Amenorrhea: **29, 84**
Androgenetic alopecia: **50**
Congenital adrenal hyperplasia: **13, 62**
Genetic counseling: **13**
Hirsutism: **98**
Hyperandrogenism: **13, 62, 98, 111**
Infertility: **84**
Irregular bleeding: **111**
Luteoma of pregnancy: **98**
Oral contraceptives: **111**
Ovarian drilling: **84**
Pituitary macroadenoma: **29**
Polycystic ovary syndrome: **62, 98, 111**
Testosterone therapy: **37**
Transgender medicine: **37**

REPRODUCTION, MALE
Anabolic steroid abuse: **7**
Androgen-deprivation therapy: **42**
Azoospermia: **7**
Congenital adrenal hyperplasia: **53**
Erectile dysfunction: **70**
Gynecomastia: **19**
Hypogonadism: **90, 104**
Infertility: **7**
Osteoporosis: **42**
Phosphodiesterase type 5 inhibitor: **70**
Pituitary adenoma: **104**
Prostate cancer: **42**
Prostate-specific antigen: **90**
Testosterone therapy: **90**

THYROID
Autoimmune atrophic gastritis with pernicious anemia: **44**
Colloid nodule: **9**
Cushing syndrome: **76**
Fine-needle aspiration: **49**
Follicular thyroid cancer: **74**
Graves disease: **27, 86**
Graves orbitopathy: **27**
Gynecomastia: **24**
Hashimoto thyroiditis: **44, 96**
Hyperthyroidism: **24, 27, 86,**
Hypothyroidism: **38, 44, 52, 58, 67, 96, 106, 118**
Lithium: **38**
Lymph node metastasis: **80**
Macro-TSH: **118**
Medication nonadherence: **52**
Medullary thyroid cancer: **58, 76**
Multikinase inhibitor: **58**
Papillary thyroid cancer: **92**
Plasma exchange: **86**
Pregnancy: **67, 92**
Recurrent laryngeal nerve injury: **106**
Subacute thyroiditis: **32**
Thyroid nodule: **49, 80, 92, 106**
Thyroid storm: **86**
Thyrotoxicosis: **32**
TPO antibodies: **96**
Ultrasonography: **9, 32, 49, 80, 92**

CPSIA information can be obtained
at www.ICGtesting.com
Printed in the USA
LVHW051912120423
744189LV00012B/465

9 781943 550111